HANDBOOK
OF
HEALTH AND MEDICINE

HANDBOOK OF HEALTH AND MEDICINE

Dr R N Kaul

MD PUBLICATIONS PVT LTD
NEW DELHI
www.mdppl.com

Published by :

MD Publications Pvt Ltd
"MD House", 11, Darya Ganj,
New Delhi-110 002
Phone : +91-11-41563325 (Customer Service)
+91-11-41562846 (Editorial)
E-mail (orders) : order@mdppl.com
Website : www.mdppl.com

ISBN : 978-81-7533-185-3

Published and Printed by Mr. Pranav Gupta on behalf of **MD Publications Pvt Ltd** at Printext, New Delhi.

PREFACE

Debates as to the nature and status of medical sociology have been an abiding theme since its inception. It is not, however, our intention to rehearse them again here. Suffice it to say that the charge of a theoretical, policy-driven discipline, in-the-service-of medicine, has now been largely dispensed with. Ideas about health and illness, as Gerhardt notes, have played a central role in the development of general sociological theory since the Second World War, including issues of order and control, 'deviance' and 'normality'. Contemporary work encompasses a variety of perspectives, from phenomenology to constructionism, and despite various 'border skirmishes' and 'internal disputes', the sociology of health and illness remains a flourishing sub-discipline, both theoretically and empirically.

Not only is qualitative sociological research formerly the 'poor relation' of social epidemiology increasingly valued in medical circles, but debates as to the relevance of theory itself, including the advent of so-called 'narrative based medicine', are now appearing in such hallowed places as the *British Medical Journal*. Tensions nonetheless remain, not simply concerning this eclectic theoretical base, but also regarding various funding crises, institutional dilemmas and the push towards more evaluative health service research (HSR), including 'evidence based' medicine and 'quality assurance' initiatives. Should medical sociologists, given these pressures, remain true to their trade, both theoretically and empirically (i.e. the autonomous, 'outsider' solution); or should they 'toil' instead under the banner of public health, HSR or some other such title in the hope of promoting 'change from within' (i.e. the 'pragmatic', insider solution)? These, to be sure, are familiar concerns, including the dilemma of 'sociological imperialism' itself. We are all, moreover, given the vicissitudes of funding and institutional constraints, called upon to be 'double-agents' at times. What has changed, however, both inside and outside the academy, are the reflexive parameters within which these and other debates are currently taking place: a dynamism in which the 'limits' of expertise, whatever its source, are increasingly exposed.

A key question here concerns whether or not we are living in a postmodern society? For some theorists the modern project—linked as it is to processes of rationality, discipline and control is all but over. Modernist notions of causality, identity, the subject and truth should, it is claimed, be abandoned in favour of a more destabilised, desedimented position which celebrates indeterminacy, contingency and flux: a postmodern carnival in which surface substitutes for depth, time dissipates into a series of ephemeral presents, the subject becomes decentred and reality itself becomes 'hyper-real'.

In a similar vein, Bauman has suggested that post modernity, properly interpreted, is really 'modernity looking at itself at a distance rather than from inside, making a full inventory of its gains and issues, psycho analysing itself'. Taken together, these critiques, alongside the emergence of critical realism as a dominant new force and promising alternative in contemporary social theory, suggest that the notion of 'postmodernity' is highly problematic, thereby encouraging the alternative view, endorsed by many contributors to this particular volume, that 'contemporary social changes are best understood as *the increased dominance of certain aspects of modernity over others,* rather than as indicators of a radical break with modernity as such'. To the extent that so-called 'postmodern' perspectives have shaken the foundations of rational thought, destabilised seemingly ossified conceptual forms, and opened up new (ethical) questions and ways of being and caring for each other, they are to be welcomed. To see this as the 'death of modernity' however, to say the very least, is premature. Rather, processes of rationality, including ongoing advances in science and technology and a resurgence of biological explanations, continue to hold sway over large tracts of society, at one and the same time as new forms of sociality, emotionality and communality begin to emerge.

It is within this context that the rationale for the present volume is located, the central aim of which is to address explicitly the relationship between mainstream sociological theory and medical sociology in the light of a number of key issues within the field of health at the turn of the century. Whilst, as we have argued, medical sociology has never been an a theoretical discipline, it nonetheless remains the case, particularly in the current economic and political climate with its emphasis on evaluation and cost-effectiveness, that bridges between mainstream theory and the sociology of health and illness need to be continually built if an instructive and *mutually informing dialogue* is to occur. Four key themes, we suggest, are central here both to current mainstream theorising and contemporary research within the sociology of health and illness. *Re-thinking of social structure,* the first of these, raises a series of issues, from debates over the future of class, to the blurring of traditional categories and distinctions concerning gender, 'race' and 'ageing' in the late/postmodern era. The *body,* our second theme, is also becoming increasingly 'contested' and 'uncertain' at the turn of the century, both inside and outside the academy. What sense are we to make of these corporeal developments, and in what ways do the embodied dilemmas of health and medicine help clarify the issues at stake? *Consumption and risk,* our third key theme, mesh closely with these arguments, from the 'rituals' of health promotion in the 'epidemiological clinic' of late modernity, to the commodification of health care in the 'marketised' state. *Emotions* are equally central here, partly through this upsurge of interest in the body, consumption and risk, and partly through the broader debates, postmodern or otherwise, they engender concerning the project of rationality itself.

Within medical sociology the debate about the relationship between social structure and health has focused, at least until recently, on the inverse relationship between social class position, health status and longevity the so-called 'inequality in health' debate. Social class position, in this respect, has tended to be conceptualised 'atheoretically', measured as it is through occupational class. Much of this research has been empirical in nature (mainly from a social epidemiological perspective), including the identification and description of more or less 'patterned' statistical relationships between indicators of occupational class, indicators of ill health and mortality and factors that might mediate between the two.

A central issue here has been the extent to which the relationship between occupational social class and ill health can be explained by social selection or by structural (material) factors. As MacIntyre points out in her review of developments since the report's publication, the debate has tended to become polarised, confusing what she sees as the 'hard' and 'soft' versions of the four different explanations proposed: artefact, natural/social selection, cultural/behavioural and materialist/structuralist. The Black Report accepted the hard version of a materialist/structuralist explanation (i.e. material, physical conditions of life associated with the class structure are the complete explanation for class gradients in health), but rejected the explanatory power of hard versions of the other three.

I am very grateful to Mr. Pranav Gupta, Director of MD Publications Pvt Ltd, New Delhi for his cooperation and support for this book.

Dr R N Kaul

Contents

1

Better Health and Greater Longevity

Introduction

The 75 percent accuracy that you will die of heart attack, hypertension, stroke, cancer, diabetes, kidney failure, or complications arising from osteoporosis. It's sad but safe to make this prediction because three out of four Americans do indeed succumb to these major killer diseases. Fortunately, you can do a great deal to cut your chances of being struck down by any of them. But avoiding them is just part of what you must do to live longer and better.

Even if you avoid all of the killer diseases, still you will grow old, and at about the same rate. Your skin will dry out and wrinkle, your hair grow thin and turn gray, your sight will dim, your hearing capacity will decline. You'll get heavier and a bit shorter. Your muscles will shrink, your joints stiffen. Your heart will pump blood less well your lungs will take in less oxygen, and your tissues will use the oxygen less efficiently. Your kidney function will diminish and your endocrine glands will secrete a lower level of hormones. Your breasts will sag or your erection flag. Your resistance to infection will be less than a fourth what it was in youth. There will be slowing of your reaction time to a stimulus, such as the sight of a car hurtling toward you. Some phases of your learning process may slow down, with a lapse in memory for recent events, such as what movie you saw three nights ago. You may not come down with a major disease, but your vulnerability to changes in your environment, the weather, and in your personal life will markedly increase with age. Finally you will die from what for a young person might not be a serious problem at all: a mild attack of the flu will become the big sleep, or you won't manage to jump out of the way of that speeding red Pontiac.

It's like a lion at the door,
And when the door begins to crack,
It's like a stick across your back,
And when your back begins to smart,
It's like a penknife in your heart,
And when your heart begins to bleed,
You're dead, and dead, and dead indeed.

—Nursery Rhyme

Even if we avoid disease, we age just about as I've described, because aging is not itself a disease but the last stage of development. I am going to tell you how this unpleasant process of aging can be slowed down and even postponed to a much later time in life than it would otherwise occur. The method mainly involves losing weight gradually on a carefully selected diet that is high in nutrition but low in calories, or what I shall refer to henceforth as the CRON diet, where CRON stands for calorie restriction with optimal nutrition.

In conservative scientific circles, what I recommend may be regarded as "controversial". That's another way of saying "not completely verified". Whether one should recommend measures to prevent disease and retard aging for which there is strong evidence that they do indeed work, but which are not too percent verified, will evoke different and sometimes (in fact, usually) heated opinions from biologists and medical doctors. Nevertheless, it is safe to say that far less skepticism exists today about the age retardation promised by a CRON regime in humans than in 1986 when the first edition of this book was published. Continuing research is proving me right, as we shall see.

Proof and Probability

For many years, firm but not conclusive evidence suggested that lowering the amount of cholesterol in the blood would help prevent heart disease. Populations with high blood cholesterol levels experienced more heart attacks than those with low levels. But this neat correlation was not considered absolute "proof", and rightly not, because other differences between the populations might show a similar correlation but have nothing to do with susceptibility to heart attacks. The population with more attacks might be mostly blue eyed, and the other one brown eyed, but it wouldn't necessarily mean that to be blue eyed was to carry a time bomb in your chest. Correlation is not the same as proof of causation! It tells you where to look, but you have to be careful about drawing conclusions.

Despite population data and other "correlation" evidence, the only way to obtain scientifically acceptable proof of the association between blood cholesterol and heart disease would be to take a large number of persons from *the same population*, put half of them on a cholesterol-lowering regimen, and see if that half develops less heart disease than the rest. This critical test was performed in a seven-to-ten-year, $150-million study conducted by the National Institute of Health. It provided formal evidence that lowering blood cholesterol will substantially decrease the chance of a heart attack. There have been further refinements of this yardstick in that the cholesterol/HDL ratio in the blood, and more recently the triglyceride/HDL ratio yield even better predictions, and possibly (most recently) the level of blood homocysteine.

Years before the proof of the importance of the blood lipid levels in heart disease was published, many very creditable physicians, including professors at major medical schools, recommended measures aimed at lowering blood cholesterol. They did so on the basis of inferential, or "probable", evidence gained from observations in humans and experiments in animals. Other equally prestigious doctors didn't agree that the evidence was enough to act upon. Until formal proof is established, matters like this remain legitimate questions of judgment, which varies from one physician to another, and even between panels of experts. In 1980, for example, the Food and Nutrition Board of the National Research Council was unwilling on the basis of available data to recommend much at all in the way of nutritional change in the American diet, whereas in the same year and *on the same body* of data a committee of the American Heart Association advised lifelong adoption of a considerably altered diet. This illustrates our situation concerning many aspects of preventive medicine, including ways to slow down the aging process. Should we wait for "conclusive" evidence, which may be years away and too late for some of us? Can we, in some instances, accept probable evidence?

Physicians, patients, and bodies of experts alike should realize that not taking a stand, insisting on waiting until all the evidence is in, is itself a position and a recommendation. Not taking a stand is not really the neutral position it is made out to be.

We cannot easily run a $150-million seven-to-ten-year conclusive study, on every promising assembly of probable evidence about preventing disease and retarding aging, so we must either stay neutral and do nothing or take a stand on the basis of imperfect evidence. Physicians like to pretend, and many have kidded themselves into believing, that whatever they espouse has been "scientifically proved", Nonsense! A great deal of what established medicine recommends with good conscience is not formally "proved", The health benefits of exercise, for example: the *formal* proof on that is not yet in, yet practically all physicians recommend it. And they are right to do so, because the probable evidence is excellent.

Recommendations about disease prevention and life extension are only as good as the ability of the recommending person to analyze and judge a wide assortment of important but inconclusive evidence. In this book I undertake to explain and rate the evidence, analyze it, judge it, and make specific recommendations. My credentials in relation to age retardation are among the best in the world. In the matter of disease prevention, they are less, but they reflect extensive reading on the subject, plus my experience as a teacher and practitioner at the University of California School of Medicine.

By rating the evidence I mean stating whether any case in point can be considered to display a very high order of probability (almost certain), a high order of probability, a moderate order, or less.

I judged it highly probable 14 years ago (for the first edition of this book) that a diet super high in nutritive quality but low in calories (the CRON diet as described herein) would retard the basic rate of aging in humans, greatly extending the period of youth and middle age; postpone the onset of such late-life diseases as heart disease, diabetes, and cancer; and even lower the overall susceptibility to disease at any age. In the intervening time, much additional evidence has accumulated, not only from further rodent investigations but also now from monkey and human studies, to support all of these assertions.

Principles of the CRON Diet

The CRON diet is based upon many years of animal experimentation in my own laboratory at the UCLA Medical School, and in other laboratories in other major universities in the United States and Europe; in more recent studies of calorie-restricted monkey colonies at the Universities of Wisconsin and Maryland; at the National Institute on Aging; and my own studies on humans inside Biosphere 2 for two years.

There is no doubt at all that the life span of animals can be extended by up to 50 percent by dietary means, corresponding to humans living to be 150 or 160 years old. I don't actually expect to achieve quite this much life extension in humans. The necessary regimen would be too tough; but a less rigorous regimen will still add many years to your life, as well as life to your years. The former without the latter would not be so good, but the CRON dietary program promises both.

The CRON diet emphasizes food combinations and menus arrived at by computer techniques so that the Recommended Daily Allowances of all important nutrients are approximated with *minimal caloric intake*. The program calls for *gradual* weight loss over six months to a year or so, until you reach and remain at a new weight point substantially below your "set point", Your set point is the weight toward which you naturally gravitate if you neither over-nor undereat. Your new weight point, if you are on the proper nutritive program, is your point of maximum metabolic efficiency, maximum health, and maximum life span.

I will also tell you how to determine fairly soon after beginning the diet whether markers of your health status have been improved, and to estimate (over a longer period) your individual aging rate, as well as can be done with present techniques. You can then determine how well the program is working for you. And you will soon observe, if you stick to the program, that you simply feel better. You will need less sleep, have more energy, enhanced vitality, and a clearer head than before.

The CRON diet is well founded scientifically. But evidence that taking fairly large amounts of certain vitamins, drugs and chemicals will give an added boost to health and longevity varies from very good (for increasing health and *average life span*) to less than moderate (for increasing *maximum life span* see below for definition of this important term). It does exist, however, and we must at least consider supplementation as a part of our program. The proper types (more than one) and amounts of exercise may yield additional advantages.

We shall thus be discussing evidence at every order of probability. In consultation with your personal physician, you must finally decide which recommendations you want to adopt.

Interacting With Your Chosen Physician

Don't use this book just to strike out on your own, regulating your diet, testing your progress, and swallowing a lot of chemicals and pills. My recommendations may apply to an average across-the-board person but still not be appropriate for a particular individual like yourself. You should discuss the book with a physician qualified to establish your current health status and supervise your longevity and health program. Such qualifications are more easily asked for than found, although the situation has greatly improved in the last dozen years as experimental gerontology and geriatrics have become important medical disciplines. Nevertheless, modern medical training, while strong in disease treatment, remains weak in disease prevention. Nutrition, for example is still a woefully small part of the medical-school curriculum. The average physician may be vaguely familiar with much of the evidence I cite in this book, but will recognize that *some* of my recommendations are not in line with what establishment medicine preaches. He (or she) is apt to feel safe in hiding his ignorance of the subject behind his doctoral authority. That's not what you need.

Establishment medicine is in general excellent, but as pointed out by medical historian P. Starr, it maintains its status and authority by two maneuvers: consensus, and the assumption of complexity. By *consensus* is meant that biologists and doctors may squabble among themselves, but they try to present a unified front to the public. Assumption of complexity means they behave as though arguments about health care were too complicated for even a reasonably educated layperson to understand. The acceptance of doctors as all-wise authority figures (which, believe it or not, dates only from about 1920) signifies "a surrender of private judgment" on the part of patients. In considering what I say in this book, I ask you not to surrender your private judgment.

Warped into the habit of consensus viewing, your physician may not be willing even to consider evidence and recommendations contained in a popular book such as this one. In that case, he or she will find the hard-core scientific evidence for much of what I say here more extensively and rigorously documented in a book my former UCLA colleague Dr. Richard Weindruch (now at the University of Wisconsin) and I have written, *The Retardation of Aging by Dietary Restriction*, published by Charles C. Thomas in 1988, plus other, rigorous scientific monographs. What I say here may well be debatable, but it is based upon sound scientific investigations carried out at numerous recognized universities by many different investigators.

The National Institute on Aging and the National Center for Toxicological Research have maintained colonies of more than 30,000 rats and mice, about half of which are on an animal version of the CRON diet and the other half on a traditional diet. These colonies were established so that investigators throughout the country could test the hallmarks of this life span-prolonging, age-retarding regimen without the enormous trouble of setting up their own animal groups, as nutritional scientists have had to do until recently. The regulation of aging by diet, an area in which I and my associates have done some of the pioneering work, has become a major field of investigation into the aging process. If your doctor does not know about it, he or she should do some reading.

To establish the best interplay between yourself and your physician, you must take an active participatory interest. Anyone either layperson or physician can easily see from his two fine books *Anatomy of an Illness* and *The Healing Heart*, that Norman Cousins mastered the technique of the patient/physician interplay. Because of that, he received more careful, informed care from his doctors than if he had blindly followed their authoritarian advice. His books portray a new kind of patient/doctor relationship. Be guided by their example.

Of course you should seek advice from your personal physician. Still, in preventive medicine you must assume a large measure of responsibility for your own health. This means knowing or learning how to evaluate evidence. Even respectable medical journals contain a great deal of hogwash, lay journals a lot more, and television commercials almost nothing but. But hogwash is not hard to recognize, wherever occurs, if you have the key concepts of what constitutes good evidence. Finally, to hold up your side of the patient/physician interplay, you must acquire a basic knowledge about the major killer diseases of late life, and about certain critical aspects of the biology of aging. This knowledge is provided by the book you have in your hand.

Average and Maximum Life Spans

To begin to understand aging and how to retard it, you must understand survival curves, in particular the significance of the average and maximum life-span points on those curves. Figure 1.1 shows four curves, A, B, C and D. Curves A, B and C are from actual populations; D is hypothetical. The vertical axis on the left indicates the percentage of the population that is alive at any age.

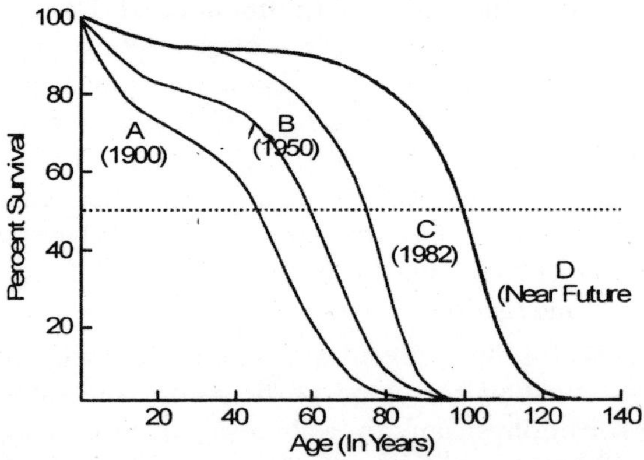

Figure 1.1. Survival curves for the United States in 1900 (curve A), 1950 (curve B) and 1982 (curve C) and for a near-future subpopulation (people on the CRON diet) whose aging rate has been slowed (curve D).

At birth all these population members were alive, so we start with 100 percent. In population A, half the people were dead by the age of 44; in population B, by 60; in population C, by 74; in hypothetical population D, by 100 years of age. All these 50 percent survival points express *average life* spans (also known as *life expectancies at birth*) for the four populations. Curves A, B and C are the survival curves for the United States in 1900, 1950 and 1982. The average life span has been increasing since the turn of the century.

This largely reflects our conquest of many infectious diseases and to some extent other diseases in First World societies. But it can be shown mathematically that if *all* known diseases were cured no heart disease, no stroke, no cancer, no diabetes—the average life span would move up to 85 years of age, but no further, unless the aging process itself were brought under control. The remarkable increase in average life span since 1900 does not reflect any retardation of the basic aging process!

Notice in Figure 1.1 that the maximum life spans are the same for curves A, B and C. Maximum life span reflects the genetically determined longevity potential for our species. At the same time, it's a good measure of the basic aging process. It has remained at about 110 years not only since 1900, but even since the time of ancient Rome-and even before that. (There are of course a few outliers: two persons have lived to 113, one to 119, and the recently deceased French woman, Jeanne Calment, to 122). According to Genesis 6:3, "man also is flesh: yet his days shall be an hundred and twenty years", That's close enough to the observed 110-year maximum! No matter how off base His devotees have portrayed Him with respect to evolution, God shines through, at least in this passage, as an excellent gerontologist.

The survival curves A, B and C teach us that we cannot influence maximum life span just by curing diseases. Even if all the major diseases were eliminated, the disease-free, older-growing population would simply become vulnerable to smaller and smaller environmental assaults, and still die off by 110 years. Only measures that truly retard biologic aging and stretch out the periods of youth and middle age will budge the shoulder of this maximal survival point and create a long-living society like the one represented in curve D. That's what the CRON diet will do.

I shall tell you not only how you can jump from curve A onto B or C, or from B onto C thus increasing your average survival potential but how you can jump onto curve D itself, becoming a member of the longest-living society that has ever existed. There is already an Internet-connected group of long-livers on this regime. Many of them will be around to celebrate the twenty-second century.

So we have two goals in this book. They are related, but not quite the same. We want to learn how to improve our survival chances in terms of average life span. That means preventing as much as possible those diseases most of us would otherwise die of. Second, we want to learn how to slow down the rate of aging, so that while we avoid the diseases, we also do not age so rapidly. In other words, we will not only *live* longer we will stay *younger* longer. We will neither sag nor flag nor forget where we are or where we have been or where we are going in this fast-moving and exciting world.

Nature of Evidence

If you get nothing out of this book except what I say in this section, you're way ahead. I'll be focusing on the biology of aging, but what I say will have general applicability to how you should evaluate any scientific or material claim, whether it be about your body, your automobile, your rose garden, or whatever but not necessarily ethical, aesthetic, or religious claims, which are of course separate areas.

Throughout much of this book I'll be presenting you with evidence followed by recommendations. I want you to be informed and then to make up your own mind, remembering that you should seek guidance from your own doctor but not be dominated by his or her assumption of authority. The frequent bamboozling of the public by health faddists is partly the fault of medicine itself, which has taught people to rely on someone else's judgment, rather than teaching them how to examine evidence.

Evidence falls into four categories: testimonial, argumentative ("make the case for"), correlational, and experimental. *Testimonial* evidence is the principal type coming from the faddists, charlatans and know-nothings. They will give you a list of people who took the treatment and say it did them good. If the list includes movie stars and professional athletes, or Olympic athletes, so much the better.

Testimonial evidence (related closely to "anecdotal" evidence) is highly unreliable. The list rarely includes people who took the treatment and did not receive any benefit. It almost never includes people who did not take the treatment but got better anyway, spontaneously. And testimonial evidence is abundantly available for almost every claim, from the benefits of Christian Science to experience with spiritualism, herbalism, black magic, faith healing, ghosts, Scientology, UFOs, Bigfoot you name it. If you accept testimonial evidence, you will end up believing just about anything and everything. Testimonial evidence isn't necessarily and inherently wrong, but it's almost impossible to evaluate.

Interestingly enough, establishment medicine is also sometimes guilty of too much reliance on testimonial evidence, but it gives it another name: the "clinical anecdote", Dr. X has seen 35 patients with a certain malady and on the basis of his experience thinks that treating them with compound Z has been beneficial. He has no controls. His opinion represents a subjective guess. He will usually say, "My impression is . . ." or "My clinical experience is" and then give the guess. This medical version of testimonial evidence is often wrong.

Argumentative evidence consists in marshaling known facts or experimental results and reasoning from them that something else ought to be so. Exercise, for instance, increases the level of high-density lipoproteins (HDL) in the blood, and these are usually associated with a lower degree of arteriosclerosis, so exercise *ought* to increase resistance to heart attacks. That's a logical argument. But do people who exercise actually experience fewer heart attacks? Maybe so, but you cannot stop with a plausibility argument! You have to test your hypothesis in the real world of what is happening.

Examples of argumentative evidence in gerontology concern the antioxidants: substances like vitamin E and the mineral selenium. These, it is argued, neutralize the damaging so-called "free radicals" that are by-products of normal metabolism. You can make an excellent case for the idea that free radicals cause aging, and that including antioxidants in the diet ought to retard it. But sad to say, including antioxidants in the diet, while it may to a certain degree indeed be health enhancing, has not so far been shown to extend the maximum life span of any species. Antioxidants so far have failed this critical test. Making a plausible case for something is not enough! Most of the Pearson/Shaw book relies upon this lower-order category of evidence, and upon the testimonial posturing of Pearson and Shaw themselves.

Sandy Shaw takes antioxidants and bends horseshoes on television, thus proving that antioxidants retard aging! Bah!

The two final types of scientific evidence, and the only really solid ones, are correlational and experimental. *Correlation* implies that when two things occur together all or most of the time, there may be a direct causal relationship between them, or that perhaps both are caused by some third (not necessarily apparent) phenomenon. Correlation can be seductive, but it's not actual proof. Nations whose citizens eat a high-fat diet generally display a higher incidence of heart disease than nations with low-fat diets. That sounds reasonable, but it's not proof. When the Santa Ana wind blows in California, a lot of people develop hay fever. The wind also causes an elevation in barometric pressure. Does elevated barometric pressure, then, cause hay fever? The wind blows pollens around; that's what leads to the hay fever. Barometric pressure is irrelevant. Yet the correlation exists.

In this book we shall be concerned a great deal with correlational evidence. In fact it can be very useful, but one has to be careful. It was observed on examination of the data from a large number of insurance companies that people who are slightly overweight seem to enjoy a better average survival. This data might well be accurate, but the true biological interpretation may be quite different from what the data *seem* to indicate that is, that it's intrinsically healthy to be slightly overweight. More on this later, but here's another interpretation, just to illustrate possibilities: perhaps the modern U.S. processed-food and junk-food diet is so poor that the average eater must consume excess calories just to get enough vitamins and essential nutriments to remain healthy and not be *mal*nourished.

The only kind of scientific evidence acceptable as genuine "proof" of a hypothesis is that of repeatable experiments, usually accompanied by what are called "control" data. Under appropriate conditions you do something, and that changes something else. And this something/something else always happens! When another investigator repeats the experiment on the other side of town or in Uttar Pradesh, the same result is obtained. The experiment, if done well, establishes the causal nature of a relationship between two phenomena. It constitutes *experimental evidence*.

Repeatedly confirmed experiments in my laboratory and in many other university laboratories have proved that cutting down calories, plus increasing the quality of the diet, produces very lean, extremely healthy animals, greatly extends their maximum life spans, markedly lowers their susceptibility to disease, and keeps them young in outward appearance, in their physiology and biochemistry, and in their physical and intellectual performance.

Correlation, if extensive enough, and experiment, if well conceived and carried out, constitute good evidence. Argument, or plausibility constructs, are the building blocks of hypotheses. They are good for pointing the investigator in what he hopes is the right direction and for suggesting how to proceed in testing his hypothesis, but if acted on directly, because they "sound reasonable", they can lead you astray. Jumping on the latest supplement bandwagon might be a case in point. Testimonial evidence is the least reliable of all, but the most frequently used in advertising.

Having categorized the evidence, you have to *interpret* it. What does it mean biologically? American insurance company statistics seemed at one time to indicate that it's better to be slightly overweight; experiments in animals, that it's better to be underweight. The correlational evidence in one instance and experimental evidence in the other were both correct, but they seemed contradictory. Why? I've just given you one hint, and we'll be discussing these matters at some length in a later chapter. But when two sets of data both seem valid in fact but directly opposed in meaning, it often turns out in science that both are correct, and you have just not found the right interpretation.

I cannot teach you the fine points of interpretation of scientific evidence. That takes years of training and lots of experience. But you should be able to recognize the *category* of the evidence being presented to you: by me, in discussions with your friends, by other writers or lecturers, by popular health magazines, by newspapers, and of course by the 30-second flash-ad media blitzes. If your barber, hairdresser, or favorite celebrity tells you, "I went to Mexico and they shot me up with XYZ and I feel great. My cancer melted away, my arches rose, my bunions decamped, and lights went on in my head," you can recognize the statement as testimonial evidence.

I hope you will look just as critically at all the evidence in this book. That's your first step toward a super-healthy and extended life.

2

Treatment and Understanding Disease

Introduction

It can be treated very successfully. Treatment for diabetes varies from person to person and will depend on the type of diabetes you have.

"Years ago it was really restrictive having diabetes, but I think there is a greater understanding now, not so restrictive as before, things are more easily related to every day life."

"Diabetes is not such a problem now because you can control it, I feel that insulin kinda takes away the diabetes."

"I felt so ill on tablets but now I'm on insulin and things are much better."

This chapter will focus on understanding and managing the different types of treatment available, including medication, healthy eating, increasing physical activity levels, and discuss the goals that people with diabetes should aim for when they undertake treatment.

Understanding and Managing Treatment with Medication

Type 1 diabetes is treated by injections of insulin and a healthy diet, and regular exercise is recommended. Type 2 diabetes is treated by a healthy diet and exercise or by a combination of a healthy diet, exercise and tablets. Eventually people with type 2 diabetes may also need insulin injections, although they are not totally 'dependent' on the insulin. If you have just been diagnosed as type 2, it is bound to take you some time to adjust to the idea, but with the right information and back-up from your diabetes care team, you will soon realise that you will be able to cope and keep yourself well. They will show you how to give injections, and take time to teach you how to manage your condition effectively. Do not worry if you need to see them several times to clarify certain points, no one will mind, and would prefer you to ask questions and come back until you feel comfortable with all the new information you have to cope with.

Tablets

There are four main kinds of tablet treatment for people with type 2 diabetes: sulphonylureas, biguanides, acarbose and thiazolidinediones. They all come under the general name of oral hypoglycaemic agents (OHAs), and any of them may be taken alone or in combination. Many people with type 2 diabetes find that these medications, together with a healthy eating pattern, keep their diabetes under control, although it may take some time to find out which combination or dose suits you best.

The tablets all work in different ways: some help your pancreas to produce more insulin; others help your body to make better use of the insulin that your pancreas does produce; and yet others slow down the speed at which your body absorbs glucose from the intestine. Your doctor will decide which kinds of tablet are going to work best for you and may prescribe more than one kind. Your doctor or diabetes nurse will tell you all about the tablets, when to take them, and how to monitor your blood or urine glucose levels.

"Going on to insulin, I found this really upsetting – felt I was doing well and it was a reflection on me to say going on to insulin."

Eventually even several types of tablet may not be enough to keep your blood glucose levels within the normal range and you may be advised to take insulin as well as, or instead of, your tablets. This is quite a usual thing to happen and is not a reflection on you or on how well you have been looking after yourself.

Insulin

People with type 1 diabetes need injections of insulin for the rest of their lives and also need to eat a healthy diet that contains the right balance of foods. In addition, a minimum of exercise is recommended for overall health and to prevent diabetes complications.

'Why do I have to inject the insulin?'

This is the only effective way of getting it into your bloodstream. Insulin cannot be swallowed because the digestive juices in the stomach destroy it.

'What types of insulin are there?'

The basic difference is in how quickly they take effect, so they can be divided into short-medium or long-acting varieties. The short-acting insulin is always clear or colourless, whereas the other two are cloudy because they contain additives to slow down the absorption of insulin from under the skin. It is possible to mix short and medium-acting insulin in the same syringe, but care must be taken not to contaminate the clear insulin with any cloudy insulin. For this reason the clear insulin is always drawn up first.

If you find it difficult to mix the insulin yourself, you may be able to use one of the ready-mixed kinds which contain short and medium-acting insulin in different proportions.

All three types of insulin may be produced from animal sources—pig or beef—or from genetically engineered human hormone. Some so-called human insulin is in fact derived originally from pigs but altered so that it is indistinguishable from the human version. The human type is the most widely prescribed insulin in the UK.

'Why do I have to inject insulin several times a day?'

The object of insulin therapy is to imitate the body's natural supply of insulin as closely as possible. In a person who does not have diabetes, insulin is released by the pancreas in response to food. As the blood glucose level falls between meals, so the insulin level drops back towards zero. It never quite gets there, however, and there is no time in the 24 hours when there is no detectable insulin in the bloodstream. What you are trying to do when you give yourself insulin injections is to reproduce the normal pattern of insulin production from the pancreas.

There are several ways of doing this using different types of insulin and numbers of injections per day. For example, many people follow a system which comprises three injections of short-acting insulin before the three main meals of the day, plus a night-time injection of a medium-or long-acting insulin to control blood glucose while they are asleep. Another popular and equally successful system involves two injections a day of a mixture of short-and medium-acting insulin. The idea is that the short-acting component covers the meal you are about to have for example, breakfast or the evening meal while the medium-acting component covers you at lunchtime or overnight. Many people have been using one or other of these systems very happily for years, and the choice between them is often simply a matter of personal preference.

If you are one of the relatively few people who simply cannot get used to giving yourself several injections a day, or if you have only a partial failure of your insulin supply, you may be able to make do with just one or two daily injections of medium or long-acting insulin.

'How and where do I inject myself?'

Your diabetes care team will show you how to do the injections and explain the various types of equipment available. Many people today use disposable plastic syringes and needles. Insulin injection pens are also very popular, largely because of their convenience and portability. Although the pens themselves are free, the needles still have to be paid for, although there is currently an active campaign to try to persuade the Department of Health to allow free prescription of pen needles. There are several types of pen to choose from, but the principles of the device are much the same. It is simply a matter of which one suits you best.

You inject insulin under your skin rather than into a vein or muscle. Recent research has suggested that many people may have been getting the depth wrong so that insulin is going into the muscle beneath the skin by mistake. Judging the depth accurately can be a problem, especially if you are slim, but it is important to master the technique because insulin can be absorbed from muscle more rapidly than expected. Your diabetes care team will show you how to do it properly, but many people find that the simplest way is to pinch the skin and inject the bunched up area at an angle of 90 degrees. Don't pinch too hard, however, or it will hurt when the needle goes in! For people who may be having difficulty with inadvertent muscular injection, there are different lengths of needle available and this problem should be discussed with your diabetes care team.

You will be given advice about the best sites for injection. The tops of the thighs, buttocks and abdomen are the most common sites, and it is best to avoid using the same area every time, otherwise you could develop a small fatty lump, which could affect the smoothness of insulin absorption. It is probably a good idea to inject medium-or long-acting insulin into your thigh or buttock and use your tummy for short-acting injections, but the most important thing is that you should be reasonably comfortable about the sites you are using.

'Will the injections hurt or mark?'

People who have been giving themselves injections for years say they do not feel a thing, but many beginners may find it slightly painful at first. Try to be as relaxed as you can and follow the technique you have been shown. Some people find that it helps to rub the skin with ice for a few seconds beforehand to numb it, and you might like to try this method. As you get more practice, you should find that the injections rarely hurt, but if things do not improve, it is worth asking someone at the diabetes centre for advice on what is causing the problem.

The needles are very fine and usually do not leave a mark. Sometimes you may get a little bleeding after an injection or even a bruise, but this is nothing to worry about. It just means that you have probably punctured one of the tiny blood vessels under the skin, which happens occasionally. There is virtually no chance of insulin directly entering the bloodstream, so do not worry if you notice some bleeding.

Understanding and Managing Healthy Eating

What you eat has an effect on your general health and well-being. Many people think that they already have a healthy diet but, on average, people in the UK eat too much fat and too many calories. This can result in high cholesterol levels and weight problems and lead to many heart attacks each year.

Whichever type of diabetes you have, your food choice helps to balance your blood glucose levels and your diet is therefore an essential part of your treatment. However, the sort of diet you should follow when you have diabetes definitely does not mean a future of self-denial on all tasty foods. Changing your eating habits does not mean that you need to follow a special diet, but just a healthy diet as recommended for everyone.

"It's all changed now – makes a huge difference not to have to weigh every piece of food. Everything had to be counted before."

Eating more healthily can reduce your risk of developing:

- Complications of diabetes.
- Heart disease by reducing cholesterol levels, blood pressure, weight.
- Some cancers (two-thirds of cancer are related to what we eat).
- Arthritis.

To eat healthily, what are you aiming for?

"My friend's grandfather was diabetic. She said I should never touch starch. Fatal, you see, for a diabetic. Makes sugar. So I'm always very strict. No bread, no biscuits, no potato ever."

The Balance of Good Health shows the types and proportion of foods you need to eat to achieve a well-balanced and healthy diet. It is based on the five commonly accepted food groups. It shows that you do not have to give up the foods you most enjoy for the sake of your health. A healthy eating pattern includes the correct balance of foods from the four main food groups every day, plus an allowance for extras from the fats and fatty sugary foods group. All your nutritional needs will be met if you choose foods in these proportions. Remember, however, that everything you eat snacks as well as meals counts towards the balance of what you eat. The basic message is:

- Base your meals on starchy foods – fill up on these. This means such foods as bread, potatoes, rice, pasta, noodles, oats, crackers, breakfast cereals. These all provide starch, fibre, vitamins (especially B) and minerals.
- Eat at least five servings of fruit and vegetables daily. Choose from fresh, frozen, or canned fruit and vegetables – and do not forget juices and dried fruit. Add in some to each meal or snack from breakfast to bedtime. These contain vitamins, minerals and fibre. Eating them may help to protect you against heart disease and cancer as they contain antioxidant vitamins (vitamins A, C and E).

- Eat moderate amounts of milk and dairy foods, and lower fat versions whenever you can. These contain calcium, protein and vitamins A and B.
- Eat moderate amounts of meat, fish and alternatives and choose lower fat versions. Lower fat choices include lean meat, chicken, fish, eggs, beans and pulses. These foods contain protein and iron. Try to have fish at least twice a week and use beans and pulses to make meat go further or for a meat-free meal.
- Reduce your intake of fats and fatty and sugary foods. Fats in the diet is the main problem as far as heart disease, high blood cholesterol and weight gain are concerned. They are of limited nutritional value and you can obtain all the fat you need from the milk, dairy, meat and meat alternatives groups. Use spreading fats and cooking oils sparingly. Keep fatty and sugary dishes and snacks as occasional rather than everyday foods. Choose low fat methods of preparation and cooking.

Intake of Fats

Two main types of fat are normally consumed:

- Saturated fats (or 'saturates'). The more saturates we eat, the more cholesterol the body produces. This builds up in our blood and increases the risk of developing heart disease. Saturated fats are found mostly in animal products such as dairy products and meat. They are also found in some vegetable oils such as coconut oil and palm oil, in hard margarine, ghee and cooking fat and as 'hidden' fats in cakes, biscuits, chocolate and puddings. They may be in the ingredients list as 'hydrogenated vegetable fat/oil'.
- Unsaturated fats (or 'unsaturates'). This group includes polyunsaturated fats and mono-unsaturated fats. In very small amounts these are essential to the body to provide certain vitamins and make foods more pleasant to eat. These fats are still high in calories. Unsaturated fats are found in vegetable oils, such as sunflower, corn, soya, rapeseed and olive oils, in soft margarine labelled 'high in polyunsaturates', in nuts and in oily fish such as sardines, herring mackerel, trout and pilchards.

Ways to substitute unsaturated fat for saturated fat :

- Use a low fat poly/mono-unsaturated spread.
- Use a poly/mono-unsaturated fat in cooking.
- Try not to use blended vegetable oil (may be high in saturated fat).

Making a Start

Making changes to your eating patterns usually means changing long-established habits related to shopping, cooking and eating. When you are planning such changes to your lifestyle, you can therefore help yourself to be more successful by thinking it through beforehand. This can help by drawing your attention to problems or difficulties that you may be able to prevent in advance.

How can you set yourself up so the changes you make are successful?

Below are some suggestions. Tick those that you think will be helpful to you. If you can think of any others, add them to the list:

- Stock your food cupboards with foods that do not trigger eating 'the wrong things'.
- Plan your shopping in advance so that you only buy suitable things.
- Carry suitable snacks with you.
- Plan eating times daily in advance.
- Have suitable snacks available in the car.
- Ask a friend, partner or work mate to encourage you.
- When cooking, avoid tasting as this may result in over-eating.
- Avoid unnecessary exposure to food.

What do you do when the going gets tough?

At times it can be quite difficult to maintain changes. It will take time for the changes you are making to become part of your everyday life. All those who try to change their behaviour occasionally find that they have done something that does not fit in with their plans. These one-off slip-ups, or lapses, often lead to feelings of guilt, which makes the individuals more susceptible to other slips and can eventually force them to abandon their changes altogether. To help you to maintain new changes, or when things get difficult, it can help to think about what you can use to motivate yourself. Below are some suggestions:

- Talk to the friend or partner who agreed to encourage you.
- Remind yourself of the short-term and long-term benefits to your health.
- Review your achievements up until the present.
- Find healthy ways to treat yourself because of your achievements.

Changing your Diet

- *Eat regular meals:* Try to plan your meals around starchy foods (such as bread, potatoes, rice, pasta and cereals) from day to day. This will help to keep your blood glucose in the normal range.
- *Try to cut down on fat*: Cut down on fried and fatty foods such as butter, margarine, cheese and fatty meats. These foods are high in calories and can make you gain weight. Choose reduced fat spreads and cheeses instead. Try skimmed or semi-skimmed milk.
- *Eat more high-fibre starchy carbohydrate foods:* The fibre in beans, peas, lentils and fruit is particularly good because it slows down the rate at which your body absorbs carbohydrate.
- *Aim to reduce your sugar intake*: Cut down on sugar, confectionery and sugary drinks. You can use artificial sweeteners such as saccharin, diet drinks and reduced sugar preserves.
- *Cut down on your salt in take*: Reduce salt added in cooking by using more herbs and spices instead. Gradually cut down on the salt you add to your food at the table.
- *Try to drink alcohol only in moderation*: People with diabetes should try to limit their intake of alcohol. Never drink on an empty stomach and always have something to eat with your drink, or shortly afterwards.
- *Avoid special diabetic foods:* They can be expensive and offer no special health benefit.

In changing your diet, it is important to set realistic goals that are actually achievable. There is nothing like success to increase motivation and enthusiasm. Look on changes as a positive opportunity to increase the enjoyment of eating and the variety of your diet—and appreciate any health aspects as an additional bonus.

What about eating out and holidays?

"Of course, the fact that I have diabetes needs to be taken into account if I eat out or change jobs but it's not at the forefront of my mind. Anyway, you're always learning when you have diabetes."

"At first, eating out and diabetes seemed like such a minefield. I thought 'what can I eat now that I have diabetes?' but I found that just making small changes to begin with really helps you."

"I was a bit afraid to eat out with my friends at first, afraid I might embarrass them."

Eating Out

Increasingly, we have more and more meals away from home eating in restaurants and pubs or grabbing sandwiches and takeaways on the run. However, food made away from home tends to be higher in fat and salt and lower in fibre than the home-made equivalent. As long as eating out is not the usual thing you do, then it should not be a problem, but if you eat out regularly look out for lower fat options, avoid items that are served in butter or cream, and are fried or battered. These are often loaded with fat because of the way they are prepared.

It is sometimes difficult to know what to do when eating out with friends who have made a special effort to prepare delicious food for you, which then turns out to be quite unsuitable. However, if you warn your friends in advance that you have diabetes and want to avoid food containing high concentrations of sugar, you will probably find it less embarrassing all round.

Holidays and Travelling

If you are going abroad on holiday the same rules apply but obviously you may have to be extra careful if you do not understand the menu or are unfamiliar with some of the dishes. Some airlines offer 'special diabetic' meals on the plane. It is actually better to avoid them because they can be low in carbohydrate caterers often do not realise that balance is the main thing, not cutting down on carbohydrate. Also it is a good idea to take extra carbohydrate in your hand luggage.

Parties and Special Events

With a little thought and pre-planning, you can feel free to go to any party and enjoy yourself as much as ever. The main considerations are that you will probably be eating later than usual, having different kinds of food and possibly dancing late into the night. When you are on insulin or on tablets, you will need to make certain adjustments to take account of these factors. You will need to eat more to allow for extra activities such as dancing. Dancing will mean that you have to have extra carbohydrate—the amount depending on how much energy you put into your performance!

HELPFUL TIPS! HELPFUL TIPS! HELPFUL TIPS! HELPFUL There are various ways of 'handling' parties and special events:

- *Plan ahead*: Think about the event before you go. Try to anticipate the types of food you will face and the actions of other people. Think about your own desires to eat and the external pressures from others. Have a general idea of what you will eat. You can phone beforehand and ask what will be [trianglerightsld] served. If you pre-plan your food intake, you will decrease the strength of your desire to eat what may not be best for you.
- *Eat before you go*: Do not go hungry to a party or special event. Everything will look good and you will forget that you only want to sample special foods. Have a salad or other low-calorie food before you go. (It is just like shopping for groceries: if you eat before you shop, you will not buy as much!) Furthermore, when you know you are going to be having a meal several hours later than normal, have a light snack before you go, then delay your injection until the food is ready.
- *Eat only special foods*: Stay away from the chips, crisps, dips, nuts and other foods that you can have any time. Use the chance to try new foods or foods you rarely have. Remember to make the best use of your calories.

- *Be the slowest eater*: Keep your eye on others and be the slowest eater at the event. Be the last to start and the last to finish. You will enjoy the food more and will feel satisfied with less. Pay attention to the texture, smell and subtleties of taste. This will stop the rapid and automatic eating that consumes so many calories.
- *Keep a proper perspective*: If you do eat more than you intend to, keep a positive attitude. Do not turn an event into more than it really is—just another day with meals and calories. In the scheme of a month or year's worth of eating, what can one day mean? One day's indiscretion should not ruin any eating plan. The trick is to bounce back. Your reaction to the eating is more important than the eating itself. Your attitudes are central to your ability to control your eating, both during and after the event.

Understanding and Managing Increasing Physical Activity

When a person who does not have diabetes takes exercise, the release of insulin from the pancreas is shut down, while other hormones are produced which cause the blood glucose level to rise. When you are taking insulin or sulphonylurea tablets, however, your insulin level continues to rise, and if you have had an injection into one of the limbs you are exercising, the insulin may be absorbed faster than usual.

Why is exercise important for people with diabetes?

Exercise is important for everyone. It helps us to look good and feel better about ourselves; it increases physical fitness; it reduces the risk of heart disease; it helps with weight control; and it improves muscle tone. Besides improving the body, exercise can also promote a positive, healthy outlook on life.

For people with diabetes, exercise offers even greater benefits. Most importantly, regular exercise can help to improve blood glucose control. Daily physical activity reduces the body's resistance to insulin and increases the body cells' sensitivity to insulin. Therefore, people with type 1 diabetes can keep tight control over their blood sugar levels with smaller amounts of insulin. The same applies to individuals with type 2 diabetes who need to take insulin or oral diabetes medications. Another benefit of exercise is that it can help to reduce blood fat levels, decreasing the risk of heart attack or stroke.

During moderate exercise, glucose stored in muscles is used up first. The muscles then begin using blood glucose, thus gradually lowering the blood glucose level. Even after exercising, the blood glucose continues to fall as the muscles replenish their glucose stores. It is also believed that some body cells respond better to insulin for up to several days after exercising. Since part of the problem in type 2 diabetes is inadequate insulin utilisation (inability of cells to respond to insulin), it is likely that regular exercise can help to keep body cells responsive to insulin continuously so that swings in blood glucose levels can be avoided.

How much exercise should you do?

In order for exercise to be effective, it usually must be practised vigorously for at least 15 minutes, three times a week. Daily exercise, of course, is better. However, consult with your diabetes team before starting any exercise programme so that you can develop one that will work best for you.

Why bother?

Many people avoid exercise because it is uncomfortable, takes time, or they feel embarrassed or unskilled. There are, however, great benefits from even small amounts of increased activity without the necessity for 'aerobics'. Physical activity and exercise are positive aspects of health they generally involve doing something constructive. Activity is for everyone; our bodies are made to move and unless we keep moving the capacity for physical functioning becomes greatly reduced. Indeed many of the concerns associated with growing older are quite often more to do with inactivity.

It is not uncommon for people who are older or overweight to think that because they cannot run six miles or do an advanced level of aerobics, anything less is worthless, and they therefore do no physical activity. However, every bit of activity is important, even the odd few minutes can help to get you going. You can then build up by gradually extending the time you can sustain the activity, within your daily routine.

Still not convinced?

'It's too much like hard work. I'd never keep it up'.

It will not seem to be hard work if you choose an activity you enjoy and build up slowly and gradually. As you get better you will enjoy it even more and you will not want to give it up.

'I haven't got time. My life is too busy'

Just 20 minutes two or three times a week can keep you feeling young and active. Once you start feeling the benefits, and your new activity becomes a habit, it will be much easier to fit into your routine.

'What I need is relaxation'

Exercise can be just the thing to help you to relax. It relieves stress by taking your mind off your problems. After a session of vigorous exercise, you will feel warm, comfortable and relaxed. You will notice the relaxing effect of some kinds of exercise even while you are doing them. Recent studies have shown that exercising can also help with depression, and you will probably find that it also helps you to sleep better.

'But doesn't it have to hurt to do you any good?'

No! If it hurts, then you are pushing yourself too hard. If you are in any pain, stop. If you feel uncomfortably out of breath, slow down or stop.

'It's too late for me—I'm past it!'

It is never too late. Anyone can get fitter. Whatever your age you can find a form of physical activity that will suit you. And the less fit you are to start with, the sooner you will notice the benefits.

'But isn't it bad for my heart?'

On the contrary, it helps to protect your heart. When you exercise, your muscles need more oxygen than usual, so your heart has to beat faster to pump more oxygen-carrying blood to them. Also, if you exercise regularly, your muscles get better at using oxygen and your heart pumps more blood with each beat, so it does not need to beat so quickly. As you get fitter you can exercise harder without overtaxing your heart. Regular exercise has other benefits too. It can help to control high blood pressure. It can also help to stop your arteries furring up, and over the years your risk of having a heart attack will be reduced.

'I'm not the sporty type'

Even if you did not like sport at school, there are now so many different activities, you are sure to be able to find one you enjoy. Just try different ones until you find the one that is right for you. Remember, walking is a very good form of exercise.

'I'd be too embarrassed'

Do not let embarrassment put you off increasing your physical activity you would be missing out on too much! People of all shapes and sizes enjoy exercising and you will not feel uncomfortable or out of place if you choose an activity that is right for you.

'I couldn't bear all the sprains and strains'

You will only get these if you push yourself too hard, too soon. Or if you do an occasional session of hard exercise and nothing in between. If you start off gently and build up slowly, your risks of sprains and strains are very low. Exercise builds up strong muscles, which protect you from injury. When muscles are not used, for example when a broken leg is put in plaster, the muscles waste away and the leg gets thin and weak. But if muscles are used more than usual, for example for exercising, they get stronger and more efficient.

'If I can't do it properly, then what's the point of doing it at all?'

You do not have to go into serious training and get super fit or play competitive sports to gain benefits from exercise. Regular activity for just 20 or 30 minutes, two or three times a week, will go a long way towards helping you to stay in good shape.

'I'm too fat for that kind of thing'

Then you are just the type of person who will benefit most from some regular physical activity, especially if it is the stamina-building type. Exercising helps you to control your weight by burning up calories. If you burn up more calories than you eat, your body will start using up its own energy stores and fat will start to disappear. There is evidence that some people may still be burning up more calories than usual sometimes for up to 24 hours—after they have finished exercising.

HELPFUL TIPS! HELPFUL TIPS! HELPFUL TIPS! HELPFUL
There are various ways of increasing your physical activity:

- To get moving, increase activity in your day-to-day routine. Increasing lifestyle activity is easy, takes little time, is not painful, does not require special clothes/equipment and helps you to feel better.

- Use more effort than usual. Find a more active way to do the things you usually do; for example, lose the remote control for the television, and get up and change the channels every time you want to watch another programme! Remember, every bit of activity counts!
- Use the stairs instead of the lift. Climbing stairs is a good way of keeping your leg muscles strong.
- Walk more! If you are not very active now, your first step to getting fitter is simply to walk more. When you walk, walk faster. Walking briskly for 20 to 30 minutes, two or three times a week, will soon build up your stamina. It is an ideal exercise.
- Build up gradually. It takes time to get fit. Work hard enough to make yourself a bit sweaty and out of breath, but not uncomfortably. That way there will also be less risk of sprains and strains.
- Keep it up! You cannot store fitness.

Are you struggling?

Sometimes becoming more active seems difficult to do because there are too many things stopping you and not enough things helping you.

- Identify the main things that are making it difficult to become more physically active:
    - Are they to do with yourself, for example, 'I haven't got the time?'
    - Are they to do with other people, for example, 'No one will come with me?'
    - Are they to do with your surroundings, for example, 'There is nowhere suitable to walk?'
- Can you remove any of these or make them less important?
- Tackle the ones that seem easiest to deal with first.
- If you can release the brake a little, then you are more likely to be able to move forward.

Understanding and Managing the Main Goals of Treatment

The main goal of any treatment programme is to bring glucose levels down to as close to normal as possible. By keeping blood sugar levels within the normal range, you can prevent short-term complications such as hypoglycaemia (low blood sugar) and hyperglycaemia (high blood sugar), and greatly reduce your risk of developing long-term complications, including kidney disease, cardiovascular disease and nerve damage.

Understanding Your Role in Treatment

You are the most important member of your treatment team because you are the one who lives with diabetes every day. It is up to you to monitor your blood glucose levels and to take any medications necessary to keep these levels within a normal range. It is up to you to make healthy food choices and to follow your physical activity programme. Ultimately, you are the person responsible for making important decisions about your care. Regardless of how many professionals are on your side, if you do not take steps to effectively manage your diabetes, you will be putting yourself at a greater risk of developing complications.

Monitoring your Blood Glucose Levels

There are four essential components in all proper diabetes management treatment programmes:

- Monitoring your blood glucose levels.
- Following a healthy diet.
- Implementing and following a physical activity programme.
- Knowing how and when to take any medications that you are prescribed.

The point of all treatment for diabetes whether it is diet, tablets or insulin is to keep the levels of glucose in your bloodstream as close as possible to normal. The nearer you get to achieving this, the better you will feel, especially in the long term. There are two ways you can monitor glucose levels and your doctor or diabetes nurse will advise you about which one you should use and how often to do the checks. The two methods available are blood tests and urine tests, and neither is particularly difficult once you understand them.

The development of simple finger-prick blood-testing methods in the last few years has transformed life for patients taking insulin. Keeping a close check on your glucose levels is very useful when you are on insulin because it means that you can make adjustments to your dose depending on the results. When your diabetes is controlled by tablets and/or diet, urine tests can give you nearly as much information as blood tests and may be more convenient. There are also blood tests that can be performed in hospital, which measure an average blood glucose level over a period which may be from two to eight weeks before the test. We will now consider each of these approaches in turn.

Blood Tests

There are two systems available for self-blood glucose monitoring (or SBMG as you may hear it called). Both give accurate results, and as well as helping you to improve your blood glucose control, they can be useful if you suspect you may be about to have a hypoglycaemic reaction. Taking an exact reading will either reassure you that all is well or confirm that you need to take action. Blood-testing strips are available on prescription but the special meters for reading them have to be purchased separately.

Urine Tests

Glucose appears in your urine when your kidneys can no longer reabsorb the amount being filtered. The problem with urine testing is that this 'overflow point' is not the same for everyone. The correct term for this overflow point is the kidney (or renal) threshold. Some people who do not have diabetes have a low threshold, and they often need the glucose tolerance test described earlier to confirm the fact and explain why glucose has appeared in their urine.

The normal threshold is around a blood glucose level of 10 millimoles per litre (mmol/l), so for a person with diabetes, a negative urine test can mean that your blood glucose level is anywhere between 0 and 10 mmol/l, depending on your personal threshold. A positive test, on the other hand, does not tell you the exact level of blood glucose or by how much it exceeds your own personal threshold.

Despite this relative lack of accuracy, testing your urine and getting mostly negative results may be all you need to confirm that your diabetes is well under control, especially if you are being treated with diet and/or tablets.

What do the results tell you?

When you do either a blood test or a urine test, you are really measuring how effective your previous dose of insulin or tablet treatment has been. In other words, doing a test just before lunch will tell someone on insulin the effect of his or her early morning injection of short-acting insulin. In the same way, a pre-breakfast test will reflect the effectiveness of the previous night-time dose. The same interpretation applies in principle to tablets.

When the test result shows a high level of glucose, you may have to increase the size of your next dose of medication to restore the balance. This solves the problem in the short term, but ideally you want to prevent the problem arising in the first place by adjusting the dose that preceded the test. It is a good idea to vary the time of day when you do your test, and also to wait for a series of results over a period of, say, three to five days, before making too many adjustments. That way, you will see whether there is any pattern to the changes in your blood glucose level.

Until you have more experience of handling your diabetes, it would be better to consult your GP or someone in your diabetes care team before altering your insulin or tablet dosage. Later, when you have learned more about your body's reactions, you will be able to make the necessary adjustments on your own because you will know what works best for you.

Hospital Monitoring

If you have type 1 diabetes, there may be situations where your medical advisers feel that it would be useful to assess the effectiveness of your treatment by means of more sophisticated blood tests. They are not a substitute for your own routine testing, but can give additional information that will help the doctor to decide whether your treatment needs adjustment. Both tests require a blood sample to be taken from a vein.

HbA1c—Glycated Haemoglobin

This measures your average blood glucose level over a period of some six to eight weeks. Like all averages, however, it could be the result of lots of small variations or much larger swings in either direction. For this reason, it is not useful for making day-to-day adjustments of insulin treatment, but is a good guide as to whether your treatment is working well overall.

Following the Treatment Plan

It is very important that you follow the treatment that your doctor or diabetes nurse has advised. You will feel much better if you keep your blood glucose levels as near to normal as possible. You should aim for a level of 4–7 mmol/l before meals, rising to no higher that 10 mmol/l two hours after meals. Your diabetes team will advise you on what is best for you.

Conclusion

- Treatment for diabetes varies from person to person and will depend on your type of diabetes.
- Type 1 diabetes is treated by injections of insulin and a healthy diet, and regular exercise is recommended.
- Type 2 diabetes is treated by a healthy diet and exercise or by a combination of a healthy diet, exercise and tablets. Eventually people with type 2 diabetes may also need insulin injections.
- Whichever type of diabetes you have, your food choice helps to balance your blood glucose levels and your diet is therefore an essential part of your treatment.
- For people with diabetes, increasing daily physical activity levels can help to improve blood glucose control, reduce the body's resistance to insulin and increase the body cells' sensitivity to insulin.
- The main goal of any treatment programme is to bring glucose levels down to as close to normal as possible.
- You are the most important member of your treatment team because you are the one who lives with diabetes every day. It is your responsibility to monitor your blood glucose levels, to take any medications necessary to keep these levels within a normal range, to make healthy food choices and to follow your physical activity programme.
- It is very important that you follow the treatment that your doctor or diabetes care team has advised.

3

Principles Parameters of the CRON Diet

Introduction

With a high order of probability such a diet would produce the same beneficial results in humans. Subsequent work in animals, now including monkeys, and my own human studies in Biosphere 2 have further strengthened that belief. Most contemporary scientists conversant with the field now largely share my views, although there is much disagreement over whether a calorie-reduced diet of this nature is "practical", which reflects the viewpoint that most people cannot follow it. Of course, since the rate of *long-term* failure on weight loss programs is over 95 percent, most people can't stick with any diet; they yo-yo back-and-forth and end up where they started. Americans, in the process, collectively spend about $40 billion per year on weightloss treatments. There is at least much greater incentive to stick with the CRON diet than merely the desire to look better, although that's included. If followed for a long period of time, the CRON diet will retard the rate of aging from whenever in life it is begun and even rejuvenate the functions of some (not all) of your bodily systems. It will greatly extend maximum as well as average life span, help maintain mental function, enhance health, increase vitality, improve looks, and cut disease susceptibility by at least half. I will show you not stories and anecdotes and testimonials hard evidence, published in leading scientific journals, to back up all these claims.

My application of the CRON diet principles to humans is based in part upon extrapolation from years of extensive work with nutritional modulation of the aging process in animal populations, knowledge of what others have done, data from a few published human studies, and the specific investigations I performed during the two-year experiment inside Biosphere 2. These records must all be taken into account in structuring how to implement the diet. Simply launching oneself on a hit-or-miss, long-term, low-calorie diet would not work well. It might even shorten your life span.

The program calls for gradual weight reduction over a period of six to nine months or longers, in short slowly, avoiding the danger of malnutrition inherent in most weight-loss regimes that continue this long. You should proceed until you reach, stabilize, and remain at a weight 10 to 25 percent below your personal set point, where set point is measured in pounds. Or, if set point is measured in Body Mass Index, proceed until you are three to four index points lower than your personal norm; and you must do this on a nutrient-dense diet that provides, with limited but targeted supplementation, all essential nutrients, known and to the extent made possible by the broadness of the diet not yet known. It's a strenuous regime, but it's clear-cut, quite doable, and the rewards are extraordinary.

The eventual degree of leanness required depends on where you begin. When fully fed, the genetically "ob/ob" obese mice I described in Chapter 3 weigh on the average 60 to 65 grams. A fully fed genetically normal mouse weighs only 35 to 45 grams. If we put normal mice on a severe calorie-restriction program and cut their weights down to 25 grams, their life spans will be greatly extended. On the low-calorie regime an "ob/ob" mouse will not become obese but will level off at about 40 grams. It will have a very extended life span, because it is weighing in at less than its set point, even though it weighs as much as or more than a normal fully fed mouse. Below *their* set point, normal mice look razor thin; "ob/ob" mice, below their set point, just look normal, or even slightly obese, but their life spans are greatly extended.

Set point is a critical concept in weight control. Heredity and early feeding experience fix a set point for each individual, which is then defended by adaptive processes within the body. Multiple feedback loops maintain the body at its set point by shunting messages through the blood and the nervous system, between the brain, digestive tract, muscle, and fat. Fat itself secretes hormonal signals. Unless he or she grossly overeats or undereats, each person tends to maintain a particular characteristic weight, which may be considerably above or below the actual "average weight" for that person's height. The body defends its individual set point by shifting the efficiency of its metabolic machine. Take in fewer calories and your body increases its metabolic efficiency; up your intake and your efficiency decreases. This tends to stabilize your weight, although your set point can gradually change (increasing with age, for example). The average American adult gains about 20 pounds between the ages of 25 and 55. Formerly regarded as "normal", this weight gain is now seen as an unhealthy trend, according to insurance company statistics.

The underlying control mechanisms for metabolic efficiency are not entirely known. However, there are so-called "uncoupling proteins" (UCPS) that dissociate the reactions that break down food from those that produce the body's chemical energy. By so doing, they raise the body's metabolic rate. Originally thought to be present only in the specialized brown fat that hibernators use to maintain core body temperature in frigid weather, UCPs are now known to be present in humans. Measurements of the amount of oxygen that humans consume when they metabolize food show that anywhere from 25 to 35 percent is being used to compensate for the "uncoupling" that is going on at all times. It is caused by the UCPS. Decreasing food intake decreases the UCPS, "coupling" is tighter, and metabolic efficiency is increased. *Increasing* the UCPs increases the metabolic rate. That may tend to reduce obesity, but it probably generates more free radicals. That's not the way to go.

Evidence exists that a high fat diet may turn up the production of UCPS, and protect mice against obesity by increasing the metabolic rate. If that's in part how the high fat diets now being touted function to cause weight loss, they are not what you want. "Burning it off" as a substitute for a low calorie intake may be okay for cosmetics, but not for life span.

Efficiency, then, refers to the percentage of your caloric intake that goes into making usable energy. The rest is simply burned off as heat. *Usable* means providing energy for manufacturing proteins and other bodily constituents, for doing muscular work, or performing fundamental processes like transporting calcium or sodium atoms across cell membranes. Normally, metabolic efficiency is about 33 percent. The top efficiency that we can possibly reach is 50 percent. We can approach this upper limit by holding our weight 10 to 25 percent below our "natural weight" or set point. Like an "ob/ob" mouse on the CRON diet, one can be well below one's personal set point and still not be razor thin.

A study of 54 farmers in Java revealed that metabolic efficiency, expressed as work done in relation to energy intake, was actually 80 percent higher for the ten farmers with the lowest intake (1,535 calories) than for those with the highest intake (2,382 calories). Heights and weights did not differ, and the two groups performed the same amount of labor. The one group had "adapted" to the lower intake and were metabolically more efficient.

A major secret of health and longevity is to be always below your set point, maintaining yourself on a high enough quality diet that you are not deficient in any essentials, and to operate at maximum metabolic efficiency. This is, in fact, the central idea of my longevity program.

Reaching for Maximum Metabolic Efficiency

From the most primitive cell to the most advanced organism, living matter needs energy to do its work and to make and maintain the structures giving form to life. It also needs energy to move itself about, to procreate, and to compete with other life forms. Life depends upon energy.

In the early days of our planet, before oxygen was freely available in the atmosphere, life forms derived energy from what is called glycolysis, the conversion of sugar into lactic acid in the tissues. We still derive part of our energy this way. When you become sore and ache from vigorous exercise, it's because lactic acid has built up in your muscles.

Chemically, glycolysis is not a very effective way to generate energy, so when oxygen started percolating into the earth's early atmosphere, mutant organisms that could derive energy from oxygen by means of respiratory metabolism had an evolutionary advantage. The term *respiratory metabolism* does not refer to breathing, but to a collection of processes, mostly taking place within the energy factories (mitochondria) of our cells, and resulting in the formation of a high energy compound known as ATP (short for adenosine triphosphate). This basic source of energy for the process of life has come down more or less unchanged since remote geologic time.

Thus our human bodies do not obtain energy directly from food, but mostly from ATP formed by respiratory metabolism. (A little still comes from residual glycolysis.). And we must manufacture ATP from carbohydrates, fats and proteins before our cells can use the ingested food for energy. A specific amount of energy remains locked up in the chemical bonds of carbohydrates and fats. Only some 50 percent of this "potential" energy can be converted into KFP. The rest is dissipated as heat or stored as fat. When you overeat, less of the energy from your food is channeled through the body-building ATP, and *more* when you undereat. For an average adult American or European male, the 50 percent maximum of "potential" energy that can be converted or the *energy efficiency*, is probably reached at about 1,800 calories daily. At 2,500 calories, the so-called "caloric RDA" for average adult males, the efficiency drops to 37 percent; at 3,300 calories to 30 percent.

This existence of so-called "futile cycles" is also important in energy regulation. A futile cycle is one in which the ATP stored in the body can be degraded without actually providing any body-building energy. It produces heat without work (that is, without usable energy). Metabolic efficiency is lowered. Of course, futile cycles can be useful! If it's cold and we need to generate body heat, increasing the futile cycles will act like an internal furnace. Futile cycles may also be turned on when we overeat on junk food, serving as additional safety valves to drain off excess food energy.

By appropriate studies one can determine how much energy a person is using at rest (the Basal Metabolic Rate), how much goes for the thermal effect of feeding, what the overall energy cost of physical activity is and the efficiency at which the person converts chemical energy into physical work. All these make up the total energy expenditure. When people drop their weight by 10 percent, their energy expenditure declines by 15 percent. The majority of the change occurs in the energy cost of physical activity itself. In terms of energy output, it costs less to run a mile if you are below your set point.

To summarize all the above: maximum metabolic efficiency means achieving the highest possible initial conversion of carbohydrates and fats into ATP, minimizing both fat storage and the breakdown of ATP by futile cycles and doing your physical activities at a reduced energy cost. The CRON diet is designed to achieve all of these goals.

Concept of Nutrient Density

An important feature of the CRON diet is that every calorie must be nutrition packed. Otherwise, gradual weight loss on a long-term basis may cause deficiencies in essential nutrients, and of course that will not prolong life span but shorten it. And do not suppose you can reach your goal by eating a low-calorie mediocre or even nutritionally poor diet supplemented with vitamins and minerals. That would be dangerous and foolhardy. Too much remains unknown about essential nutriments what forms they should be in, how they interact, how many are still undiscovered but you can bet you are not going to find acceptable combinations simply in refined white flour, hot dogs and cola drinks plus a handful of pills. Calcium in the form of a calcium carbonate pill, for example, has value as a supplement, but it exerts a partially suppressive effect on bone remodeling; the same amount of calcium in milk has no suppressive effect. Certain forms of fiber in the diet will help lower blood cholesterol, but only if it is a component of the actual food or else carefully mixed with the food. Just taking the fiber as an extra supplement may have no effect. According to a *Consumer Reports* study of vitamin fortified cereals, the added vitamins' availability to the body is questionable. Supplementation has a place in the CRON diet program, but good nutrient dense food selection is essential.

The average American diet is anything but nutrient dense. The calorie level is inflated, 2,400 to 3,200 for men (depending on age) and 1,650 to 2,150 for women but it is often deficient in essentials. Large surveys have been run of what Americans eat: the National Food Consumption Survey of 7,500 families conducted by the U. S. Department of Agriculture and the National Health and Nutrition Examination by the Department of Health and Human Services. They found that meat, fish or poultry was consumed daily by 90 percent of the families, dark green vegetables by only 9 percent, yellow vegetables by 8 percent, fruit by 33 percent and whole grain cereals by 16 percent. Fully half of the 7,500 families were below what the National Academy of Sciences has set as the Recommended Daily Allowances (the RDAs) of one or more nutrients, especially calcium, vitamin A, vitamin C, iron, thiamine and riboflavin. The RDA for magnesium was reached by only 25 percent of individuals; of vitamin B6, 20 percent; of iron, 43 percent; of vitamin A, 50 percent. Magnesium levels in the average diet have dropped from 475 milligrams per person per day in 1900 to 245 milligrams today. One survey revealed deficiencies in iron, copper, zinc and chromium. According to another, the vitamin B6 content of meals served in 50 American colleges averaged 1.43 milligrams per person per day; thus, over 80 percent of the meals served in these colleges were below the vitamin B6 RDA of 2.0 milligrams per day. It is shocking to realize that even on the high-calorie diet of the richest nation in the world, our own United States, borderline nutritional deficiency is widespread. The average American diet is not nutrient dense, but the opposite.

Simply eating less of the same old things would restrict calories, but it would also bring on malnutrition as a potentially devastating side effect. This is the danger of many weight-loss diets, including most of the popular ones.

Even well-educated, financially comfortable people may show nutritional deficiencies. Protein, vitamin C and various B vitamins (folic acid, niacin, pyridoxine, riboflavin, thiamine and vitamin B12) emerged as the nutrients most often deficient in 5 to 10 percent of a population of 256 affluent individuals surveyed by scientists at the University of New Mexico. And those persons deficient in water-soluble vitamins tested lower than nondeficient partners on tests for abstract thinking and memory! Either borderline malnutrition affects brain function or else dumber people select worse diets.

Vitamin and mineral deficiency is even more common among the elderly. In one study, fully 50 percent of elderly patients consumed less than two-thirds of the RDA for zinc. Iron and possibly chromium have also been found deficient in the diets of the elderly. Intake of vitamins C and A and niacin has been reported to be less than twothirds of the RDAs in over 25 percent of subjects in more than 50 percent of published reports on nutrition in the elderly. Even as conservative an authority as the late pioneer-physiologist Dr. Nathan Shock of the National Institute on Aging recommended for the elderly, supplementation with RDA amounts for vitamins and trace elements.

Parable of Ross's Rats

Many people suppose that animals would instinctively select what is good for them nutritionally if given the chance and that humans would too, if they were not heavily influenced by advertising and cultural and ethnic conditioning. This is a delightful idea. Rousseau would have loved it. But Dr. Morris Ross's introduction of dietary selfselection into the study of aging and disease showed it to be quite naive. Among four populations of rats, one received a diet of 10 percent protein throughout life; a second, 22 percent protein throughout life; a third, 51 percent. The rats of the fourth population were allowed to select what they wanted from among the three available diets. Dr. Ross measured growth rates, body sizes, life spans and frequencies of different diseases in all four populations. The rats that self-selected—that is, the fourth population—grew more rapidly and attained a greater body size than all the rest. They instinctively selfselected food combinations that would optimize growth and development; but—and here is what made the experiment unique and fascinating that very self-selection resulted in a far higher incidence of tumors and other diseases. The actual data are striking. Note that the prevalence of disease was considerably greater than 100 percent if you add up most of the columns. By the time of death many animals had multiple afflictions. Indeed, 66 percent of those on the self-select diet had at least three of the four diseases listed. (Notice, incidentally, the difference in tumor incidence between the low percent protein and both higher protein diets.

Now here's my parable. Given free choice, an animal will instinctively choose a diet that leads to quick growth and development and to reaching sexual maturity as soon as possible. This tendency promotes survival of the species in the wild, but is at the same time highly counterproductive for individual long life. In terms of innate self-selection hungers, the welfare of the species and of the individual are in murderous conflict. Animals are instinctively programmed to choose what will make them grow fast and have lots of offspring, even if that choice brings them frequent disease later on. This direct conflict between species and individual survival may be unprecedented in biology.

Table 3.1. The frequencies, by percentage, of diseases in male rats kept on either fixed or free choice (self-selected) diets

	Fed throughout life on one diet containing either 10%, 22% or 51% protein			Free choice daily from 10%, 22% or 51%
Disease	**10%**	**22%**	**51%**	**Protein diets**
Cancer	26	29	28	62
Kidney disease	38	56	73	90
Heart disease	11	42	48	67
Prostate disease	5	10	12	62
TOTALS	80	137	161	281

The behavior of Ross's rats suggests that some of the crazy and selfdestructive things we do are the result of species-survival instincts acting through us without our knowing what is really going on. These instincts were of course formed in prehistoric times, during the process of evolution and they may not be appropriate at all in today's world, even for species survival itself, much less our long-term personal survival. Whatever the value of these speculations, it seems most unlikely that we can trust our instincts to select what is good for us as individuals.

Nutrient-Dense Food Combinations

It's difficult to devise low-calorie menus that are not deficient in essential nutrients. If you think it's easy (and many dietitians and physicians do seem to think so, judging from such bland offhand advice as "Select items from the five food groups."), just try it.

Initially, about 14 years ago, I fed nutrient information on hundreds of foods into a main-frame computer and asked for combinations containing less than 1,500 calories but approximating or exceeding the RDA levels recommended by the National Academy of Sciences for each major nutrient, with calories derived from fat between 8 and 20 percent of the total and total protein 60 grmas to go per day. My original diet was based on these computer-optimized food combinations. The computer programming was carried forward to become the software package known as *The Interactive Diet Planner* we used to chart our meal planning inside Biosphere 2.

Because it permits such a ready and graphic comparison of the nutrient values of foods (without eyeballing of endless pages of tables), the computer approach can be instructive and surprising. For example, we hear a great deal these days about the nutritive value of pasta, cereals and grains, from the Pritikin program, the macrobiotic enthusiasts and conventionally qualified academic nutritionists. These constitute the base of the famous "food pyramid", and are what you are advised to eat the most of. But calorie for calorie and especially if you wish to restrict fat intake, vegetables are far and away the most nutritious foods. Table 3.2 tells the tale. On both a weight (3.2A) and a calorie (3.2B) basis, it compares nutritive values of some of the most nutritious vegetables with top candidates from the legumes, cereals, grains, red meat, fish and even yeast.

I definitely do not recommend that anyone begin a CRON diet until they are fully grown. After that, the sooner the better. Beginning the program halfway through life should yield about half the degree of life extension as starting in young adulthood and proportionately for other time periods.

Caloric restriction beginning in childhood would yield the greatest extension of maximum life span, but remains an unacceptable option for humans. Substantial restriction in very young animals may cause an increased infant or early age mortality, even though the survivors do go on to enjoy remarkably long lives. We could not sacrifice a small percentage of young humans to ensure long lives for the survivors. Also, restriction during the growing years in animals is often associated with a smaller final body size. In humans, this could mean being six to ten inches shorter than you otherwise would have been.

Do not take these caveats to mean that a somewhat lower-calorie, higher-quality diet would not potentially increase life span for today's children. Indeed, translating this animal data into human terms, Dr. Morris Ross estimated that a difference in daily intake of merely 100 to 125 calories during the period of human growth would influence the duration of life by 2.5 years. Empty calories for children socalled "energy snacks" and the like are bad news for their health later on in life.

Table 3.2A. Comparative nutritive components of selected high-quality foods on a weight basis

Weight basis percentage of RDA per 100 grams	Turnip greens	Kale	Broc-coli	Soy beans	Lima beans	Brown rice	Mil-let	Buck wheat	Liver	Beef	Sal-mon	Hali-but	Yeast
Amino acids													
Tryptophan	26	27	25	291	102	46	122	81	166	144	125	111	388
Isoleucine	14	20	19	279	163	41	77	55	138	159	156	149	333
Lysine	21	18	22	326	190	41	47	62	201	266	272	244	458
Valine	16	23	22	238	153	47	71	92	142	145	142	127	321
Methionine	5	6	9	87	55	30	40	30	75	90	108	98	133
Threonine	22	26	27	262	171	53	71	75	160	173	173	158	410
Leucine	21	29	18	302	177	67	160	71	182	187	176	156	333
Phenylalanine	23	17	18	348	180	70	46	76	171	171	159	134	395
Vitamins													
A	152	178	50	1	0	0	0	0	450	0	6	8	0
D	0	0	0	0	0	0	0	0	3	0	38	11	0
K	928	0	285	271	0	0	0	0	128	0	0	0	0
C	231	208	183	0	0	0	0	0	60	0	15	0	0
E	22	53	4	153	4	13	0	36	13	1	13	8	0
B1	14	0	7	78	34	24	52	42	14	6	12	5	1142
B2	23	15	13	17	9	2	22	8	158	11	4	4	235
B6	13	15	10	40	30	27	37	15	35	20	35	21	125
B12	0	0	0	0	0	0	0	0	2000	61	133	33	0
Niacin	4	11	5	12	10	27	12	24	61	28	38	46	222
Folic acid	23	15	17	42	27	4	0	0	55	1	6	3	975

Pantothenic acid	9	25	30	42	25	27	0	37	200	12	32	7	300
Biotin	0	0	0	60	9	12	0	0	100	0	5	8	110
Minerals													
Calcium	20	15	8	19	6	2	1	9	0	1	6	1	17
Magnesium	15	9	6	66	45	22	40	63	0	5	7	5	57
Copper	4	4	0	5	9	18	42	21	250	2	10	11	265
Zinc	0	0	1	24	18	12	12	5	26	27	6	4	73
Chromium	0	0	60	0	120	0	0	0	120	60	0	0	320
Potassium	4	20	20	90	81	11	22	24	14	18	22	23	401
Iron	10	12	6	44	43	10	37	17	50	17	5	3	94
Manganese	56	22	2	112	21	68	76	83	6	0	0	0	16
Selenium	0	4	0	120	0	78	0	36	86	0	0	0	142
Calories per 100 gm.	28	38	32	403	345	356	327	335	140	143	217	100	283
% calories from fat	10	19	8	40	4	5	8	6	32	38	54	11	3

Table 3.2B. Comparative nutritive components of selected high-quality foods on a calorie basis

Calorie basis percentage of RDA per 100 calories	Turnip greens	Kale	Broc-coli	Soy beans	Lima beans	Brown rice	Mil-let	Buck wheat	Liver	Beef	Sal-mon	Hali-but	Yeast
Amino acids													
Trytophan	93	73	78	72	29	13	37	24	118	101	57	111	136
Isoleucine	52	54	59	69	47	11	23	16	98	111	71	149	116
Lysine	77	47	69	81	55	11	14	18	142	186	125	244	160
Valine	57	62	68	59	44	13	21	27	101	101	65	127	112
Methionine	19	17	28	21	15	8	12	8	53	63	49	98	46
Threonine	80	70	86	65	49	15	21	22	114	121	79	158	143
Leucine	78	76	57	75	51	19	49	21	129	131	80	156	116
Phenylalanine	84	46	57	87	52	19	14	22	122	120	73	134	138
Vitamins													
A	542	468	156	0	0	0	0	0	319	0	2	8	0
D	0	0	0	0	0	0	0	0	2	0	17	11	0
K	3315	0	894	67	0	0	0	0	91	0	0	0	0
C	827	547	573	0	0	0	0	0	42	0	6	0	0
E	78	140	14	38	1	3	0	10	9	0	6	8	0
B1	51	0	22	19	9	6	15	12	10	4	5	5	400
B2	83	40	42	4	2	0	6	2	112	7	2	4	82
B6	46	39	31	10	8	7	11	4	24	14	16	21	43
B12	0	0	0	0	0	0	0	0	1420	43	61	33	0
Niacin	15	30	15	3	3	7	3	7	43	20	17	46	77
Folic acid	84	39	54	10	7	1	0	0	39	1	2	3	341

Pantothenic acid	33	65	93	10	7	7	0	11	142	8	14	7	104
Biotin	1	1	1	15	2	3	0	0	71	0	2	8	38
Minerals													
Calcium	74	39	26	4	1	0	0	2	0	0	3	1	6
Magnesium	53	24	18	16	13	6	12	18	2	3	3	5	20
Copper	16	11	1	1	2	5	13	6	177	1	4	11	92
Zinc	0	0	5	6	5	3	3	1	18	19	2	4	25
Chromium	0	0	187	0	34	0	0	0	85	42	0	0	111
Potassium	14	53	63	22	23	3	7	7	10	13	10	23	35
Iron	35	32	19	11	12	2	11	5	35	12	2	3	33
Manganese	202	57	7	28	6	19	23	24	4	0	0	0	5
Selenium	0	12	0	30	0	21	0	10	61	0	0	0	49
Calories per 100 gm.	357	263	313	25	29	28	31	30	71	70	46	100	35
% calories from fat	10	19	8	40	4	5	8	6	32	38	54	11	3

Loosing of Weight

The CRON diet works very well for rapid weight loss. In fact, because of its nutrient density, it is probably the best of all diets for that purpose. At an equivalent caloric intake, it will leave you better nourished than other diets. But a word of caution is needed here. In Western societies, enormous subliminal and not so subliminal pressure is exerted on everyone to be as slim as starlets and models. We are made to feel we should be not merely "not fat" but positively slender. Responding to this pressure, people plunge desperately into quick weight reduction regimens. A popular diet book promising rapid, painless slenderizing comes out almost every other month. No checkout-counter tabloid is without one. From the standpoint of health and longevity, quick weight loss is harmful.

It had been known since 1935 that if you kept animals on a lowcalorie diet from time of weaning, you could dramatically extend life span and decrease susceptibility to disease. But nobody could make the method work if it was started in adulthood. Indeed, in the early experiments this actually *shortened* the life span. Studying these early experiments, Dr. Richard Weindruch and I noted that the investigators had put the animals suddenly, or over a very short period, on the lower-calorie diet. This sudden switch, we reasoned, may have injured them metabolically. Then, in our own investigations we found that if a CRON diet was begun very gradually in adult animals, leading to a very slow weight loss (equivalent to weight loss in humans over a four to six-year period), life span could be greatly extended and disease incidence reduced. If this applies to humans, then the quick weight loss promised by most modern diet books may be dandy for your immediate cosmetic appeal, but across-the-board bad for your ultimate health, and even for the long-term cosmetic appeal of looking younger than you are. Anyway, almost everyone knows that all these diets don't work very well. You lose weight and then you gain it back. Then you buy another highly promoted diet book and do it again. The whole cycle is discouraging, irrational and unhealthful.

Based on further work in animals and on the Biosphere 2 experience, I now believe the time period for weight loss in humans can be reduced from four to six years to six to nine months or better still, up to one or two years. You may ask, "What's wrong with going faster?" There are two reasons not to! The first is that the Biosphere 2 crew members sustained the major part of their substantial weight loss during the first six to nine months, yet remained healthy; so one to two years seems conservatively safe for humans in terms of what we learned from the animal experiments. Thus, one to two years is ample to allow for metabolic adaptation. Less might also be all right, but I am not entirely sure.

The second reason for losing weight slowly concerns the release into the blood of toxic materials, such as pesticide residues, out of your own stores of bodily fat. Certain pesticide residues like DDE (from DDT), as well as dioxin and the PCBs, plus others, are not broken down very rapidly by the detoxifying enzymes of the body. However, because they are fat soluble, they are prevented from doing harm by being absorbed into the body's fat. It's a bit like storing nuclear wastes in underground salt domes, only in this case it's in fat. Because Biosphere 2 was a totally closed system and there was no chance of DDT or PCBs blowing in with the dust or other sources and influencing the pesticide levels in the crew's blood, we were able to follow those levels under constant environmental conditions. We discovered that with the rapid loss of weight (and therefore fat mass) the levels *increased*. Furthermore, because the body's detoxification system does not handle fat-soluble residues very rapidly, they *remained elevated* for a year or longer. Therefore, you should lose weight slowly enough for the released toxins to be cleared without getting too high. And yo-yo dieting is particularly bad, as it may wash toxic material in and out of the blood stream.

What level of toxic residues is too much? The answer is, any level is too high, but a certain amount cannot be avoided because of the environment in which we live. The government has established so-called "allowable limits". These seem generally okay. On the other hand, in 1996, 11-year-olds in Michigan exposed in the womb to only slightly higher levels of PCBs than the U.S. average were found to have measurably lower IQs.

What calorie range suffices to enable you to lose weight slowly over a one- to two-year period, placing you below your set point? It will vary from person to person. For example, the caloric RDA for a 120pound woman is given as 1,700 to 2,500. That means that *some* 120pound women will stay at that weight on a 1,700 calorie intake, but others will require 2,500. The amount is very individually specific. Nevertheless we can form a general idea from a study performed not long after World War 2 by scientists at the University of Minnesota. They placed 32 young male conscientious objectors on a strict 1,600 calorie per day diet for six months. The subjects lost weight fairly rapidly, and the loss levellled off to a maintenance value of 75 percent of the original weight. Once lost, the weight was not regained unless more than 2,000 calories per day were given.

Start your own program with about a 2,000-calorie CRON diet if you are an average-size man, 1,800 calories if a woman and see if this induces gradual weight loss and at the same time enhances your sense of physical well-being. If so, continue. If you are losing weight too fast or too slowly or not at all, adjust your intake accordingly. Unless you have a medical reason for wanting quick weight loss, add about 300 to 500 calories of intake to any of these daily regimens. Choose whatever you like for these extra calories, but keep in mind what I shall outline in the next chapter about susceptibility to the major killer diseases.

What should be the quantities and ratios of the macronutrients (protein, carbohydrate and fat) in your diet? This question has evoked great and continuing controversy, particularly about the proper percentage of fat in the diet. The low-fat enthusiasts are supported by the following: obesity is rare in experimental animals kept on a low-fat diet and common in animals maintained on high fat diets. In numerous studies in humans, total energy intake and therefore obesity was higher when the subjects consumed high fat diets. The amount of body fat is also higher when the excess energy comes from fats rather than from proteins or carbohydrates. However, it is difficult to separate the fat effect from an energy density effect. People tend to eat a constant weight of food and the energy density of fat is over two times that of the other macronutrients. The picture has been complicated by the fact that an increasing number of processed "low-fat" foods have because of low fiber and water content and addition of sugar – an energy density per weight as high as fat.

On the other side of the question: not all experts agree that dietary fat promotes development of obesity. On a population basis, obesity prevalence has greatly increased in the last decade whereas the percentage of energy intake from dietary fat has decreased. Studies of diabetes and diabeteslike syndromes suggest that when high-carbohydrate diets are compared to high mono-fat diets, subjects show better physiologic responses with the latter.

However, it is noteworthy that most of the above information, especially that from humans, comes from relatively short-term studies, and it is well established that long-term calorie reduction may yield results different than short term. For our purposes the best cohorts to study – unfortunately, they are few in number – are those reduced obese individuals who have stayed reduced for five years, i.e., the small percentage of really successful dieters. They report that their success in weight-loss maintenance stems from consumption of a low-fat, low total energy intake, accompanied by high levels of regular physical activity.

Fasting

One should be aware that while total fasting *increases* UCP (uncoupling protein) activity in the rat, merely restricting food intake by 50 percent actually *decreases* UCP expression. When totally deprived of food, the body acts to maintain temperature by turning up the UCPs, thereby decreasing its metabolic efficiency and burning its fat. On the other hand, responding to *partial* food deprivation, it may just turn down the thermostat. Indeed CRON humans, as well as monkeys, tend to display a body temperature one or more degrees lower than normal.

It's acceptable to cut caloric intake by frequent fasts, if that's the easiest way for you to go, as long as the fasts are short, no more than one or two days. Some of the animal studies have entailed "intermittent fasting", giving the animals as much as they want of a high-quality diet, but only every other day and on alternate days they receive nothing. The overall weekly caloric intake turns out to be less, slow weight loss ensues and life span is extended.

In human societies fasting has an extensive history, dating back to antiquity. Many cultures and religions have incorporated it into their writings and practices. North American Indians and Eskimos fast prior to being ordained for their priesthood. Muslims fast for many reasons (before prayer, when ill, or when they wish to conjure). Eastern yogis fast to achieve spiritual enlightenment. Jesus fasted forty days and nights.

Technically, you are "fasting" only if you consume nothing but water. Such fasting is short-term starvation. Fasting under proper supervision (especially if long-term, which for the reasons given I do not recommend) differs from actual starvation in that the diet is supplemented with vitamins and minerals. Without this, symptoms of frank vitamin deficiency develop in totally fasting individuals in considerably less than two months. On the other hand, very obese people have gone without food (properly supplemented and in a hospital, where they could be observed) for as long as 249 days without apparent harm.

Short-term fasts of one or two days per week, with more generous amounts of high-quality foods on the eating days, are just as effective in inducing gradual weight loss as simply eating less each day. It depends on what is comfortable for you. An occasional short-term fast is also good because it will change your perceptions of hunger and energy. Hunger is partly habit. And skipping or cutting down on meals does not rob you of energy: in fact, the reverse. In one study, five men were subjected to five two-and-a-half day fasts at five to six-week intervals. Their ability to undertake hard physical labour during the fast periods was measured. Between the first and final periods, reaction times and pattern recognition (a test of intellectual function) actually improved. Glucose-tolerance tests showed an increased ability to regulate blood sugar. Short-term fasts may aid metabolic adaptation; however, they are not a necessary part of the CRON diet program.

Appetite and its Control

Following weight loss resulting from low calorie intake, the concentrations of the hormones insulin and leptin (a recently discovered hormone released from fat tissue itself) decrease and glucocorticoid concentrations increase. This combination of changes activates pathways that stimulate appetite and promote weight gain, while inhibiting pathways having the opposite effect. This so-called "lipostatic model" is currently favoured to explain appetite and the set point. It links food intake to the amount of stored energy (fat mass) in the body. Animals modify their eating pattern so that sufficient calories are consumed to maintain a constant amount of fat stores. Other gut-derived "satiety factors" can alter the size of individual meals, but they have limited influence on overall adiposity. Resting levels of insulin are proportional to total fat mass.

By contrast, posteating insulin levels are proportional to the rise in glucose following a meal. Glucocorticoids secreted by the adrenal cortex antagonize the actions of the fat-derived hormone leptin and of insulin in the control of energy balance. Glucocorticoid increase (as occurs to a mild degree in people on a CRON diet) decreases the ability of insulin and leptin to promote appetite suppression and weight loss. The interaction of these various factors makes losing weight difficult, which is why most diets don't work.

In any long-term dietary program leading to gradual, substantial, and sustained weight loss, appetite control is a problem. You will ask, "Am I going to be famished all the time?"

You won't feel as full as a gorged lion, but on a CRON diet you won't be as hungry as you might imagine. The type and quality of food itself also influences appetite. Rats on a low-protein, high-carbohydrate diet voluntarily restrict their intake and live longer. Rats fed a high-fat, "junk food" diet gain a great deal more weight than normally fed rats. A study at the University of Alabama revealed that volunteer humans allowed to eat as much as they liked achieved full satisfaction from as little as 1,500 calories a day from whole foods, but it took 3,000 calories of refined and processed foods to satisfy them. The "whole" foods included fruit, hot cereals, skim milk, soups, salads, non-meat sandwiches, pasta, fish, chicken, rice, vegetables and whole-wheat toast and rolls. The "refined" foods included bacon, eggs, juice, buttered toast, fast and fried foods, roast or steak, buttered vegetables, whole milk, cake and ice cream.

One hypothesis of appetite regulation maintains that unrefined foods with a low energy density will induce a feeling of fullness at a low energy intake. *Low-energy density* means a lot of bulk per calorie. There is no contradiction between high *nutrient* density and low *energy* density: turnip greens, for example, are bulky, packed with nutrients but low in calories.

Fiber material such as guar gum added to a meal significantly prolongs the time after eating before hunger returns. An addition of 10 grams of guar gum to meals twice daily decreased appetite by delaying gastric emptying time, with a significant weight loss over ten weeks in obese persons, accompanied by a decrease in LDL fats in the blood and an improved glucose-tolerance curve.

Refined sugar in the diet stimulates appetite. Persons eating highly refined and processed foods have been shown to consume 25 percent more calories than persons on a more natural diet.

The CRON diet is a high-nutrient density/low-energy density formulation. As such, it will give you greater satiety per calorie than any other diet.

Drugs that decrease appetite are not a good answer for long-term gradual weight loss. A number of complex events occur in the body that result in its asking, "What's to eat?" These involve metabolic rates, the energy enzymes of the body, insulin, blood sugar, and a portion of the brain called the hypothalamus. Trying to handle all these events with a pill doesn't make sense. Like suppressing a toothache with codeine, it'll work for a while . . . but your tooth will rot.

You can make a rat eat by pinching its tail. The pain causes the release of chemicals (opioids) in part of the brain (the hypothalamus) that block the sensation of pain, but also stimulate hunger. Like opium or morphine, these opioids (also known as endorphins) are addicting. Pinch a rat's tail frequently for ten days and it will release opioids and overeat. That's one way (not a very nice one) to get a fat rat. Suddenly stop pinching its tail, opioids are not released, and the addicted rat will go into a fit the same reaction as a heroin addict. Mental pain or stress may also augment endorphin or opioid release and so stimulate hunger. Avoidance of stress will aid in appetite control. In this sense, weight gain and obesity may be thought of as a kind of auto-addiction.

Translatability

Granted that the CRON diet works well in animals, how do we know it will work in humans? Of course the final, absolute proof will not come until people on a CRON diet are seen to live extraordinarily longer than the norm and the outlook of traditional, conservative medicine would be to wait for this ultimate demonstration. But, of course, if we do wait before going on the diet, we probably won't be around to see what happens. We'll have died before the final answer comes in.

However, in medicine it is not uncommon to recommend measures not yet "proved" but for which substantial evidence exists.

As mentioned earlier, many doctors have for years been recommending the lowering of blood cholesterol because this would probably help prevent coronary heart disease, but this was not "proved" until 1984 and then for only a selected category of patient. And only in early 1985 did a panel of 13 experts convened as part of a National Institutes of Health "consensus conference" conclude "beyond a reasonable doubt" that lowering elevated blood cholesterol levels would reduce the risk of heart attacks. "Beyond a reasonable doubt" in fact means "with a high order of probability." Surely this is not *formal* proof. It's a consensus decision. Many more examples could be cited. The key question for much good medical advice is not whether proof is at hand, but what is the order of probability that the advice is correct.

Existing evidence indicates not absolutely but with a very high order of probability that the same CRON diet that extends life span in all the varieties of nonhuman species so far tested will do the same for man. One reason for thinking so is that we are dealing with a very general process. Experiments involving the overall operation of the immune system, the nature of DNA repair, and the various types and causes of cancer indicate that these *general* phenomena are quite similar across the species barrier. Nutritional modulation of the aging process seems to be such a general phenomenon, involving common processes across wide species barriers. In my view this animal work is entirely translatable to humans.

It is occasionally asserted, as evidence against translatability of calorie-restriction experiments, that in underdeveloped countries or situations where people are underfed, there is no increase in longevity. I find it astonishing that those who express this view never pause to consider that these underfed populations are also malnourished. Their caloric restriction is often accompanied by inadequate vitamin, mineral, protein and other intake. Nobody claims that undernutrition with malnutrition increases life span.

Direct Evidence

Aside from the question of translatability, there is in fact a modest amount of *direct* evidence beyond what I have already set forth, that the CRON diet will exert the same effects in humans as in animals.

Long-term (three to nine months) low-calorie supplemented diets have been investigated in the treatment of obesity and diabetes. These diets yield metabolic effects in humans that closely resemble some of those seen in animals on similar diets: a decrease in cholesterol, an improved insulin response and a better regulation of blood sugar.

Anorexia nervosa is a dreadful, sometimes fatal psychological disease in which (usually) young women, often overachievers, develop a compulsive urge to control their weight. They literally starve themselves slowly, sometimes even unto death, as did the popular singer Karen Carpenter in late 1982.

Despite the disastrous nature of the disease, certain things about it are interesting for our purpose. Anorexics typically restrict their intake of fat and carbohydrates but allow themselves relatively more protein in vegetables and low-fat cheeses. They undergo drastic weight loss but with considerably less comparative malnutrition than is seen in typical semistarved individuals from famine or poverty areas. So it's a bit like a high-quality low-calorie diet except it's carried to excess. And for a while, anorexics do remain surprisingly well despite their growing emaciation. They do not usually get into serious problems until up to 30 to 40 percent of their body weight has been lost. Despite an extremely low calcium intake, they do not experience an automatic increase in parathyroid hormone levels and reabsorb calcium from bone. They do not show any increased susceptibility to infections. And quite unlike the results of malnutrition caused by famine or poverty, the immune system in anorexics is generally preserved until weight loss is far advanced. Indeed, in early stages the immune responses may be better than control values. The same phenomenon of heightened immune response is of course found in rodents subjected to caloric restriction commencing in adulthood.

In *Maximum Life Span* I discussed two populations world famous for fabulous longevity, the people of the former Soviet Georgia and the villagers of Vilcabamba, Peru. Alas, they are not really long-lived! They possess no secrets of longevity at all and their maximum life span is no longer than anybody else's. Yogurt advertisements notwithstanding, in the absence of reliable birth records, no knowledgeable gerontologist believes the Georgian myth. The same is true for the villagers in Vilcabamba, who for about a dozen years received a great deal of press coverage because they supposedly had many super-centenarians in their society. But it's just not true. According to the most recent evidence, the oldest person in Vilcabamba is only 96.

But there is one population today who just might be breaking the maximum life span barrier, and it is not in a mysterious place, but on the Japanese island of Okinawa.

Okinawan Experience

In Japan, large-scale and quite accurate nutritional surveys have been conducted yearly since 1946 by the Ministry of Health and Welfare. Accurate information is available about weight, body size, health, and disease incidences of the different areas of Japan. The numbers of centenarians are also known throughout Japan, since accurate legal birth records have been kept there since 1872.

On the island of Okinawa and in a few other areas of Japan, there are 15 to 37 centenarians per 100,000 persons over 65 years of age (the highest incidence is in Okinawa!), whereas in most of Japan the number ranges from one to nine. One way to estimate maximum life span of a population, besides finding the age of the oldest tiny cohort of survivors, is to calculate the average age of the last surviving 10 percent of the population. This is called the *tenth decile* of survivorship. With so many more actual centenarians in the population (and therefore also a lot more people over 90) than elsewhere, it seems likely that the tenth decile is significantly higher in Okinawa than elsewhere in Japan. It's not just average age that's longer there, but maximum survival too.

Now, the daily caloric intake of Okinawan schoolchildren, though adequate in vitamins and animal protein, is only 62 percent of the "recommended intake" for Japan. Average sugar and salt intake for Okinawans is lower than the national average, while consumption of green/yellow vegetables and meats is higher. Although it is not nearly so rigorous as the one spelled out in this book, the Okinawans, compared with the rest of the Japanese, seem to be on a CRON diet.

The frequencies of cancer, heart disease, high blood pressure, diabetes and senile brain disease are lower by 30 to 40 percent in Okinawa than elsewhere in Japan. And the average heights and weights of the population are lower.

The increased number of centenarians among Okinawans, the quality and caloric content of their diet, the lowered incidence of the major diseases of aging and their smaller body size are exactly what one finds in laboratory animals on a CRON diet since early life. Professor Yasuo Kagawa of Jichi Medical School, who has studied the Okinawans, attributes their longevity and health to caloric restriction.

Dr. Vallejo's Experiment

The high-low diet idea was tackled in an experiment performed in Madri. An over-65 population of 180 men and women in an oldage home were divided into two equal groups. One group was placed on a diet of 2,300 calories one day and 885 calories the next. The control group received 2,300 calories every day. Over the three years of the experiment, the subjects receiving the fewer calories spent only 123 days in the infirmary, compared with 219 days for the fully fed subjects. And their death rate was only half that of the control group. While Dr. Vallejo's experiment was not large enough, long enough, or careful enough to be regarded as definitive proof, it is still of considerable interest.

Two Venerable Gentlemen

The Renaissance Italian gentleman Luigi Cornaro, a member of the minor Italian nobility, led a gluttonous life that resulted in dangerous ill health by age 37. Then, on his doctor's advice, he adopted a very temperate dietarily restricted regimen, which seems to have been equivalent to about 1,500 calories per day. The diet was also of good quality, considering the primitive state of nutritional science at that time. We know all about Signor Cornaro because he wrote a famous autobiography called *The Art of Long Living*. He died in 1567 at the age of 103. A few hundred years later Dr. A. Guenoit, president of the Paris Medical Academy, elected to follow a similar regimen. He died in 1935 at the age of 102.

Conclusion

You will recognize, I hope, that the histories of Cornaro and Guenoit constitute merely anecdotal evidence. Does it really mean much that among historical figures who followed a (for their times) carefully selected high-quality, low-calorie diet, two out of two lived to become centenarians? No, not a great deal by itself. But note carefully where we now stand, even leaving aside the pleasant histories of our venerable gentlemen.

Overwhelming evidence proves the CRON diet will increase maximum life span in animals, and the biology involved is of such a general nature it ought to apply to humans. In humans and their close neighbors, the monkeys, low-calorie nutritious regimens yield biomarker changes similar to what a CRON diet produces in rodents. And while the experiments have not gone long enough to assess long-term survival, in the monkey populations a decrease in the diseases of aging is already being observed. One existing well-documented human population on a low-level approximation of the CRON diet appears to show an excess number of centenarians and less disease. In an experimental human population, and even beginning in old age, three years on intermittent calorie deprivation seemed to decrease the rates of illness and death.

4

Exercises, Stretching and Fitness for Good Health

Introduction

It accomplishes this largely by inhibiting the development of a number of diseases, most notably (in humans) cardiovascular disease. However, exercise has several potential downsides if not properly done. On the CRON diet you are going to be inhabiting your body for a lot of additional years. There are circumstances that may be damaging to it, changes that are not secondary to "aging" but to the mere passage of time and the effects of constant use. You don't want to live to be 150 years old but suffer from severe traumatic arthritis for the last 50 from having engaged in hard-impact sports for 70 out of those first 100 years. While cancer, heart disease, diabetes, and other such illnesses will be much less prevalent in a long-living CRON society, or among a long-living cohort within a traditional society, other maladies will likely pop up if one simply lives a 150-year life span with an 80-year attitude. Let us give thought to these issues.

Exercise

Joggers, 20 million strong, an army of the fit, fanatically striving for Perpetual youth and good health, along with hordes of tennis players, Cross-country skiers, Nautilus pumpers, aerobic dancers, long-distance walkers, and swimmers: millions of Americans have for some time been pursuing one of the great lay religions of today physical fitness.

There is good evidence to back up part of this faith. But like much else in the lay health field, the value of exercise and fitness has ballooned into a sky-high, free-for-all, no-questions-asked ride. Exercise makes you healthy and sexy, and the more you exercise, the healthier and sexier you grow. In the movie Pumping Iron, champion bodybuilder Arnold Schwarzenegger declares, "I'm *coming* all the time" .

The value of exercise depends on what you want to optimize. Regular sports competition has nothing necessarily to do with health as a primary aim. But exercise can be fun; it generally makes you feel good; it helps relieve stress and depression, improves blood-sugar metabolism, and increases cardiovascular fitness.

The goals of the CRON program include some of these but differences do exist. CRON goals are to optimize longevity, health, and freedom from disease. Does exercise actually promote all of these fully? What kinds of exercise? Is a certain amount helpful, and too much not helpful in relation to longevity? How do diet and exercise compare in importance? And what is the interplay between diet and exercise?

We know that dieters generally do better when they exercise fairly vigorously following or during weight reduction; but let's look at the evidence in some detail. It derives from animal studies; from humanpopulation studies; from studies of the effects of exercise on the biomarkers of aging in humans, on "risk factors for disease" in humans, on actual disease incidence, on human longevity; and from studies of the interplay between diet and exercise.

Animal Studies

In old rats, the diaphragm muscle, which is actively used in breathing, shows little or no change with age in the number and diameter of its fibers. In contrast to the active diaphragm, the leg muscles of inactive (caged) rats deteriorate as they grow old. It's a "use it or lose it" physiology. In rodents, exercise begun in youth or middle age (12 months) and continued throughout life yields a 10 to

15 percent increase in average life span, but if it is not started until 24 months, an actual decrease occurs. Lifelong exercise benefits cardiac function in rats as judged by enzyme patterns (they stay at a younger level.) However, at a certain point in life (over 24 to 27 months in the rat, equivalent perhaps to 70 to 75 years in humans), a "threshold of age" appears. When previously sedentary 24- to 27-month-old rats are put on a vigorous exercise program, cardiac function may be damaged.

Aerobic exercise in mice and rats fails to decrease the accumulation of age pigment in their hearts, and such pigment is a biomarker of aging. In mice started on a running schedule at 14 and 24 months of age, no difference was noted in the amount of age pigment in their hearts compared with that of sedentary mice. And in another study, a greater accumulation of age pigment occurred in the hearts of old exercised rats than in sedentary controls. By this particular biomarker, exercise does not do well.

The overall animal data suggest that while exercise protects against certain diseases, such as arteriosclerosis, increasing average life span, it may fail to retard the basic process of aging. Certain kinds of exercise might even accelerate that process.

Both animal and human studies indicate that very strenuous physical exercise (exercise to exhaustion) leads to considerable oxidative stress (free radical generation) characterized by lipid peroxidation and DNA strand breakage. In humans at least, this can be inhibited or prevented by taking vitamin E (800 to 1200 milligrams daily) for three to 14 days before the exercise. Persons engaged in marathons and other exhaustive sports might wish to consider this, although the main lesson here for life-extenders may be not to undertake this kind of sport at all. The data also suggest that starting exercise in youth or middle age and keeping it up throughout life is productive, but beginning vigorous exercise too late in life may be counterproductive. This is in line with the rodent data.

Human Population Studies

In a variety of occupational groups (indoor versus outdoor workers, skilled versus unskilled labourers, active compared with inactive post office workers), a greater incidence of heart disease has been found among the more sedentary. On a normal diet, sedentary persons run more than two times the risk of heart disease as active people.

That sounds straightforward, but in fact there are problems with such data as to its true significance. People in different occupational groups have different habits. Businessmen generally have more sedentary jobs than manual labourers, for example, but they also eat differently. They eat more fancy cheese, hollandaise sauce, and marbled red meat. And people of different physical types (genetically obese versus genetically slender) tend to enter different occupations in the first place, and maybe it's the physical type rather than the occupation itself that influences the disease susceptibility. So we cannot conclude much of anything from such human population studies. There are too many variables.

Effect of Exercise in Humans on Biomarkers and "Risk Factors for Disease" Biomarkers and risk factors relating to heart function and susceptibility to arteriosclerosis are favorably influenced by aerobic exercise. Exercise promotes a higher level of the beneficial HDL in the blood and lowers LDL as well as the total cholesterol-HDL/LDL ratio one of the better indicators among the blood-fat factors of risk of cardiovascular disease. Increase in blood HDL has been demonstrated in middle-aged male and female runners, young elite distance runners, Norwegian skiers, middle-aged Finnish runners and skiers, joggers and male marathon runners. In both sexes, the beneficial effect on HDL levels is reached only when a person exercises until his pulse reaches 70 to 85 percent of its theoretical maximum rate (estimated very roughly by subtracting his or her age from 220) for at least 20 minutes three times a week.

Exercise increases the insulin sensitivity of the tissues and improves carbohydrate metabolism. And the physically fit person has only about 60 percent as much chance of developing high blood pressure as a sedentary person. It also increases the body's generation of so called "heat-shock proteins". These proteins are induced by most any kind of physical or metabolic stress, including those of hyperthermia and exercise, and they serve to repair other proteins injured by the stress, and to participate in new protein synthesis. They are important engines of maintenance and repair.

Exercise works against the slowdown in reaction time that occurs with age. Men in their sixties who have exercised vigorously for 20 or more years display reaction times equivalent to or better than those of inactive men in their twenties. And in both young and older ages the more fit individuals have been reported to display a higher level of "fluid intelligence" a term that refers to the ability to reason, to think things out, as opposed simply to memory. Thus, very possibly the aging organism can postpone, by chronic exercise, the decline in oxidative capacity of the brain that usually occurs with aging. A study was conducted recently to determine if aerobic exercise (walking) versus anaerobic exercise (stretching and toning) in 60- to 75year-old adults would result in selective improvement in "executive control processes" including planning, scheduling, and working memory all known to be supported by the frontal regions of the brain. Substantial improvement was noted in those who walked. Performances in other, nonexecutive control processes were not affected. The mental improvements following aerobic exercise may be selective, but they clearly do exist.

The above results were derived mainly from studies of aerobic exercise, like running or swimming. What about resistance training, such as weight lifting or body building. Resistance training for 45 minutes three times per week has been found to lower cholesterol and LDL. Weight training can of course be done both aerobically and anaerobically in what is referred to as "circuit training" (little or no resting between the handling of the weights), and exert combined benefits.

This measurement of your "aerobic capacity" is one of the very best measurements of "physical fitness". The lowered VO2 max with age is due in part to diminished capacity of the tissues to extract oxygen quickly from the blood and partly to a lower maximal heart rate with age. Aerobic exercise will boost the VO2 max of a sedentary person to a substantially higher level. Some men in their sixties and seventies are able, for example to increase their VO2 max levels above those of healthy untrained younger men. One can thus argue that while exercise increases physical fitness and therefore resistance to certain types of disease (cardiac disease especially), it may actually slightly accelerate the rate of aging. The boosted VO2 max declines from a higher point, but does so more rapidly, and eventually reaches the same level as for an old, sedentary person.

Effect of Exercise on Actual Disease Incidence and Longevity

In a large follow-up study of 16,936 Harvard alumni from 1962 to 1978, it was found that habitual postcollege exercise rather than amount of athletic participation as students coincided with a lower death rate from heart disease. Sedentary alumni, *even former varsity athletes*, were at higher risk. But while the death rates declined as the amount of exercise increased from less than 500 to more than 3,500 calorie expenditure per week beyond 3,500 the death rate *increased* slightly. In a more recent study, among 2,500 men aged 71 to 93, those who walked more than two miles a day had half the risk of heart disease as those who walked less than one mile.

The Pritikin group have presented evidence that their program of diet and exercise inhibits the progression of peripheral vascular disease, coronary arteriosclerosis, and adult-onset diabetes. But their studies do not differentiate clearly between the benefits of diet and those of exercise.

A common public fallacy about exercise and heart disease holds that exercise is more effective than diet in preventing an attack. That's decidedly not true. The idea that diet is rather irrelevant as long as you exercise strenuously is a myth. Jim Fix, author of the 1977 best-seller *The Complete Book of Running*, who transformed himself from a chubby 214-pound, two-pack-a-day smoker into a sleek 160-pound marathon runner, died at the age of 52 from a heart attack while pounding the road in Vermont. He paid dearly for his expressed belief that running all by itself would suffice to prevent heart disease.

Do not fall so deeply into the myth of exercise that you neglect other preventive health measures. Diet is the most important, even for heart disease, although exercise provides additional benefit. But there is no evidence in either animals or humans that exercise influences the incidence of cancer, the second major cause of death after cardiovascular disease, and we know that cancer is very heavily influenced by diet.

Interplay Between Diet and Exercise

Studies on this interplay in mice and rats have given confusing, indeed conflicting results where calorie restriction is concerned. At the time of my first edition in 1986, it seemed clear from reports by scientists at the National Institute of Aging, and confirmed by the eminent exercise physiologist, John Holloszy, that when fully fed, completely sedentary rodents were compared to similarly fed rodents allowed a wheel to run on, the latter lived longer; but that when calorie restricted rodents were subjected to a similar comparison, the sedentary ones lived the longest. However, in later studies Holloszy seems to have reversed his position. Wheel runners on a normal diet still enjoyed an average survival longer than sedentary rats on a normal diet, although their maximum life spans were the same; but when the restricted wheel runners were compared to restricted sedentaries of comparable body weights, the life spans and survival curves were identical, and both were substantially greater than those of the nonrestricted animals. It appears from these (and other) studies that once calorie restriction is instituted, the degree of restriction can be a little less if one is exercising as long as the same degree of weight loss is maintained and maximum life span extension to the same degree will occur.

I want to reiterate, however, that exercise alone, without calorie restriction, will not increase maximum life span. It may therefore seem paradoxical that evidence reveals that being unfit confers an even greater risk of death than being obese, in that lean sedentary men (BMI < 25) showed twice the risk of mortality from all causes than fit overweight men with BMIs > 28 but in neither case were these subjects on a calorie-reduced diet, in which a different metabolic set-up prevails. Similarly, the extent of decline with age in respiratory chain function in the mitochondria is greater (50 percent) than anticipated from the low levels of mitochondrial DNA mutations (1 percent) that occur with age, and reduced physical activity makes a major contribution to this decline, while physical activity ameliorates and may even mask such mitochondrial "aging, at least in muscle tissue.

One careful study in humans compared the results of eight weeks of calorie restriction (a 1,000-calorie reduction from an originally 2300-calorie intake) combined with resistance weight training (bench press, biceps curl, triceps extension, leg press etc. in all, eight exercises with three sets of ten repetitions each), to calorie restriction alone, to weight training alone. Calorie restriction alone was associated with decline in lean body mass, but addition thereto of weight training prevented the decline; nevertheless, the same amount of weight was lost indicating that the combination led to fat loss but not muscle loss. This is good news for those CRON dieters who want to maintain their lithe and muscular California bodies.

Recommendations for Exercise

The overall evidence suggests that aerobic exercise considerably increases cardiovascular fitness and substantially decreases the susceptibility to heart attack, and improves some features of carbohydrate metabolism. At the same time possibly owing to an increased generation of free radicals or a temporary increase in body temperature and metabolic rate it may slightly accelerate the basic rate of aging. Exercise definitely has a good effect and possibly a mildly bad effect.

The fitness effect increases rapidly up to a certain point as you exercise more and more, but beyond that point benefits may level off. According to Dr. Kenneth Cooper, Dallas, running tops out its aerobic benefits at fifteen miles a week. He says, "If you run more than that, it's for something other than fitness". Others agree with this assessment.

I will not lay out specific programs, but state simply what I myself do, and urge you to do the equivalent in whatever form you find most acceptable. Having been a gymnast in my youth, I find it simple and pleasant to spend four periods of one to one-and-a-half hours per week at a local gymnasium where I alternate aerobic workouts of 20 minutes each on a stair climb and two other types of aerobic exercise equipment, with circuit workouts on various types of Nautilus machines. In short, I engage in both aerobic and weight resistance exercise. If you wish to follow such a routine but don't know how, the gym owner or personal trainer will be glad to guide you.

Stretching

Flexibility exercises were not included in earlier editions of the above guidelines; but the College now recommends static stretches held ten to 30 seconds to the point of mild discomfort, repeating them four times per muscle group two to three times per week. The excellent book by Marilyn Moffat and Steve Vickery, reflecting the views of the American Physical Therapy Association on posture, gait, body mechanics, exercise and flexibility is well worth consulting.

On the subject of stretching, however, I have sought the input of my daughter, Lisa Walford, coauthor of *The Anti-Aging Plan* and a nationally recognized expert on restorative yoga. You will find a complete set of stretching routines plus other information on yoga on the Internet by clicking on Lisa's Section of the Walford web site, www.walford.com. An abbreviated treatment by Lisa, including eight stretches, is as follows:

> *In the last few years, Yoga has entered into our mainstream vocabulary, and is commercially successful in health clubs all over the country. According to a recent Roper poll, there are now approximately six million people practicing yoga in the United States.*

Hatha Yoga features movement and meditation to eliminate pain, reduce stress, encourage a full range of motion in the body while strengthening synergistic muscle groups, and improving coordination and balance, perfect for any anti-aging plan. Unfortunately, there is little documented research on what, until recently, has been deemed esoteric. However, additional benefits to a Yoga practice include some prevention of osteoporosis; decrease in severity of symptoms related to menopause; and other effects of the relaxation response on health.

There is currently no uniform standard regulating Yoga instructors. Differences between styles and even between teachers varies greatly. You should sample several classes and styles before you settle in and then schedule several classes a week, at least for a while. Yoga postures and movements are subtle, and you will profit greatly by taking a few good classes.

There are four main factors that may adversely influence your body over time, which yoga specifically addresses: the effect of gravity on the spine, posture, a sedentary lifestyle, and a poorly designed or imbalanced exercise regime. By contrast, the stance of water bearers in third world countries is light, long, composed, even as they balance heavy loads on their heads. Through proper alignment of their skeleton they maintain a plumb line that gives them great strength with the least amount of exertion and effort. This alignment is integral to Yoga. It often implies a restructuring of the body's patterning and changing postural habits.

In addition to posture, the wear and tear effects of any repetitive motion, and particularly asymmetrical ones such as tennis, carrying a baby on the same side of the body, getting in and out of a car, etc., lead to such common complaints as bursitis, tendinitis, sacroiliac imbalances, and general low-back pain. In fact, low-back pain is the fifth most common complaint resulting in a visit to a physician; after hypertension, pregnancy, general check-ups and colds.

A well-balanced exercise program should increase the range of motion in the hip joints and shoulder girdle (ball and socket joints); and strengthen the corresponding and more vulnerable lumbarabdominal (lower back and abdomen) and thoracic-cervical (upper back) component parts of the torso. In addition, it is imperative to stretch the hamstring muscles, as they are, if tight, a major culprit in weak lower backs. High impact exercise programs, often highly repetitive within a narrow range of motion, such as running, may more readily result in joint problems if not accompanied by stretching exercises.

A basic anti-aging movement routine should have the following aims: to increase extension in the spine and lengthen the erector spinae muscles; strengthen the deep abdominal muscles to protect the integrity of the lower back; lengthen the iliospoas muscle to promote optimal support and length in the lower back; stretch the hamstrings to align the pelvis level with the ground; strengthen the upper back muscles (rhomboids, trapezius,) to prevent slumping; open and stretch the chest to reduce pressure on the neck and upper back; reverse the effect of gravity on circulation in the legs and abdomen. The following eight exercises touch briefly on these areas:

To stretch the hamstring and buttock muscles:

(1) Lie on your back with your legs outstretched. Relax your shoulders down to the floor, so as to avoid tension in the neck and diaphragm. Bring one knee to your chest and wrap your arms around your shin. Firmly extend the straight leg, through the heel, so that you feel the entire length of your body elongate. Do not clench your stomach or push the lower back into the floor, as this will overextend the lower back muscles rather than target the hamstrings and buttocks. Hold the pose for six to seven breaths, and repeat several times.

Variation with belt: As above, only clasp your big toe and straighten the bent knee up toward the ceiling. Place a belt around the foot and hold on to the belt as you straighten the leg, so as to put tension on your hamstrings. Extend the floor leg as above, and hold the pose, keeping both sides of your torso long and free of distortion.

To stretch the lower and upper back:

(2) Lie on your back and draw both knees up to the chest. Keep the diaphragm relaxed. Lower both legs to one side of your body. Gently hold the bent knees to the floor and twist away from the legs. As you inhale, lengthen the spine and the sides of your torso. As you exhale, as if you are wringing out a washcloth, revolve your abdomen away from the bent knees. Continue to coordinate your movements with your breath, and allow time for your back muscles to release and to lengthen.

Variation: If you have strong stomach muscles and no back problems, you may practice this with straight legs. This will strengthen the oblique abdominal muscles and relieve tension in the shoulders and upper back. Begin from the bent knee position and extend your arms out to either side. Relax the shoulders away from your neck. Extend your legs up to the ceiling. Keep the torso long and your weight balanced on the lowest portion of the lower back, just above the tailbone. Lower the legs towards your hand on one side, and revolve your abdomen away from the weight of your legs. Initially, bend both knees to roll back onto your back before extending the legs vertically again. As you build strength in your stomach muscles and upper back, you may draw the legs back to vertical with straight knees.

To strengthen the buttocks, stretch the front thighs and lengthen the lower back:

(3) Lie on your back with your knees bent, feet flat on the floor, hip width apart, parallel to each other and close to your buttocks. Extend your arms overhead on the floor. If your arms do not reach the floor, and you feel any restriction in the neck or shoulders, then place a blanket underneath your forearms so you can lengthen your torso without straining your shoulders. Then, without tensing your stomach muscles, exhale, lengthen your lower back and lift your hips up off the floor. As if there were a leash attached to your tailbone, draw your tailbone up towards the ceiling, pressing your heels into the floor as you lift your hips. Hold this position for thirty seconds, then exhale and roll down vertebra by vertebra, lengthening your lower back.

To strengthen and lengthen the lower back:

(4) Lie down on your stomach on a rug or mat. Place your hands on the rug underneath your shoulders. Lift your upper body up and pull with your hands as if you wanted to crawl forward. You should feel the shoulders rolling back and down away from your ears, and the spine in between the shoulders drawing in toward your chest. Look straight ahead. Keep your pubic bone on the floor and lift your chest further up off the floor. Hold the cobra pose for several deep breaths, and release down. Repeat several times, and then draw your buttocks to your heels into a fetal position with the arms extended out in front of you. Relàx your back.

To stretch the chest, shoulders and abdomen:

(5) Get on your hands and knees, your feet hip-width apart and hands shoulder-width apart, then move your hands a few inches in front of your shoulders. Curl your toes under, exhale, lift your knees off the floor, and straighten your legs. Draw your weight off your hands and back onto your legs. Keep elbows and knees straight. Breath deeply, lengthening your back through your shoulders, waist, and hips. To release from the pose (called downward-facing dog), come back down onto your knees.

To stretch the deep hip flexors and front thigh muscles and to lengthen the iliospoas muscle:

(6) Facing a wall, place your legs very wide apart, one in front of the other as though you were taking a long stride. Inhale and extend your arms up overhead so that you feel the entire spinal column and torso lengthen. Square your hips and torso with the wall in front of you so that waist and rib cage are parallel to the wall. Press the back heel firmly down into the floor. Exhale, continue to stretch the pelvis up from the legs, and bend your front leg until your thigh is parallel to the floor. Your knee should be directly above your ankle. Keep your back leg straight as a rod, and realign your torso to parallel the wall once more. You should feel a big stretch on the front of your back leg and over the front of your pelvis. Stretch upwards! Hold this position for thirty seconds, and repeat on the other side. This pose is very helpful for those who sit, run, or stoop a lot. Repeat it several times.

To stretch the hamstrings, firm the side hips (women!) and relieve sacroiliac and sciatic tension:

(7) Stand erect and place one foot up on a stool, countertop, or

desk. The height depends on your flexibility. Keep your torso erect, and do not allow your pelvis to round in the direction of the lifted leg. Rather, press firmly into your standing foot and stretch your torso upwards. You may place your hands on the back of a chair beside you, to keep your balance if needed. Inhale and lengthen your torso more. Notice if your pelvis is parallel to the floor. If it is not, firm the outer thigh of your standing leg and drop the hip of your lifted leg until you feel that both sides of your lower back, waist, and pelvis are even. Elongate through the core of your body and both sides of the waist. It is this elongation that will stretch your lower back, so the details are important. Hold this pose for as long as you can. You may also practice this with the leg to the side. Begin as above but then turn your standing foot, your leg, and body at a 90 degree angle to its prior position. Align your pelvis as above.

Closing postures, to reverse the effect of gravity on circulation in the legs and abdomen and relax:

(8) Lying on your back, place your buttock against a wall and your legs up the wall, with a folded blanket underneath your hips and waist, and a small pillow underneath your neck and head. If your lower back rounds or comes off the floor, then your hamstrings are too tight, and you should move away from the wall slightly. Your legs will be at an obtuse angle to the wall, and your back released and relaxed. Release your arms out to the side, gently rolling the arms out, so that your chest opens. Your shoulders should be on the floor. Remain in this posture for at least five minutes.

Maladies of Wear and Tear

There are a number of potential medical problems whose incidence may increase with the mere passage of time, problems that even a thorough-going CRON diet may not protect you from, but that may be avoidable by other means. An easy example is your teeth. If they have to last 140 to 150 years instead of a mere 80 years, you should take good care of them.While again not an expert on all the matters of wear and tear, I may at least serve good purpose by calling your attention to this area, and suggesting a few illustrative, preventive remedies. In the maladies of wear and tear, of the back, neck, or joints of the extremities, the culprit is often merely the accumulated stress, strain and abuse from years of poor posture and body mechanics, of not allowing minor injuries to heal before returning to active play. My intention is not to turn you into an overcautious wimp, but merely to call your attention to this area of concern, and to suggest, as a sort of symbolic dogma, the following: "Live dangerously if it pleases you, but with good posture and well-fitting shoes"! Here's some advice:

(1) What appears to be "aging" of the skin is most often sun damage. Compare the skin of any older person's face or the skin on the back of their hands with that of their buttock, which one presumes has not seen much of the sun, and you'll prefer the relative smoothness of the latter. One hundred fifty years of unprotected, even casual sun exposure will leave you looking like Boris Karloff in *The Mummy*, regardless of the CRON diet. Always wear a hat and use sun screen if you intend to be hanging around for other purposes than multiple Halloweens.

(2) You will probably be spending a good many hours of your long life in chairs in front of desks, benches or tables. If that is so, and because bad chairs lead to bad backs, go to an orthopedic chair store—every big city has these—and buy good chairs for wherever you will repeatedly be putting your sunless buttock down. They are expensive ($500 to $1,000) but well worth the expense in preventive back maintenance.

(3) Ditto for shoes. Look into it, and buy the best for your precious 150-year feet!

Summary

The CRON diet will make you live long. Following the advice given in this chapter will substantially improve the quality, as measured by efficiency, accomplishments and enjoyments, of that long life.

5

Stages of Child Birth and Caring of Patient

Introduction

Labor is divided into three stages. The *first stage* begins when regular contractions are occurring and the cervix is dilating (opening up). The passage of a mucous plug (bloody show) or spontaneous rupture of the membranes (breaking of the bag of waters) also counts as evidence that labor is starting. In a first labor the complete absorption (incorporation) of the soft, thick, tubelike cervical canal into the body of the uterus (a taking up of the cervix, also known as effacement) is also evidence of the onset of labor. (In subsequent pregnancies the cervix usually thins out before contractions begin.) The first stage of labor lasts until the cervix is completely dilated, marking the onset of the *second stage*. The first stage is further divided into latent and active phases. I discuss these later on. The second stage, which begins with full cervical dilatation, ends with the birth of the baby, when the *third stage*, the delivery of the placenta, begins.

The progress of the first stage of labor is judged according to the diameter (width) of the cervix. The size of the opening ranges from zero (completely closed) to fully dilated, at an average of ten centimeters (just under four inches) with a full-term baby. The smallest discernible dilatation is noted as a fingertip; that is, it allows for the introduction of the tip only of the examiner's finger. The cervix may be dilated one to two centimeters before labor begins, especially in first pregnancies.

Dilatation and effacement (thinning) of cervix. Left-hand column shows cervix in a first birth; right-hand column shows the cervix after two or more births. Painful uterine contractions without evidence of cervical activity (effacement; dilatation; or the indirect evidence of cervical activity, occurrence of a bloody show, or rupture of membranes) do not constitute labor. These are common late in pregnancy and are referred to as Braxton Hicks contractions. Braxton Hicks contractions are characteristically irregular in their timing. They change unpredictably in length, strength, or frequency and often stop with a change in activity. Shifting from standing to lying down (or vice versa) or taking a warm bath will often make them stop. In contrast, labor contractions increase in regularity, duration, strength, and frequency. They grow stronger with activity.

Another important consideration in assessing the progress of labor is the location of the fetus in relation to the birth canal, that is, how far into the birth canal the fetus has descended. The level of descent is known as the *station*. The midpelvis is called station zero. When the head reaches station zero, it is said to be engaged. Above the level of the midpelvis the station is called negative; below the midpelvis, positive. Plus one, then, means one centimeter below or beyond the midpelvis; minus two means two centimeters above the midpelvis. Descent of the fetus is recorded in sequence as minus three, minus two, minus one, zero (at the midpelvis), plus one, plus two, and plus three (when the baby's head is visible).

In addition to determining the location of the fetus, it is important to determine which part of the fetus is entering the birth canal head, face, hands, or buttocks and how it is oriented to the birth canal. The presenting body part, say, the point of the head (known as the *occiput*), can usually be identified during a vaginal examination. Determining the way the head, or other presenting part, is rotated in the 360 possible degrees requires identification of its landmarks, or topical characteristics, with reference to an imaginary line or axis that follows the course of the birth canal.

In the case of the head, *sutures*, or *fontanels*, distinguish the front from the back of the skull. These sutures are the seams between the still-unknit bones of the skull. The fontanels are the triangular spaces at the junctions of the sutures, a large one in front (anterior) and a smaller one in back (posterior). Using these landmarks, it is possible to determine whether the head is facing forward, backward, or crossways. In medical terms, the location of the occiput is described as being to the left or right of center, pointing forward (anterior), backward (posterior), or crossways (transverse), ninety degrees to the right or left of the midline. Thus, LOA (left occiput anterior, the most common position), means that the occiput (the *O*) is directed left and forward.

Touching the head of the fetus reveals whether the scalp is swollen. Swelling is called *caput succedaneum*; a caput signifies that the ring of pressure exerted by the cervix on the scalp has interfered with the return of blood from the skin in the center of the ring. The presence of a caput indicates that the cervix is not yielding to pressure from the head and may mean some degree of obstruction to the descent of the fetus. At times a caput can be several centimeters thick, suggesting a greater degree of descent (a lower station) than is the case.

Another effect of pressure on the fetus's head is known as *molding*, the shaping of the head by the architecture of the birth canal. At birth a baby's head, unlike that of the adult or child, can be squeezed and elongated because the separate bones of the skull have not yet fused. The seams are open and the bones can overlap. This overlapping of the bones can often be detected in a vaginal examination. Molding is seen at birth in the form of elongation of the head and usually reverses spontaneously within a few days. The capacity of the head to mold is an adaptation of the human species to the stresses of labor. The give of the skull prevents it from cracking and permits a birth that otherwise would have been obstructed. The molding of the fetus's head is complemented by the looseness of the joints of the woman's pelvis, which also allows for some give of the birth canal to accommodate the fetus as it passes through.

During a vaginal examination the woman will usually hear the examiner report his or her observations on the dilatation of the cervix, its effacement, the station, the presenting part of the fetus, and the orientation of the presenting part. For example, "six centimeters, 80 percent, minus one, LOA" means that the cervix is six centimeters dilated and 80 percent effaced, and that the head is one centimeter inside the midpelvis and oriented with the occiput pointing forward and to the left.

These measurements are usually made during a contraction, when dilatation and descent are maximal. A variation of this principle is used to assess the roominess of the pelvis early in labor; the examiner pushes the fetus down and into the birth canal by pressing the abdomen on the top of the uterus with one hand while feeling the head in the vagina with the other. The ease with which the fetus descends reflects the fit between the fetus and the birth canal.

The first stage of labor includes two phases of cervical dilatation, the *latent phase* and the *active phase*. The active phase is further divided into the *acceleration phase* and the *deceleration phase*. The latter part of the acceleration phase and the early part of the deceleration phase are referred to as the *transition*, in which the cervix opens rapidly, from about seven centimeters to full dilatation. Transition is often the hardest part of labor, and its pain may be intense. It is often accompanied by nausea and vomiting.

Each stage and phase of labor has its own characteristics. A sensitive attendant, or the laboring woman herself, particularly if she has given birth before, can often tell the status of labor by the frequency, duration, and intensity of contractions, the presence or absence of pressure sensations in the birth canal, and the presence of associated symptoms, such as nausea or vomiting.

Early in the latent phase of the first stage, contractions are five to thirty minutes apart and last from fifteen to forty seconds. They are often described as mild cramps, gas, back pain or pressure. During the active phase, the contractions come two to five minutes apart, are forty five to sixty seconds in duration, and are stronger and more intense. In transition the contractions occur one and one-half to three minutes apart, last for forty-five to ninety seconds, and are the strongest they will be during the whole labor. Often, one contraction follows another so rapidly that resting between them may be impossible. Once full dilatation is achieved (the beginning of the second stage of labor and the end of the first), the contractions may space out to three to five or more minutes apart, so that some women are even able to doze off between them. As the fetus descends to the perineum, many women report a burning sensation. The contractions are now less intense, and discomfort shifts from the uterus to the rectum and vagina and includes a sense of pressure and an urge to push. This urge should be followed to the extent that it feels comfortable to do so. (See discussion later in this chapter on pushing during birth).

The configuration of the birth canal varies along its course. It is not like a curved tube or tunnel with a constant diameter throughout. At the entry to the birth canal the widest measurements are the oblique distances running from the right back to the left front and from the left back to the right front. At the outlet of the canal, the widest dimension is from front to back, from the tip of the spine (coccyx) to the juncture of the pubic bone in the front. As the fetus descends in the birth canal, it turns and twists to accommodate to these shifts in dimension. The fetus apparently plays an active role in moving along. In the LOA position, the head approaches the perineum at an angle and then moves to a direct front-to-back orientation just as the baby is being born, while the shoulders and back, following behind higher in the canal, are still at an angle. When the head fully emerges, it immediately turns back into alignment with the rest of the body. As the shoulders are born, they move into a direct front-to-back position with one shoulder under the pubic bone as the other emerges over the coccyx. As the shoulders turn, the head turns with them and the baby's face looks directly to the side.

Although the posterior position (occiput pointing to the back) is a normal, but minority, presentation from which babies are safely born, it is often associated with the prolongation of labor and the experience of back pain. If a fetus is posterior and progress in labor is slow, efforts are usually made to help the head (and the fetus) to rotate forward, either by having the woman change position or by having the attendant turn the head manually in the vagina.

Timing your Contractions

Place your hands on your uterus and feel for its tightening and then relaxing. You will usually experience some pain at the same time. In early labor, contractions last between twenty and sixty seconds and the tight

Birthing Center or Birth Attendant

For a first labor, call if you can no longer talk through contractions or when your contractions come regularly every three to five minutes over one hour, last at least forty-five to sixty seconds, and are much stronger when you walk. For second or subsequent labors, call when contractions occur every five to seven minutes, last forty-five to sixty seconds, and become stronger when walking.

Also call if your bag of waters breaks or if you have bright red vaginal bleeding, not to be confused with the bloody show, which is the dark, blood-tinged mucus passed from the cervix as it dilates.

Approaches to Labor and Birth

There are two major approaches to labor and birth, which I call the *active* and the *unhurried.* Each approach has its own solutions to the central problem of pain in labor. The active approach is often called the *medical model of childbirth* because its interventions are drugs and surgery, which only doctors are licensed to use. These interventions, discussed in detail elsewhere, include medical pain relief, drugs that contract the uterus, episiotomy, forceps and vacuum extraction, electronic fetal monitoring and cesarean section. The unhurried approach is most commonly referred to as *natural childbirth,* which is a perfectly adequate term. I prefer calling it the unhurried approach only because in my analysis its distinguishing feature is the absence of an expectation for how long or in what way a woman should labor or give birth and the presence of an expectation (call it confidence) that a woman has the capacity to handle the pain of labor without being traumatized in the process. She sets her own pace and finds her own way. In the unhurried approach interventions include patience; lots of hands-on, one-on-one care; psychological support and encouragement; relaxation; changes in position; a soothing environment; body contact with attendants and close ones; and, more recently, immersion in a warm tub for labor and delivery. Labor pain is managed rather than eliminated. An essential part of managing this pain is the mind-set that in the right environment and with the right support, it can be done. Although critics of the active approach describe the unhurried approach as noninterventive, I do not agree; it is just that the interventions used are different.

Although the two approaches are very different, they are both safe and they both work. Both are being refined and improved. For example, the active approach now offers the dual spinal-epidural anesthetic, a major advance in pain relief and the unhurried approach now includes water birth, also a major advance. Which approach is best for you depends on individual preferences, availability (of birth attendant and facility), and cost. In general, the active approach is practiced by physicians and the unhurried approach by midwives. Some physicians are also skilled practitioners of the unhurried approach. You will need to select a birth attendant based on your preference, assuming that you have a choice. If a medical complication develops in a labor using the unhurried approach, as occurs in a minority of circumstances, a physician (and often an anesthesiologist and pediatrician) will be needed.

The goals of the active approach are that no woman should suffer from pain in labor and that labor should be handled with whatever tools are needed to accomplish delivery within a defined number of hours, usually twelve. Enter the hospital at a certain time and leave at a predictable later time, baby in arms. The active approach is usually applied to first labors because they normally last longer than subsequent labors, but it can be used with subsequent labors as well. (For many women, second and later labors seem to take care of themselves). A quick delivery and shortened hospital stay are perceived as using scarce hospital resources efficiently and as fitting in with the widely accepted goal of containing health-care costs, although the active approach is probably more expensive than the unhurried one. The active approach can also be viewed as fitting better into the busy parents' schedule.

The unhurried approach is based on the observation that women normally vary in the durations of their labors, just as they do in their heights and blood pressures, and that there is no exact figure for how long a labor should be. As long as there is no expectation about how long a labor *should* last, the fetus and the woman are doing well, and the woman and her birth attendant both believe things are going well, there is no need to do anything other than provide support, in all of its many forms, to the woman throughout the process. In these conditions well over 90 percent of women will give birth without most of the interventions that are a part of the active approach.

There is evidence that the unhurried approach is less costly. Statistics compiled in 1995 on charges in birthing centers, which offered only the unhurried approach, show that the average birth cost $3,241, whereas a hospital birth in the same community at the same time averaged $6,378. The estimate of annual savings for just 100,000 births in birthing centers (a small fraction of all births in the United States each year), including savings resulting from performing fewer cesarean sections, was a sizable $1.4 billion. However, this estimate is probably high because the costs of hospital care for uncomplicated births include paying, in part, for the standby resources needed for complicated births operating rooms, specialized equipment, highly trained personnel, and so on. Because of these unavoidable built-in costs, which birthing centers do not have, exact financial comparisons are difficult, if not impossible. Nonetheless, it does appear that the unhurried approach has economic benefits.

The differences experientially between the two approaches can be startling. They certainly were for me as an observer. Having been educated only in the medical model, my first exposure to the unhurried approach, with care provided by midwives at the Booth Maternity Center in Philadelphia in the mid-1970s, was a real eye-opener, nothing short of astonishing. Women of all backgrounds and ages simply had their babies, without any of the high-tech devices to which I was accustomed and did perfectly well in all respects. I had to question the need to do anything different for any women at low risk for labor problems.

Between the pure examples of the active and unhurried approaches as I have presented them, there are gradations that combine elements of each. Because the active approach is in a sense easier and less demanding, the woman who wants the unhurried approach needs to consider the setting in which she will labor very carefully and the extent to which the institution (or home) and her attendants will be supportive of her preferences. For example, repeatedly asking a woman in the second stage of labor whether she would like an epidural anesthetic, as is sometimes done in hospitals, instead of simply providing, matter-of-factly, nonmedical methods of pain relief implies that the pain will sooner or later become unbearable.

My concern is that of access and choice. Support for the active approach can easily be found anywhere in the United States, whereas support for the unhurried approach is limited or nonexistent in many communities. Although the percentage of births attended by midwives, the primary practitioners of the unhurried approach, increased from 1.7 percent in 1980 to 9 percent in 1998, midwives still attend only slightly less than one in ten births in the United States. The active approach remains dominant. Consider recent statistics showing that labor inductions are up 14.0 percent, as many as 30 percent of women may receive oxytocin to stimulate their labor contractions, more than 80 percent of labors are monitored electronically, epidural anesthesia use has increased, and about 10 to 15 percent of women need assistance from forceps or a vacuum extractor in delivering (or, more to the point, being delivered of) their babies.

Many women do not even know that there is a way to labor and deliver other than by the active approach. It is the only choice available in their communities, which means, in essence, they have no choice. Judith Rooks , in her book *Midwifery and Childbirth in America* (which is also an excellent history of how we have come to have the maternity care system we have), expresses this concern very well when she links (correctly, in my opinion) the availability of the unhurried approach (she uses a different term) to the supply and distribution of midwives: "Given the examples of other countries; given the safety, effectiveness and benefits of midwifery care; and given the importance of the qualitative aspects of the childbearing experience to many women and families, it is wrong to deny any American woman the option of choosing to have a midwife as her primary-care provider if her pregnancy is normal".

In the same vein, doctors Murray Enkin, Marc Keirse, James Neilson, and midwife Mary Renfrew, authors of the second edition of the highly respected and influential book, *A Guide to Effective Care in Pregnancy and Childbirth* (see Appendix), which is derived from the Oxford database of clinical trials, include in the category of "Forms of Care That Are Unlikely to Be Beneficial" the following: "Involving *obstetricians* in the care of *all* (my emphasis added) women during pregnancy and childbirth" and "Not involving obstetricians in the care of women with serious risk factors". Under the category of "Forms of Care That Are Likely to Be Beneficial" they list "Midwifery care for women with no serious risk factors". Pointedly absent in this category is care by physicians of such women. Clearly these editors recognize that the great majority of women will do very well if offered the unhurried approach with midwives as their attendants.

There is some evidence that more women would like to have the *option* of the unhurried approach. For example, a 1995 survey of the largest HMO in the state of Washington found, according to Rooks, "that 8% of reproductive-age women were interested in the idea of a midwife-attended home birth and might choose that option if the cooperative would provide the same benefits for a home birth that it provides for a birth in one of the H.M.O. hospitals".

Elements of the Active Approach

The packaging of them as the active management of labor has been achieved and popularized by the Royal Maternity Hospital of Dublin. In that institution active management involves (1) a strict definition of labor onset that includes regular and painful uterine contractions at least once every five minutes in association with, in first labors, complete effacement of the cervix, bloody show, or spontaneous rupture of membranes or, in all labors, progressive dilatation of the cervix (in many second and subsequent pregnancies the cervix is dilated before labor onset); (2) purposeful rupture of the membranes of all women in labor in whom such rupture has not occurred spontaneously (this intervention alone has been proved to shorten labor); (3) use of oxytocin in first labors (only) when the cervix dilates at less than one centimeter per hour; and (4) cesarean section if delivery does not occur within twelve hours. The primary birth attendant in the Dublin program is a midwife who gives one-on-one care to the laboring woman.

Elements of the Unhurried Approach

The following list summarizes the major elements of the unhurried approach:

1. Choose a midwife as your birth attendant or a physician who is skilled in midwifery (hard to find). Unhurried births are the stock-in-trade of midwives. Also consider having a doula with you. Don't look to your significant other to play the role of doula. Your partner, who inevitably is too emotionally involved with you to provide the *professional* input you need, does have an important contribution to make, however.

2. Don't start the labor clock ticking by going to the hospital or birthing center too early and then staying there if you're not in active labor even though you're experiencing contractions. Otherwise, expectations of how long you should be in labor will come into play, and if you don't meet these expectations you are more likely to become disappointed and lose your nerve and the odds that medical interventions will be proposed and accepted will increase. If you're not in active labor, go home. (The criteria used in Dublin are good ones to use in determining whether you should stay or leave). Then, stay at home until you are in active labor. Stay in phone contact. Make it a point to be on the phone with your attendant *during a contraction.* As obstetrician Alan Schapker pointed out in a talk at the 1995 annual meeting of the National Association of Childbearing Centers, if you can talk through a contraction, it's not time to head out. If possible, have the doctor, midwife, or nurse check you in the office, as the hospital, for many people, raises anxiety levels because of its association with illness. The less anxiety the better in labor.
3. Avoid having your membranes deliberately ruptured. Because of concerns about infection, the clock really starts ticking loud and clear after this procedure is performed and puts pressure on all to achieve delivery within a certain time. Spontaneous rupture of the membranes at term has almost the same implications for duration of labor as does amniotomy.
4. If possible, do not use an electronic fetal monitor strip, often standard procedure on arrival in the labor and delivery unit. Use of a fetal monitor can increase anxiety, symbolizes the medical model and has no evidence-based rationale. It puts you in the mind-set for an active-management approach.
5. Don't ask for predictions on the duration of your labor. Expectations will then be set, which, if not met, will increase your concern that something may be wrong and that something has to be done about it.
6. Labor is one situation that you can't control, so don't even try. Go with the flow. Surrender.

7. As midwives Susan Melinkow (of Sharpthe Birth Place, San Diego) and Holly Schochat (of Northwest Hospital, Tucson) suggest, when labor stalls, consider psychological as well as physical factors. For example, when encouraged to talk, a woman whose labor is going nowhere might identify and express a fear that she won't love this baby as much as her first, that her husband won't love the baby, or that she feels guilty about having this baby because she had an abortion with her last pregnancy. The mere communication of such concerns, no matter how silly or embarrassing they may seem, has unblocked many a labor. The woman lets go of her resistance and the baby is born.
8. Keep your environment simple and relaxed. Labor is not the time to host a party for your friends and relatives, particularly during the first stage. Wait until the second stage of labor if you want a few close friends and family members with you.
9. Find the positions that work best for you. In general, avoid giving birth while lying flat on your back; avoid the use of stirrups; and keep control of your legs.
10. Take advantage of the benefits of being massaged and stroked, of being held and hugged, of having your hair combed. Counterpressure against a sore back can be a blessing. A cup of tea, dim lights, and music all have their place. Also consider nontraditional methods of pain relief, such as foot massage, acupuncture, and guided imagery and visualization (for example, of waves on the ocean). Labor is the time of times to be soothed, praised, babied, accepted, heard and not criticized.
11. Consider a water birth.

Research on the Active Approach

Active management has resulted in excellent outcomes, including a cesarean delivery rate of less than 6 percent, which is remarkably low by U.S. standards even when allowance is made for possible differences in the populations of women served. Further, 30 percent of the women seen in the Royal Maternity Hospital require oxytocin and about 20 percent have epidural anesthesia, both of which are used only in first labors.

The Dublin experience has attracted much attention in the United States as a possible approach to reducing the high C-section rates. Two well-conducted studies have tested the results. In both studies the control group received many of the interventions received by the active management group, but did not receive them as consistently or under the same guidelines with respect to the time elapsed from the onset of labor. As reported in 1992, Jose Lopez-Zeno and colleagues at Northwestern University conducted a controlled trial of active management during first labors and achieved a cesarean-section rate of 10.5 percent, compared with 14.1 percent in the control (usual-care) group. In this study, not using midwives, the average length of labor was shortened by 1.66 hours and significantly fewer infections occurred among the women who were actively managed. Almost three-fourths of the women at Northwestern in both the active management and the control groups received epidural anesthesia.

Another controlled trial of active management was conducted under the direction of Fred Frigoletto at Brigham and Woman's Hospital in Boston in 1995. This study used one-on-one nursing, with the nurses changing only at shifts. The average duration of labor was shortened by 2.7 hours and there was no difference in the C-section rate of 19 percent in each group. Fifty-four percent of the women in the active management group and 64 percent in the usual-care group requested epidural anesthesia.

With the active-management approach using epidoral anesthesia the woman may well be able to watch television during labor and delivery will usually involve the use of stirrups, washing of the perineum and the covering of the woman's legs and lower abdomen with sterile drapes. Unlike unhurried labors, which are often noisy and spontaneous, actively managed labors tend to be neat and orderly.

Why the differences in results between the Dublin and the U.S. versions of active management? A major element in the care provided in Dublin was the one-on-one attention by a midwife using the midwifery approach to labor and delivery. This is very likely a crucial element. This notion is echoed by the authors of Active Management of Labor, The Dublin Experience, who conclude that "No form of management of labor can be really effective unless it can be practiced by nurses independently, almost, of doctors. This requires a level of mutual confidence between nurses and doctors which is not too often found".

Research on the Unhurried Approach

Research data on the unhurried approach are limited. The best sources of data are birthing centers, which emphasize the unhurried approach. Another source of data on the unhurried approach is home births. Although less common in the United States than in other countries, home births are still popular among a small segment of the U.S. population (about 1 percent) and holding steady. (Until the twentieth century the home was the *only* place to give birth; Richard Nixon was the last U.S. president to be born at home).

Freestanding birthing centers were pioneered during the 1970s. The Maternity Center Association of New York, under the leadership of nurse midwife Ruth Lubic, opened a center in a converted brownstone house on the upper east side of Manhattan. The Booth Maternity Center of the Salvation Army (which also included a hospital component), under the leadership of nurse midwives Kitty Ernst and Ruth Wilf and obstetrician John Franklin (and over the sometimes very strong opposition of obstetricians, especially in New York), was opened in Philadelphia. In the United States freestanding birthing centers now number 145, with 85 more under development. Most centers are certified by the National Association of Childbearing Centers (see Appendix), an organization that maintains very high practice standards and collects statistics on every birth at its centers. Nurse midwife and researcher Judith Rooks reported the association's statistics in the December 28, 1989, issue of the New England Journal of Medicine. The data came from the 84 centers certified at the time and involved 11,814 women admitted for labor and delivery. Overall, the outcomes were excellent and comparable to or better than the best achieved in a hospital setting among similar women. The intrapartum and neonatal mortality rate was (a low) 1.3 per 1,000 births—0.7 per 1,000 when infants with lethal malformations are excluded from the statistics. Using very conservative indications, slightly over 16 percent of the women were transferred during labor to a hospital, and 2.4 percent were transferred as emergencies. Women with first pregnancies were more likely to be transferred than those with later pregnancies (29 versus

7 percent). The rate of cesarean sections (all performed in hospitals) was (a low) 4.4 percent and no women died. Seventeen percent of the women had episiotomies. Of the rest, 34.0 percent had no vaginal tears, 45.7 percent had minor tears, and slightly over 2.0 percent had deeper tears. Internal continuous electronic fetal monitoring was used in 1.1 percent of the labors (the rest were monitored by intermittent listening to the fetal heartbeat), and 95 percent of the women drank liquids or ate while in labor. Forty-three percent of the women took showers, baths or both. Twenty-four percent of women in their first labor and 6 percent of women in a later labor received analgesics for pain relief.

Freestanding birthing centers emphasize continuity of care by nurse midwives and, more recently, lay midwives (physicians usually participate as consultants to the midwives or in some cases, as birth attendants); secure transport services and backup arrangements with hospitals and obstetricians; strong prenatal education; and treating pregnancy, labor and delivery as normal, happy experiences. They do not administer oxytocin to augment labor, nor do they (with few exceptions) use electronic fetal monitors or epidural or spinal anesthetics. They place great emphasis on helping women find *what works best for them* in labor, drawing on each woman's own strengths. They encourage laboring and delivering in an upright position. Their excellent outcomes probably reflect the combined effects of these policies and practices, which differ from the standard hospital-based approach and offer a revealing comparison. As a model of care, the birthing center that meets the standards of the Commission for the Accreditation of Birth Centers (based on the nationally recognized Standards for Birth Centers published by the National Association of Childbearing Centers) has much to recommend it, including reaching women in need of services who have fewer financial resources and reducing the costs of care by as much as 30 to 50 percent. More and more hospitals are adopting a birthing-center approach within their own walls or grounds (side by side with the active approach as an option) and achieving similar results, with an added advantage of easier access to facilities and personnel in case of complications.

I find it intriguing that the results of midwife-attended birth in birthing centers are not that different from midwife-attended birth using the active-management rules followed in Dublin (I do not have access to data on duration of labor in the birthing centers). What this seems to say is that if you want these kinds of results, use midwives, doulas or nurses who provide one-on-one care.

The classic setting for the unhurried approach is the home. The best natural laboratory for research on outcomes of home births has been the Netherlands, where national health policy, a nonactive intervention philosophy of birth, and an excellent support system, including maternity aides who stay during labor and the baby's first week, have enabled midwives and general practitioners to continue to attend many births at home. A study that analyzed data compiled by the Central Bureau of Statistics found no significant differences in outcomes between cities with an almost 100 percent rate of hospital births and cities of similar demography with a 50 percent rate of hospital births.

Following international trends, in the Netherlands between 1960 and 1990 the proportion of deliveries occurring in the home declined from 70 to 35 percent and is continuing to drop. However, birth at home continues to be very safe. In a 1990 report of almost 9,000 births, the perinatal death rate was 0.14 percent, and only 3.1 percent of infants were admitted to the hospital in their first week. (Data on mothers transferred to hospitals are not available). The overall cesarean-section rate in the Netherlands, including births for which labor began at home, is less than 5 percent. Studies from the United Kingdom, Switzerland and the Netherlands reported in 1996 showed similar excellent results. In these countries, home birth is a recognized and supported option with a defined transport and transfer system in place if hospitalization is required. These elements are crucial.

Home birth in the Netherlands has benefited that nation's entire system of maternity care. Through the repeated experience and highly visible model of successful normal births in the home, as well as through the prominent role of midwives in hospitals as well as at home, a philosophy of nonintervention in maternity care (relative to other countries) is maintained even for hospital births. The rate of cesarean sections in the Netherlands was 2.0 percent in 1969, 3.0 percent in 1975, 5.0 percent in 1980 and 6.0 percent in 1987. In the United States the rate was 5.3 percent in 1969, 10.2 percent in 1975, 15.2 percent in 1978 and 24.0 percent in 1988.

In the United Kingdom, the National Birthday Trust Fund's survey of 6,044 planned births in 1994 and the 1996 study of the Northern Region Perinatal Mortality Survey Coordinating Group found no evidence to support the claim that the safest policy is for all women to give birth in the hospital. In the United States, midwives and, to a lesser degree, physicians who have attended women at home, often facing hostile opposition from the organized medical community, along with the women who have had home births, have played a critical role in establishing a beachhead for the unhurried approach to labor and delivery. For a long time, the home was the only place where unhurried births could occur.

Comparing the Active and the Unhurried Approaches

There are no comparison studies of the two approaches beyond the data already presented. There are no randomized control trials comparing births in hospitals in birthing centers, and at home. It is unlikely that there will ever be such trials, as it is highly unlikely that women would accept the randomization required. Because women who choose a particular setting for labor and birth are self-selected and may differ in important characteristics, such as motivation and attitudes toward pain, it is difficult to know whether the different outcomes observed result from care in labor peculiar to the site of birth, from characteristics of the women themselves or as is more likely, from a combination of the two.

Water Birth

Water birth (warm-water immersion for labor and delivery) is the latest and perhaps, one of the most interesting developments in support of the unhurried approach to birth. It is gaining in popularity in the United States and has had a major impact in other countries, such as the United Kingdom, where a majority of hospitals under the National Health Service are now equipped with tubs. It is estimated that well over 50,000 water births have occurred worldwide, with no reports of life-threatening complications for either the mother or the baby. A 1999 study in the United Kingdom of 4,032 water births (217 of 219 maternity centers responded to the survey) that occurred between 1994 and 1996 showed that deaths of babies and admission to the special-care nursery were no different for babies born in water than for babies born vaginally but not in water, all in low-risk pregnancies. The small numbers in this study somewhat limit the strength of its conclusions. Although these data are impressive and the enthusiasm for water birth is undeniable, no controlled trials of its effectiveness have been done to date. I hope that such studies will be carried out.

The use of water as part of labor started in Europe as a comfort measure during labor. Women liked it so much that they refused to get out to deliver their babies. To everyone's surprise, the babies did just fine being born in the water, with no risk of drowning. (They don't begin breathing until they're brought up from the water). I can just imagine the early scenes of French doctors tearing their hair out when faced down by a woman who defiantly wouldn't budge when told it was time to leave the tub and go to the delivery room ". But, but ... Madame Ladieux, please be reasonable!"

Water appears to provide enough external support to the woman to elevate (float) her to a new level of coping. A favored birthing position is on hands and knees. By avoiding bearing down with her contractions and by gently pushing between them (a practice encouraged by midwives in most deliveries), the woman eases the fetus through the birth canal while gradually stretching it. (Episiotomy rates with water birth in the United Kingdom have reportedly dropped from 60 to 10 percent). Finally, the mother reaches down to cradle the baby and pull him or her into the water and, shortly thereafter, into the air. The mother delivers her baby; the midwife is an ever-alert bystander.

A major resource for water birth in the United States is Global Maternal/Child Health Association, under the leadership of nurse Barbara Harper. As part of its educational and support services, this organization has produced a powerful and moving videotape of a woman laboring and giving birth in water. Particularly memorable are the woman's haunting sounds and twisting dance as, eyes shut and fully in control, she retreats deep into herself (defying all the rules about the importance of breathing in a certain way and maintaining eye contact), where she must be accessing all the enormous innate (and often untapped) strength that a woman brings to childbirth. What an extraordinary sense of fulfillment this woman must have experienced, one that will last a lifetime. My prediction is that just as birthing centers, rooming-in and support for breast-feeding in hospitals developed in response to public demand (women voting with their feet), so, too, water birth will become an increasingly available option.

Fluids and Food

The rationale for the traditional hospital rule that women in labor should avoid eating and drinking and rely on intravenous fluids (IVs) exclusively is that if a general (gas) anesthetic is required as part of an emergency delivery (usually by cesarean section), there is a risk that during the induction of anesthesia, the woman will vomit and breathe the stomach contents into her lungs. This is indeed a serious problem; chemical pneumonia and even death can result.

This traditional policy has been modified in light of new evidence and considerations. First and foremost, proper anesthetic technique (compression of the upper airway by pressing on the neck) can prevent aspiration of vomited stomach contents during anesthesia induction until a tube is secured in the airway. Second, general anesthesia is little used today, certainly compared with fifty or more years ago when the policy of no food or fluid by mouth was developed. Third, it has not been proved that a stomach empty of fluids and food will prevent the aspiration problem. Even in the absence of food, the acid in the stomach is highly irritating to the lungs if aspirated. Given this evidence, the policy of no food or drink has been substantially liberalized in many hospitals. In birthing centers and for home births it has never been an issue.

Early in labor it makes sense to eat easily digested carbohydrates, such as bread, fruit, rice and pasta, and light proteins, such as cheese and yogurt. As labor progresses, the emphasis should shift to high-calorie liquids. In general, water, sports drinks, iced tea and noncitrus fruit juices are well tolerated. Added honey or sugar can provide calories for women who want to drink plain water. Optimally, women should consume eight ounces of fluid and 200 calories an hour (a tablespoon of honey contains 64 calories; one cup of grape juice, 167 calories).

Some home-birth attendants have observed that citrus and apple juices and dairy products can cause vomiting in heavy labor. They advise women to freeze cranberry or grape juice in ice-cube trays to use in the event of nausea. Crushed ice from these juices, plain ice chips, or small sips of cool water tend to be kept down if taken in small amounts between each contraction. Dry toast or crackers also often help reduce nausea.

Drugs that Contract the Uterus

The drugs *oxytocin* (trade names Pitocin and Syntocinon), *ergonovine maleate* (Ergotrate), and *methylergonovine maleate* (Methergine) stimulate contraction of the uterus. Oxytocin is the synthetic form of a hormone normally secreted by the pituitary gland to contract the muscles of the uterus and the glands of the breasts, leading to the ejection of milk. In the postpartum period, the secretion of this natural hormone accounts for the afterpains of uterine contractions familiar to nursing mothers, particularly with their second and subsequent babies. The secretion of natural oxytocin is stimulated by nerve impulses that reach the brain and pituitary gland from the breasts during nipple stimulation. Thus, stimulation can initiate and augment labor as well as initiate both the letdown of milk and the uterine contractions that help prevent postpartum hemorrhage. Because synthetic oxytocin is metabolized readily and lasts but a short time in the blood, it is ideal for augmenting uterine contractions in labor. It is less effective in initiating labor, but is used for that purpose.

When used intravenously to enhance labor, oxytocin is delivered through a constant-infusion pump set to regulate the amount of hormone entering the woman to produce the right intensity and frequency of contractions. Intrauterine-pressure monitors inserted via a tube through the vagina are sometimes used to measure the intensity of uterine contractions during oxytocin stimulation.

Oxytocin is also used to initiate (induce) labor if deemed necessary to the woman's or baby's health, for example, in cases of preeclampsia or prolonged pregnancy. Finally, oxytocin is used to help contract the uterus after the baby is born, which decreases postpartum bleeding (hemorrhage). For this purpose oxytocin can be given by injection or added to an intravenous infusion already in place.

Multigravidas (women who have had more than one full-term pregnancy) are more sensitive to oxytocin than are women who are pregnant for the first or second time. They experience more cramping and pain from administered oxytocin or from the natural hormone they produce themselves. (As mentioned, their afterpains are characteristically more intense).

Ergonovine is a chemical derived from the ergot fungus found in rye and other grains or produced synthetically in the laboratory. Ergonovine causes uterine contraction. Unlike oxytocin, the effects of ergonovine last for hours, making it unsuitable during labor but useful for maintaining a contracted uterus after delivery of the placenta. Ergonovine and methylergonovine are administered by injection after the placenta has been delivered and should be given along with tocin, not alone. They can also be given by mouth to maintain the uterus in a contracted state. Both can be used to contract the uterus and prevent bleeding after a D & C. Because of the undesirable side effects of ergonovine preparations, including nausea and elevated blood pressure, they are less frequently administered today.

Prostaglandins are another widely used group of naturally occurring chemicals that cause uterine-muscle contraction and can be used to initiate labor. They are placed in a gel base and inserted into the vagina or into the cervical canal. They ripen the cervix for labor and stimulate contractions of the uterus. (Once labor is under way, oxytocin can be administered as needed). Prostaglandins, given intravenously, are also used to contract a baggy (hypotonic) uterus after delivery of the placenta.

Medical Pain Relief

The elements of the unhurried approach, which I described in some detail, are mainly directed toward this goal. Here I will discuss the role of drugs and of various ways of administering them.

Analgesics

Analgesics and anesthetics are medications used for pain relief. Analgesics reduce pain to make it tolerable, whereas anesthetics are intended to eliminate it completely. Analgesics in everyday use include aspirin, ibuprofen (Advil, Motrin) and acetaminophen (Tylenol). Moderately strong analgesics include codeine and oxycodone-aspirin (Percodan). The strongest analgesics include morphine, meperidine (Demerol), alphaprodine (Nisentil), nalbuphine (Nubain) and fentanyl.

The analgesics most commonly used in labor are meperidine, fentanyl, nalbuphine and butorphanol. To counteract the nausea associated with them, these drugs are sometimes combined with the antihistamine promethazine. These analgesics are given by injection or intravenously; if given intravenously, the dose is controlled by the woman, within certain safety limits. In addition to relieving pain, analgesics produce some drowsiness and euphoria. Many women find that these drugs help them regain their strength during a long, difficult early labor.

Analgesics pass through the placenta to the fetus, where they can depress the centers in the brain that drive respiration, an effect of clinical importance only when, after birth, the baby must breathe on his or her own, not in utero when the work of respiration is being done by the woman. Analgesics can also sedate the fetus, resulting in drowsiness that can interfere with the baby's responsiveness and feeding during the first few hours after birth or even longer. Because of their depressant and sedative effects, these drugs are used mainly in the first stage of labor. Barring an unexpectedly rapid birth, as in an emergency cesarean section, their effect on an infant's respiration should be over long before delivery. If the effect is not over, and if the baby's respiration is depressed, assistance can be provided as needed with a breathing bag and oxygen. The drug naloxone hydrochloride (Narcan) can also be administered to the baby to reverse the respiratory-depressant effects of analgesics.

Anesthetics

Anesthetics are drugs designed to eliminate rather than simply relieve pain. Two broad classes are used: blocking drugs, which disrupt impulse transmission in nerves and inhaled gases, which shut down pain transmission and perception in the entire nervous system, including the brain and put the patient to sleep. Lidocaine (Xylocaine) is an example of the former and nitrous oxide, the latter. Improvements in anesthetics over the past fifty years have been substantial and offer women almost complete pain control that is also safe.

Nerve Blocks

Nerve-block drugs are used in pregnancy to achieve local, peripheral nerve, spinal and epidural anesthesia. The names designate the site of action of the anesthetic: the peripheral nerves of the skin or vaginal surface (local anesthesia); the pudendal nerves, which supply the vagina and perineum (pudendal nerve block); the nerve roots within the spinal fluid (spinal anesthesia); or the nerve roots outside the spinal cord (epidural anesthesia). Each type will be discussed in turn, along with the recent practice of combining spinal and epidural anesthesias.

Local Anesthesia: Local anesthesia is accomplished by injecting the blocking drug directly into the site to be numbed, blocking the end branches of the nerves within that site. In pregnancy, local anesthesia is used just before an episiotomy is done, before the repair of an episiotomy, or tear, and in numbing the skin through which the needle used in spinal or epidural anesthesia will be introduced.

Pudendal Nerve Block: The two pudendal nerves are situated in the lower back corners of the vagina and are identified within the vagina by feeling (palpating), on the right and left sides, a specific prominence in one of the pelvic bones adjacent to which the nerves run. A successful *pudendal nerve block* will anesthetize much of the perineum and vagina and reduce the pain associated with vaginal stretching and tearing, whether spontaneous or by episiotomy, during birth. A very long needle is needed to reach these nerves, which are very deep in the vagina. To guide the needle to the sites, one at a time, the physician positions a fingertip on the bony landmark and slides the needle along the same finger to its destination. Pudendal block is infrequently used because epidural block accomplishes the same goals better and also eliminates labor pain.

Spinal Anesthesia: In spinal anesthesia, the blocking agent is injected into the spinal canal through a needle that is inserted between the vertebrae of the lower back. The drug bathes the spinal nerves within the canal before they exit the cord. Both sensory and motor nerves are temporarily blocked, so that the woman's lower abdomen, pelvic area, and legs are numbed and cannot be voluntarily moved. The level of anesthesia (that is, how high on the abdomen the anesthesia reaches) is largely determined by how much drug is given and by the position the woman assumes immediately following the injection. For a vaginal delivery, the goal is to anesthetize only the perineum and legs. For a cesarean section, anesthesia should reach the lowest ribs. Spinal anesthesia is given only after full cervical dilatation. Thus it is of no help with pain during the first stage of labor.

Spinal anesthetic is administered while the woman is sitting or lying on her side. First, the skin is cleaned with an antiseptic solution. Then a sterile drape with a central hole is placed over the lower back. The anesthesiologist numbs the skin with a local anesthetic, infiltrating the solution down to the spinal column so that the channel between skin and spinal column is anesthetized. The woman is then asked to curl forward to open the spaces between the vertebrae. A thin, hollow needle containing a removable stylet is pushed through the numbed channel until it passes through the meninges into the spinal fluid just below the end of the spinal cord and nerve roots. The stylet is removed, and the location of the needle in the spinal canal is verified by the return of clear spinal fluid. A syringe containing the anesthetic solution is then attached to the needle, and the medication is introduced between uterine contractions. For a vaginal delivery, the woman is asked to sit up for forty-five seconds to allow the medication to settle to the bottom of the spinal canal. For a cesarean section, the woman lies first on one side, then on the other, to allow the anesthetic to travel upward in the canal to block the nerves that supply the entire abdomen. The level of anesthesia is controlled to some extent by tilting the operating table up or down as indicated. The anesthesiologist checks the level by checking the woman's response to the prick of a needle moved up or down the abdomen.

In vaginal delivery, spinal anesthesia interferes with the woman's ability to push. The higher the level of anesthetic, the more her capacity to push is impaired. In addition, spinal anesthesia requires that the woman lie on her back with her legs in stirrups during delivery, further interfering with pushing. As a result, forceps or vacuum extraction is more likely to be needed, as well as episiotomy.

Spinal anesthesia carries several risks. The most common is a drop in the woman's blood pressure brought on by blockage of the sympathetic nerves that control the tone of the muscles within the walls of arteries. When the arteries dilate, the same volume of blood is contained in a larger volume of vessel and thus the pressure of the blood falls. This drop in blood pressure is made worse if a woman lies flat on her back to deliver; in this position, the uterus rests on the large vein in the back of the abdomen (inferior vena cava), interfering with the return of blood to the heart and the pumping of blood from the heart. For this reason, the delivery table is tilted to the side. The expected fall in blood pressure is also minimized by boosting blood volume with fluids given intravenously before beginning the procedure. If a drop in blood pressure occurs despite these measures, medication is given to contract the dilated muscles in the arteries. Because of the risk of low blood pressure, spinal anesthesia is not used when a woman's blood volume is already compromised, for example, when blood loss has occurred or when preeclampsia is present.

An undesirable consequence of spinal anesthesia, much less common today than in the past, is headache. A spinal headache is caused by the leakage of spinal fluid through the puncture site into the space surrounding the spinal cord, the epidural space. The reduced volume of spinal fluid leads to shifting of the brain, with added stress on its pain sensitive attachments to the inside of the skull. Spinal headache is minimized by using a very thin needle, which produces a very small hole and a very slow and small leak. When it occurs, bed rest and analgesics are helpful. If these measures fail, injection of a small amount of the woman's blood into the epidural space near the puncture site has proved effective in sealing it. The effects of spinal anesthesia on bladder function may necessitate the use of a catheter during the first twenty-four hours following delivery.

A dreaded but rare complication, which results from the inadvertent introduction of an excessive dose of anesthetic into the spinal canal, is blockade of all nerves below the neck, thereby producing paralysis of respiration and a precipitous fall in blood pressure. In this emergency, hypotension (low blood pressure) is treated by using the measures previously discussed and by elevating the legs to maximize the volume of blood returning to the heart. Respiration is assisted by measures ranging from bag breathing by the anesthesiologist to intubation of the airway and mechanical ventilation.

Spinal anesthesia is avoided in women who have had allergic reactions to local anesthetics, whose skin at the injection site is infected, or who have chronic low back pain, which could be aggravated by the spinal needle. While spinal anesthesia is used primarily in emergency situations, the same technique using a narcotic drug as well as an anesthetic along with an epidural anesthetic is gaining in popularity and will be discussed below.

Epidural Anesthesia: Epidural anesthesia eliminates pain in both labor and delivery. It is by far the most popular approach to medical pain relief, whether used alone or in combination with spinal anesthesia. In epidural anesthesia the nerve roots are numbed after their exit from the spinal fluid into the space in the spinal canal just below the lower pole of the meninges (which surround and contain the spinal fluid). This compartment is called the epidural space. Within it are the nerve roots that serve the parts of a woman's body involved in labor and delivery, including the uterus, cervix, vagina and perineum. In the epidural space the sensory nerves that transmit external stimuli are less well insulated and more susceptible to blockade than are the nerves that stimulate muscle contraction. Thus, when nerve roots in the epidural space are blocked, pain and other sensations are eliminated. Some voluntary movement is preserved, but not enough to permit walking. An epidural is given only after labor is well established, during the active phase of the first stage. If given too early it can dampen or even stop uterine contractions. Even when given in the active phase, an epidural may temporarily slow labor. Epidurals definitely lengthen the second stage of labor because of reduced uterine forces pushing the fetus into the birth canal. Recent studies suggest that the fatigue of the laboring woman after receiving an epidural can be reduced if she waits for an hour before beginning to push in the second stage (unless the urge is there) without affecting the duration of labor or the well-being of the baby. This delay in pushing is sometimes referred to as laboring down or passive second stage.

The procedure for performing an epidural is similar to that used for a spinal. Once the needle enters the epidural space, a thin plastic catheter is passed into it. Often the woman will experience a twinge of pain in her back or leg as the catheter touches a nerve root. When the needle is withdrawn, the catheter is left in place and the anesthetic solution is injected into the space. The catheter external to the skin is taped to the back. A major advantage of epidural block, in contrast to spinal block, which is a one-shot deal, is that additional anesthetic solution can be given as needed. The anesthetic solution can be given as a continuous infusion or, more often in practice, as a top-off every ninety or so minutes. The advantage of the intermittent-dosing approach is that less total drug is used and fewer drug-related effects occur. Studies have shown that women can successfully self-administer the anesthetic solution as they need it by controlling the infusion pump.

Epidural anesthesia is not always completely effective even when administered by an experienced physician. In one study, 85 percent of women were free of pain, 12 percent had partial relief and 3 percent experienced no relief at all. An epidural given to relieve labor pain, with the catheter pointing upward (toward the head) to direct the solution to the nerves supplying the uterus, may not effectively numb the perineum during the second stage. As with spinals, epidurals can also cause a decrease in blood pressure, which responds to the same measures used for hypotension in spinals.

A serious complication can result if the anesthetic solution is inadvertently injected through a vein into the woman's bloodstream. This risk is markedly reduced by gently pulling back the plunger of the syringe before injecting solution to check for blood and by using a small test dose to see if the woman experiences any systemic reactions.

A disadvantage of epidurals is that both mothers and babies are more likely to develop a fever. For the baby, fever raises the question of infection, which must then be evaluated with blood, urine and sometimes spinal-fluid tests. There is no evidence that use of epidurals results in greater use of forceps or vacuum extraction. Whether the rate of cesarean sections is increased cannot be answered with the data available at this time.

Dual Spinal-Epidural Anesthesia: A more recent and increasingly popular use of spinal and epidural anesthesia is to use them in combination in what is called a *dual spinal-epidural* or *walking epidural*. In this approach a narcotic drug as well as an anesthetic is used for the spinal and a lower dose of anesthetic, sometimes also with a narcotic, is used for the epidural. The great advantage is that there is no loss of muscle control and the woman can be up and about and push effectively. It is a major advance in anesthesia for labor. Undesirable side effects of the narcotic are itching, retention of urine in the bladder and nausea and vomiting. These effects can be reversed with the narcotic antagonist *naloxone.*

General Anesthesia

Although less commonly used in obstetrics today than blocking agents, general anesthesia with inhaled gas, the oldest of the anesthetic methods used in childbirth, still occupies an important place in labor and delivery. General anesthesia with chloroform was introduced by the Scottish physician Sir James Simpson in 1847 and was popularized by Queen Victoria during the birth of her eighth child in 1853. The great advantage of general anesthesia is ease of administration and rapid onset of action. Thus, in emergencies in which time is critical, usually when an urgent C-section is needed, it is the anesthesia of choice. Nitrous oxide, self-administered by the woman during a contraction, is a general anesthetic used in labor.

The disadvantage of general anesthesia used for birth, even with the improved gases available today (chloroform is no longer used), is that they pass directly to the fetus, anesthetizing it as well. This is usually not a problem during cesarean birth unless the fetus is already having problems with the oxygenation of its blood. Use of nitrous oxide during labor has no demonstrable effect on the fetus or baby. Of course, with general anesthesia for delivery the woman is not awake during birth. A more serious concern with general anesthesia for delivery is that the woman may vomit and aspirate stomach contents into her lungs, producing a chemical pneumonia. This problem is preventable with proper anesthetic technique.

Learning about Anesthesia

In some hospitals anesthesiologists meet with pregnant women and their partners to answer their questions about anesthesia and the role of the anesthesiologist. Some obstetricians routinely refer patients for these consultations, which may be regarded as part of childbirth education as they are equally informative to those who have definitely decided they want anesthesia and those who would use it only if needed. The topic of anesthesia is also covered in most childbirth-education classes. Couples should inform themselves about anesthesia prior to, rather than during, labor, when decisionmaking is more pressured.

Position during Labor and Delivery

In a traditional hospital birth, a woman lies on her back with her legs in stirrups. This supine, or *lithotomy*, position is often associated with episiotomy and the use of anesthesia and forceps. It was designed primarily to allow the physician easier access to the birth canal and perineum for the manipulations that often characterize this type of delivery. In fact, the supine position makes these interventions more likely, and it has come under criticism for several reasons.

First, when a woman lies flat on her back, the uterus rests on the large vein that runs adjacent to the spine. Compression of this vein results in a diminished return of blood to the heart and outflow from the heart to various organs, including the uterus and placenta. Thus, the fetus's access to oxygen is reduced and the margin of safety during contractions, when oxygen access is normally reduced, is narrowed. Fetal distress may result, particularly for fetuses already compromised. Moreover, the uterus, deprived of its normal circulation, is less able to contract effectively, potentially interfering with labor. Another problem is that bearing down during the second stage is more difficult for the woman and less effective when the woman is lying on her back than when she is vertical. Finally, Michel Odent, obstetrician at the famous birthing center at Pithiviers in France, claims that tearing of the perineum is reduced to a very low level when the woman gives birth in the upright position and episiotomies are rarely needed.

The position for birth in preindustrial societies is almost always either standing (by holding or being held up) or squatting, in both cases taking full advantage of the force of gravity to push the baby out. X rays of the pelvis show that the outlet of the birth canal is increased by as much as 28 percent (almost a third) when a woman squats! An increase of this magnitude can make the difference between a vaginal and an operative delivery.

The upright position (standing, sitting, or squatting), is also an excellent one in which to labor, especially if it relieves pain. There has also been an impression among some birth attendants that walking can shorten labor. Research findings on this question have been conflicting. A small controlled study from the University of Southern California showed that walking was as effective as oxytocin in stimulating labor. A larger randomized control study done by Steven Bloom and colleagues at the University of Texas in Dallas, reported in 1998, showed no effect of walking on the duration of labor.

The upright position also appears to be as advantageous in delivering the placenta as it is in delivering the baby. Although there have been no controlled studies, clinical observations suggest an advantage in expelling the placenta while squatting.

The results of a randomized control study of birth in the squatting position were reported in the July 8, 1989, issue of the Lancet. With squatting there were fewer forceps deliveries (9 percent versus 16 percent) and shorter second stages of labor (thirty-one versus forty-five minutes); there were fewer perineal tears, but more labial tears. In addition, 82 percent of the women who squatted in birth also maintained the upright position for most of the second stage. The women reported great satisfaction with being vertical during the latter part of labor and during delivery. Squatting also appears to offer advantages when the baby's head is posterior and when a small rim of cervix (anterior lip) remains as an obstacle to further progress.

Another position that is more effective than lying on the back is sitting up, at least at a forty-five-degree angle, drawing the legs up if desired to provide more effective pushing and to enlarge the dimensions of the birth canal. (The newer birthing chairs, returning to designs used for centuries and then abandoned, help women achieve this position). If the woman is seated in bed, she either brings her buttocks to the edge of the bed or elevates her buttocks with a firm object (such as an inverted bedpan covered with a soft pad) in order to provide room for the emerging baby.

Another effective position for labor and delivery, but one that has not yet been subjected to critical evaluation, is lying on the side with the upper leg held up by an assistant and the back and buttocks near the edge of the bed. The attendant stands behind the buttocks with one hand supporting the perineum and the other arched over the uplifted leg to control the baby's head. This position also helps the woman to see her baby emerging. A closely related position is kneeling on one knee with the other leg bent at the knee and the foot flat on the bed or mat.

Forceps and Vacuum Extractor

Forceps and the vacuum extractor are tools used to assist in vaginal births by pulling the baby through the birth canal. Forceps are metal instruments, which look like tongs, with blades at one end that fit around the baby's head and handles at the other that lock together. The vacuum extractor is a suction cup (usually plastic) attached to a hollow handle and air pump. The cup is applied to the baby's head during a contraction of the uterus, and a vacuum is created within the cup by the air pump to seal it to the head. The suction is released when the contraction is over.

In the United States, vacuum extraction has become the favored of these two techniques among most birth attendants. Both methods are used when progress through the birth canal has stopped or when birth must be accomplished quickly because the baby is in difficulty. One or the other technique is used in 10 to 15 percent of vaginal deliveries.

Several complications for the baby can result. A 1999 study from the University of California at Davis looked at all births in the state that occurred between 1993 and 1994 among women having their first baby. The study considered only babies who weighed between 2,500 and 4,000 grams at birth. Bleeding between the scalp and skull was increased from 2 percent for spontaneous vaginal births to 6 percent when forceps or a vacuum extractor was used. Five percent of babies with cephalohematoma also had thin (hairline) fractures of the underlying skull. In fewer than 1 in 800 vacuum-extractor- and 1 in 600 forceps-assisted births, bleeding of some type occurred within the skull (intracranial bleeding). In contrast, such bleeding was found in fewer than 1 in 900 babies born by cesarean section performed after labor had begun and in fewer than 1 in 2,500 babies born by unassisted vaginal delivery or cesarean section performed before the onset of labor. The highest rates of intracranial bleeding were found when cesarean section was performed after a failed attempt at assisted vaginal birth, 1 in 333 and when both forceps and a vacuum extractor were used, 1 in 277. Although we do not know the long-range significance of intracranial bleeding, it seems prudent to avoid it. What we can conclude from these statistics is that when the likelihood of a successful assisted vaginal delivery appears low (for which we need better predictors), it should probably not be attempted, nor should forceps or a vacuum extractor be used in sequence after one of them has failed.

Regarding long-term outcomes, a 1991 report from Israel of 52,282 infants born in Jerusalem between 1964 and 1972 is reassuring about the safety of both forceps and vacuum extraction. In this study, reported in the journal Lancet, there was no evidence of medical or mental impairment at age seventeen years among those who had been delivered by either of these methods. How to relate the two studies cited here is not clear, but certainly the data presented do not argue against the appropriate use of either forceps or a vacuum extractor.

A rare complication of vaginal birth assisted by forceps or a vacuum extractor is damage to the nerves that control the muscles of the arm, which can result in a permanent palsy. A complication from forceps is a temporary weakness of the face, usually in one side only, caused by pressure of the blade just below the ear on the nerve that controls the facial muscles. For the woman, forceps use in contrast with use of a vacuum extractor, according to a study reported in 1998 by Abdul H. Sultan and his colleagues in London, is more likely to increase the hidden tears and functional injury to the rectal sphincter muscle (affecting bowel control) that commonly occur with vaginal birth.

Episiotomy

An episiotomy is an incision or surgical cut made with (sterile) scissors or a scalpel in the perineum, the area between the lower junction of the labia and the anus. The incision may be made in the midline (median) (the more common practice in the United States) or angled to the side (mediolateral). Its purpose is to widen the opening of the vagina to ease passage of the baby's head. An episiotomy typically is repaired (sewn up) following delivery of the placenta, using absorbable sutures that dissolve and so do not require later removal. Polyglycolate sutures (Dexon or Vicryl) have been shown to be associated with less pain. If a spinal or epidural anesthetic has not been administered, a local anesthetic is injected to ease the pain of an episiotomy and its repair.

The traditional medical view of episiotomy, which once informed its nearly routine use, was expressed in a past edition of the well-known textbook *Williams Obstetrics* as follows:

It substitutes a straight, neat surgical incision for the ragged laceration that otherwise frequently results. It is easier to repair and heals better than a tear. It spares the fetal head the necessity of serving as a battering ram against perineal obstruction. If prolonged, the pounding of the fetal head against the perineum may cause intracranial injury. Episiotomy shortens the second stage of labor.

This view has to be understood in the context of the labor and delivery practices of the times. During delivery, most women lay flat on their backs with their legs in stirrups. In this position it is difficult to push the baby out. Anesthesia further compromised women's capacity to bear down. Babies often needed assistance in navigating the birth canal and often had to be pulled out with forceps. At the very least, it seemed, the barrier to birth presented by the perineum had to be removed; hence the policy of routine episiotomy.

Episiotomy is alleged to prevent vaginal and pelvic relaxation following birth and to prevent urinary (stress) incontinence, but there is no evidence to support these claims. Episiotomy is valuable in removing a barrier to progress of labor when the perineum is the barrier, especially when the baby is in distress and must be delivered quickly.

The topic of episiotomy has aroused strong feelings. In the past especially, the policy of many obstetricians was *always* to do an episiotomy. At the opposite extreme, Sheila Kitzinger, a well-known English midwife and childbirth educator, once called the procedure "ritual genital mutilation", in which males (as most physicians at the time were men a rapidly changing situation) exert power over women's bodies and deny women the opportunity to experience birth as a sexual act.

Critics of routine episiotomy point to the pain during healing of the episiotomy and its negative effects on lovemaking, urination, and defecation. These discomforts are far worse, they believe, than the pain of a natural and more physiological tear in the perineum. Indeed, in several early noncontrolled studies women who had had episiotomies reported more postpartum pain and were slower to return to full activity, including sexual intercourse. The problem with such studies is that women who had the procedure and those who didn't may have been different to start with. For example, it could be that only women who were most likely to tear badly had an episiotomy and that these women would have been worse off without it.

In one study, conducted by Adrian Grant at Oxford, women were allocated at random to either a restricted conservative or a liberal use of the procedure; in other respects the two groups had similar characteristics and the women were treated similarly in labor. The episiotomy rates were 10 percent for the restricted group and 51 percent for the liberal group. Interestingly, there were no differences between the groups with respect to the amount of pain reported after birth, the time it took for the perineum to become pain free or problems controlling urination. The only other difference in outcomes was that women in the restricted group were more likely to have resumed sexual intercourse within a month after delivery (presumably because it was less uncomfortable for them). Despite the differences in episiotomy rates, there was little difference in the frequency with which suturing of the perineum was required. The women who did not receive an episiotomy were more likely to tear on their own, so that not having an episiotomy did not spare women from tearing and being sutured.

A randomized control study from Canada under the direction of Michael Klein, professor of Family Medicine at McGill University, persuasively showed that women who had episiotomies had worse outcomes in all respects than did those who did not have episiotomies: more pain, poorer perineal tone and a slower return to sexual functior.. Vaginal tears sustained during delivery healed better than did episiotomies. This study provided convincing evidence that there is no justification for routinely doing episiotomies. The only valid reasons for doing an episiotomy are distress in the fetus that necessitates a quick delivery or an inability of the woman to overcome the resistance of the perineum to delivery, which is an unusual circumstance. More recently, a report in 2000 from the Brigham and Women's Hospital in Boston compared women who had a midline episiotomy, women whose perineum spontaneously tore during delivery and women who had neither tearing nor episiotomy. In this study, the presence of flatus incontinence (inability to control the expulsion of intestinal gas) and stool incontinence was determined at three and six months after delivery. The women who had had episiotomies fared worse than did the women in the other two groups, whose outcomes were similar, except at six months, when there was not significant difference in fecal incontinence among the groups. The findings in all these studies should allow us to take a more relaxed view of perineal tearing during delivery. A number of measures taken during delivery appear to minimize perineal tearing. (Few of these have been subjected to controlled clinical studies). What follows is based on the experience of many practitioners:

1. As long as the woman and the fetus are doing well, birth should be gradual and unhurried, allowing the perineum to stretch slowly. Women should push only if pushing increases their comfort.
2. To prevent undue stretching, the woman can respond selectively to her urge to push, according to the status of her perineum. Attendants can give verbal feedback and show her the effects of her pushing with a mirror. If pushing causes excessive stretching, the woman can stop pushing and allow her uterus to do the work alone. A gentle push between contractions can then ease the baby's head out.
3. Maintenance of flexion of the baby's head (chin to chest) results in the smallest part of the head pushing through the vulva. Flexion is supported by downward pressure on the top (vertex) of the head by the attendant's hand during contractions.
4. Supporting the perineum by maintaining constant counterpressure with the hand applied to the perineum as it gradually stretches is thought to minimize tearing.
5. Position during delivery may also be important. There is accumulating evidence that the upright position standing or squatting minimizes tearing, another good argument for avoiding lying flat on the back during delivery.
6. Water birth may contribute to less tearing of the perineum and to decreasing the need for an episiotomy.
7. Preparation of the perineum through Kegel exercises, which have a toning effect on the muscles and fascia, is believed to

make these muscles more stretchable and less likely to tear. This notion is analogous to the idea of preventing muscle strain in joggers and other athletes by stretching the muscles before running or playing a sport.

A recent and important insight pertaining to episiotomies and vaginal births in general has been provided by Abdul H. Sultan and his colleagues in London. These researchers reported in 1997 that visible vaginal damage (tearing) to the anal sphincter, the set of muscles that controls the bowels, occurred in 3 percent of first deliveries and in no subsequent deliveries. Yet testing revealed that in 35 percent of first deliveries and 44 percent of subsequent deliveries women sustained measurable sphincter damage. According to this study, an episiotomy, as well as the use of forceps, added to hidden sphincter damage, above that caused by vaginal birth alone. Although problems (symptoms) from such injury may not show up until much later in life (along with problems with bladder control), findings such as these enliven the debate on the virtues of elective cesarean birth as well as the details of the process of vaginal delivery and the rehabilitation of the perineal muscles after birth.

Delivery of the Placenta

The third stage of labor begins with the birth of the baby and ends with the birth of the placenta. To facilitate separation and delivery of the placenta and minimize bleeding (*the* major concern following birth of the baby), an effective active-management approach has been developed. This approach includes giving oxytocin to contract the uterus, cutting the umbilical cord just after the birth of the baby, and gently pulling on the cord to help the placenta separate. (The effectiveness of cord traction has not been critically studied). Sometimes oxytocin is given on the appearance (birth) of the baby's shoulder. There is some evidence that the squatting position can aid in the expulsion of the placenta. After birth of the placenta, keeping the uterus contracted to prevent bleeding is important. If oxytocin and gently massaging the uterus are insufficient, ergot drugs can be given by injection and prostaglandins can be given intravenously. If even these measures fail, the uterus can be compressed between the hands of the attendant, one in the vagina pushing up and the other on the abdomen pulling down.

If the placenta is not delivered within a half hour of birth, or if there is brisk bleeding (more than the normal sixteen ounces of blood lost at delivery), it must be removed by hand to prevent significant blood loss. (In the past, postpartum hemorrhage was a major cause of the death of mothers.) Manual removal is uncomfortable to the mother and may require anesthesia. Once removed, the placenta is carefully inspected. In the unlikely event that a large piece is missing, the uterus must be explored manually under anesthesia to identify and permit removal of the fragment left behind. In one of several thousand births (the exact incidence is not known) the placenta or a section of it grows into the wall of the uterus, making separation either difficult or impossible, depending on the depth of penetration. This situation is called *placenta accreta*. Unless the placenta can be removed manually, the only treatment is removal of the uterus (hysterectomy).

Cesarean Birth

Cesarean section (C-section) is the surgical procedure used to deliver a baby through an abdominal and uterine incision. Legend has it that the operation is named after the first Roman emperor, Julius Caesar, who supposedly was born this way, although his mother did not survive. Documentation reveals that C-sections were attempted as early as the seventeenth century, but the procedure was not performed in large numbers until the end of the nineteenth century, and even then the maternal death rate was high. Consistent success, that is, with both baby and mother surviving, did not occur until well into the twentieth century. By the time of World War II, cesarean section had proved to offer dramatic benefits in dealing with such life-threatening problems as placenta previa, placental abruption, eclampsia and severe disproportion. During the 1960s and 1970s doctors increasingly recognized that cesarean section could benefit maternal and infant health even when a life was not immediately at stake. For example, babies delivered by cesarean section were found to do much better in terms of neurological problems (that is, there were fewer cases of cerebral palsy, learning problems and so on) than babies delivered by forceps while still high in the birth canal (so-called *midforceps* delivery). With certain kinds of breech presentations babies delivered by C-section were also found to do better than babies delivered vaginally.

Some doctors, midwives and childbirth educators believe that too many of these operations are being performed. Figures for C-sections hover at one-fifth of all births and close to 1 million deliveries per year, making C-sections the most frequently performed major surgical operations. A critical reappraisal of the reasons for cesarean delivery has already led to some leveling off in the percentage of deliveries by surgery. However, we are still far from achieving the goal, set by many involved professional organizations but not agreed to by all, of a U.S. national C-section rate of 15 percent by the year 2000.

The childbirth-education movement has responded to the increased frequency of cesarean sections with a constructive critique. For example, educators have urged that the term *cesarean birth*, rather than *cesarean section*, be used to emphasize that a birth, not merely an operation, is occurring. Fathers are welcomed in the operating room and early parent-infant interaction is encouraged despite the surrounding distractions. Discussion of cesarean birth is now included in prenatal classes, and organizations have been formed to meet the needs of women who have undergone or will undergo cesarean sections and of those who contemplate vaginal birth after a cesarean (VBAC).

A Typical Cesarean Birth

In most hospitals, cesarean section is performed under spinal, epidural or dual spinal-epidural anesthesia. General anesthesia is reserved for emergencies, when there is no time for starting spinals or epidurals, or when they have not worked. Before beginning the operation, the lower abdomen is shaved from just below the navel to the pubic bone. A catheter is inserted in the bladder and left in place until after the operation. The skin is vigorously scrubbed with surgical soap, and sterile drapes or an adherent plastic covering is placed over the abdomen to leave only the lower belly uncovered. The operating table is tilted about fifteen degrees to the side to roll the uterus off the great vein in the abdomen, the inferior vena cava, so that the return of blood to the woman's heart and the flow of blood to the placenta will not be compromised. The obstetricians and surgical nurse wear gowns, caps, masks and gloves; all other people present, including the husband or partner, labor coach or doula, wear surgical scrub suits, masks and caps in the operating room. Obstetricians reserve the right to ask nonprofessional participants to leave the room during an emergency. Policies on participation by husbands or partners may vary from one hospital to another. Women are advised to clarify this issue ahead of time.

A vertical screen is usually placed above the woman's upper chest so that she cannot see the surgeons. However, she is able to hear them and can carry on a conversation with those around her. Ideally, she should feel no pain, but if she does, she should report it so that measures to stop it can be taken. She may feel some tugging and pressure, especially during the delivery of the baby. Once the amniotic sac is opened, she will hear the noise of the suction machine drawing the amniotic fluid from the uterus into a collecting bottle. Following the removal of the amniotic fluid, the obstetrician reaches into the uterus to take hold of the baby's head, which is then worked through the incision. The assistant presses the top of the uterus to help push the head out. In a breech delivery the legs are delivered first.

After the head is born, the obstetrician clears the amniotic fluid from the baby's nose and mouth with a bulb syringe. If meconium (the baby's stools) has been passed into the amniotic fluid, this suctioning is more intense and is done with a plastic catheter. As the rest of the baby is delivered, the obstetrician will usually ask the anesthesiologist to inject a dose of oxytocin into the mother's intravenous infusion to cause the uterus to contract. It is also common practice to give the mother a single dose of intravenous antibiotics to prevent uterine infection; so that the antibiotics do not pass to the baby, they are given to the mother after the umbilical cord is clamped. The cord is cut, and the baby is handed to the nurse or pediatrician, who carries the newborn to a nearby warming table. The baby may be further suctioned and examined. When clearly doing well on his or her own, the baby is wrapped, capped and handed to the father or other designated person.

Meanwhile, the surgeons remove the placenta and sew up the incisions in the uterus and the abdominal wall. From beginning to end the surgery usually takes between thirty and forty-five minutes. Afterward, the mother is wheeled to the recovery room. The baby can usually remain with the parents, though there may be a brief period during which he or she is taken to the nursery for weighing, measuring and eye treatment. Breast-feeding can begin right away.

During the postoperative period medications are administered to the mother to deal with the pain of the incision. Blood pressure, pulse, urine flow, amount of bleeding and the tone of the uterus are checked regularly.

By the day after surgery, many women can drink fluids and the intravenous infusion can be slowed and pulled out after forty-eight hours. The bladder catheter is removed after twelve hours. On the second and third days, gas pains from ineffective bowel action are common and a rectal suppository or enema can be helpful. Women can walk with assistance on the day after surgery. Early walking promotes quick recovery and prevents the formation of blood clots (thrombi) in the veins of the legs. By the fourth day skin sutures or clips can be removed. On the fifth, or even the fourth day, mother and baby can go home.

Risks of Cesarean Section

Even though the C-section has become a remarkably safe operation and death of the mother exceedingly rare, it is, nonetheless, major surgery and has risks. These risks include phlebitis, uterine infection, urinary tract infection, and the complications of anesthesia. A C-section carries all the economic costs of major surgery and also causes a delay of at least one week before a woman can return to her normal activities.

Improvements in the operation continue to be made. Some of the now-standard techniques mentioned are of recent origin, including tilting of the operating table to the side; use of intravenous antibiotics at the end of the surgery; early walking to prevent phlebitis; and the favored use of epidural anesthesia, alone or in combination with spinal anesthesia.

Necessasty of Cesareans

The cesarean birthrate in the United States increased from 5.5 percent of all births in 1970 to 15.2 percent in 1980. The rate was up to 24.7 percent in 1988, dropped to 23.5 percent in 1990 and dropped to 21 percent in 1998. The rates vary considerably from one hospital to another for reasons not well understood. Certain hospitals clearly have a higher rate in part because the women they serve are at higher risk for complications of labor and delivery. However, even when dealing with similar populations of women without risk factors for complications and using a similar, but not identical, approach to care in labòr and delivery, the rate can vary from 5 to 6 percent in the Royal Maternity Hospital in Dublin to 19 percent in a U.S. teaching hospital.

A 1980 National Institutes of Health (NIH) report that looked at ways to reduce the rate of cesarean sections concluded that the diagnostic categories that had the largest effect on the increase in the rate between 1970 and 1978 were repeat cesarean, breech presentation, dystocia and fetal distress. A category not considered at that time, still small in numbers but of growing interest, is *elective cesarean birth*.

Repeat cesarean section has been identified as the category most amenable to correction. One obvious way to reduce this category is to reduce the others; without an initial section there can be no repeat. Until twenty years ago, once one section had been done the die was cast for all births that followed. Doctors applied the dictum (first pronounced in 1916), "Once a section, always a section", because they feared that the scarred uterus would rupture during a subsequent labor. This risk is real with the classical vertical (up-and-down) uterine incision, which involves the body, or middle portion, of the uterus rather than its lower segment. The chances of tearing the scar are far less, however, with the transverse (side-to-side), lower-uterine incision now in wide use. This incision cuts through the part of the uterus that is less muscular and contains fewer blood vessels. Thus, in a subsequent labor, if a tear should occur, bleeding, which can threaten the lives of both the woman and the fetus, is less likely. Although obstetricians now make every effort to use only this transverse, lower-uterine incision, it is not always possible to do so.

The current recommendation is to forgo subsequent vaginal birth if a previous vertical incision was made into the body of the uterus or into the lower uterine segment (the risk of rupture is 1 to 3 percent). When there is a vertical, lower-uterine-segment scar, there is a good chance that the incision actually extended into the upper uterine segment, with increased risk for tearing during subsequent labors. If there is a J shaped incision (as opposed to a curved-line incision) as a result of tearing or deliberate cutting while making the transverse lower-segment incision, repeat cesarean section is also recommended.

Since the 1980s, the "once a section, always a section" rule has been challenged and overturned. Now well over half of women (between 60 and 80 percent) who have had C-sections are successful in delivering vaginally. But just how safe is labor for women who meet the accepted criteria of a previous transverse uterine incision and a fetus weighing less than 4,500 grams (9 pounds, 14 ounces) as determined by ultrasound? Performing research to address this question has been difficult. In the most recent of several well-conducted studies done in the 1990s, Michael McMahon and his associates at the University of North Carolina compared the outcomes in 3,249 women who elected labor with 2,889 who chose a repeat C-section. There were no maternal deaths in either group and no overall difference in complications (morbidity) in the two groups. However, major complications (such as the need for a hysterectomy; rupture of the uterus; or injury from the surgery), although uncommon in both groups, were *twice as common* (1 percent) for the women attempting labor and vaginal birth who eventually required C-sections. (When uterine rupture occurs, the risk of serious complications for mothers and babies is less than 1 percent in hospitals that are equipped to deal with such emergencies). Another finding of the North Carolina study was that women who were more likely to succeed in delivering vaginally were under age thirty-five, had babies weighing less than 8.8 pounds and gave birth in a major medical center.

Just as formerly doctors almost automatically recommended repeat C-sections, now they may tend automatically to promote VBAC rather than leave the choice to the woman and her partner after informing them of the advantages and risks of both approaches. The sometimes subtle and often not so subtle temptation to push VBACs is increased by managed-care arrangements for health care, because vaginal deliveries are considerably less expensive. Sometimes lost in the debate over whether to encourage VBACs is a more focused consideration of how to *prevent the initial C-section*, the event that creates the need to consider VBACs at all.

In looking at the case of breech presentations, most of which are delivered by C-section, the NIH report recommended vaginal delivery as a safe choice for full-term breech babies under the following circumstances:

- The expected weight of the baby is less than eight pounds.
- The woman has a normal pelvis.
- The baby is in a frank breech, that is, with legs extended and head flexed.
- The doctor and his or her assistants are experienced in vaginal breech delivery.

As a result of this recommendation, some doctors have been more willing to consider vaginal breech births, but for reasons discussed elsewhere, the majority of physicians still favor delivery by cesarean section. *Dystocia,* or failure to progress in labor, was also identified by the NIH report as an explanation for much of the increase in the rate of cesarean births in the United States. It seems possible to reduce the number of cesarean sections done for this reason. For example, in 1988, 7.6 percent of all births in the United States were cesarean births because of dystocia, whereas at the National Maternity Hospital in Dublin at about the same time, only 0.7 percent of all births required cesarean sections for this reason. The major distinguishing features of the approach in Dublin were the prompt use of oxytocin if labor failed to progress at a defined rate and one-on-one attendance in labor by a midwife. Aspects of the Dublin approach are now being used in the United States.

In considering *fetal distress* as a reason for cesarean birth, the NIH report recommended further studies to improve the accuracy of the diagnosis of fetal distress, the development of new techniques for making the diagnosis, and improved nonsurgical ways of dealing with this problem. In particular, more widespread use of fetal blood testing was recommended.

Elective cesarean birth was not considered by the NIH report because it has emerged only recently, and rather unexpectedly, as a consideration. The reasons women give for choosing a C-section over a vaginal delivery include simply not wanting to go through the rigors of labor, given an increasingly safe alternative; not wanting to have their vaginas sore and stretched; and not wanting to deal with what for them and their partners may be less than optimal sexual functioning. Many older women who have problems controlling their bladders and bowels have had repeated vaginal births. Now there is evidence from research studies that in measurable ways, vaginal birth, particularly when tearing or an episiotomy has occurred or forceps have been used, is indeed likely to damage the muscles that control the rectal sphincter, both in the short and in the long run. What is not yet known is how these findings relate to such factors as how labor was conducted—for example, using the active or the unhurried approach the size of the baby, and the use of prenatal and postpartum perineal exercise. Clearly, more attention must be paid to these quality-of-life issues as they relate to pregnancy, childbirth and women's overall health.

Care of the Patients

The omen now bring their babies home from the hospital or birthing center soon after delivery, and as the number of women having their babies at home remains steady, parents need to depend more on themselves and less on professionals for dealing with common postpartum concerns.

Caring for the Body

Immediately after giving birth the mother should urinate frequently. An empty bladder will help keep the uterus contracted. To relieve stinging, a woman can dilute her urine by using a squeeze bottle to spray warm water over the perineum during urination or she can urinate while in the shower with water running over her body. In contrast to stinging localized to the labia, a urinary tract infection is signified by burning on urination in which the discomfort is inside the bladder rather than on the sore perineum and possibly by fever and flank pain.

The woman may not have a bowel movement for the first several days after giving birth. There is no need to strain, for it is not necessary to defecate immediately and straining may be harmful. Prune juice, increased fiber and increased fluid intake can soften or stimulate stools. Hemorrhoids, which may have developed during pregnancy, usually improve on their own after delivery.

The uterus should be checked every fifteen to thirty minutes for the first few hours and hourly for the rest of the day after delivery. If it is not hard, like a softball (or coconut), it needs to be gently massaged until it firms up. If massaging does not work, the midwife or doctor should be informed. Nursing (through the release of oxytocin) also helps, as it results in uterine contractions, sometimes called afterpains. Through human evolution the feeding of the infant has become linked to survival by maintaining contraction of the uterus and thus preventing postpartum bleeding. The uterus should be monitored until it is too low in the abdomen to feel, about the tenth day after delivery. The vaginal flow *(lochia)* should not be greater than a heavy menstrual period. It should not be green or have a foul smell. By the tenth day the flow has usually become a light pink to brown discharge. Sanitary pads, rather than tampons, should be used for the first two weeks, since tampons may introduce germs into the vagina and the uterus.

The woman may shower when she feels steady on her feet. Tub baths have traditionally been discouraged for two weeks, in the interest of preventing infection from bacteria washed into the uterus. The validity of this precept has not been critically studied. Perineal pain may respond to hot sitz baths (one and one-half inches of water) several times a day. A strong brew of the herb comfrey (available in health-food stores) added to the water is alleged by many midwives to promote healing, but this has not been critically studied.

Ice applied to the perineum during the first twenty-four hours will help reduce labial swelling. If the woman is at home, crushed ice can be packed in a rubber glove tied at the wrist and wrapped in sterile gauze. A sterile cotton ball soaked in refrigerated witch hazel can be placed under a perineal pad over sore regions rectum, perineum and labia. Local anesthetics creams, sprays, or lotions have been proved to provide pain relief. Foam-rubber rings for sitting are popular. Acetaminophen (Tylenol) and ibuprofen (Motrin, Advil) are safe and effective analgesics.

Caring for the Emotions

Every experience is unique, all new parents pass through several developmental stages. In the first stage, which may be called *taking-in,* mothers think and talk about the delivery a great deal and in considerable detail. As they take stock, they work on resolving any mixed feelings. In this stage a mother can feel focused on herself and inwardly directed and may even welcome being mothered herself.

In the second stage, *taking hold,* a mother becomes energized to take charge of herself and her new baby. She feels less dependent on her family and wants to move quickly into asserting her new role.

Pitfalls of this stage of rising expectations and mobilized energy are fatigue and anxiety about one's competence as a mother.

Last, there is a *letting-go*, or settling-in, stage, in which the transition represented by the birth experience is resolved and put away, the baby's separateness is realized and enjoyed, and the parental role is fully incorporated into the parent's identity.

Women often report feelings of grieving after a birth. They discover that the sense of loss they experience is the loss of being pregnant. The unique feeling of fullness within, the self-conscious pride, and the attention of others can all be sorely missed once the baby arrives and steals the show. Mothers sometimes feel like a cross between an anonymous cow that dutifully supplies milk and an underappreciated maid whose job is to clean up messes, while the baby is the focus of every one's loving attention. To soften this letdown, families can provide a little extra loving and mothering of the mother for a month or so. The result will be a mother who has plenty of love to give because she is receiving much love and who is strong and more confident because she feels valued and special. During this time, when a father is called on to provide a lot of extra attention and do extra work, he, too, deserves extra love.

Mothers often find it hard to imagine a life separate from mothering. One postpartum mother described a feeling of "fluffiness in the head". It is as if they have forgotten how to do anything except care for the baby. Especially troublesome is the inability to find or remember a word or carry on a coherent conversation. This state of mind is probably related to a combination of factors, including hormonal effects, lack of sleep, and intense emotional involvement with the baby. Among the many reactions it can elicit from others in the family are amusement and annoyance. The "fluffiness" soon passes.

The very common swings (lability) in mood, from elation (euphoria) to irritability (dysphoria) that new mothers experience are usually referred to as *postpartum blues* or *maternity blues*. These mood swings are thought to result from a rapid decline in the pregnancy hormones, which have direct and indirect effects on the central nervous system. There is no specific treatment for these temporary mood changes, which must be distinguished from depression.

Sexuality

Genital sex usually is temporarily suspended late in pregnancy and early after the birth. As couples well know, however, genital sex is only one expression of intimacy. This is the time for other forms of intimacy talking, cuddling, holding, caressing, grooming, massage, mutual masturbation and showering together. Having jointly created a child will forever alter their feelings about each other.

Whether prevention of infection of the uterus should be a concern with intercourse in the weeks after birth isn't clear. Although the American College of Obstetricians and Gynecologists recommends waiting for four weeks, there is no evidence to support this precaution. Simply doing what feels comfortable (what most couples do anyway) appears not to have any dire consequences.

If on the resumption of intercourse the vagina is dry or has tender spots, a water-soluble lubricant, such as K-Y jelly, will help relieve irritation. Adjustments in position will reduce pressure on sore areas. Milk ejection may occur spontaneously with arousal and seem bizarre or humorous to both partners. Although breast-feeding suppresses a mother's ovulation, it is *not* a foolproof form of contraception. Since ovulation occurs *before* the return of menstrual periods, menstruation is not a reliable guide to resumed fertility. The combination of a condom and foam or jelly is a very effective contraceptive that can be used indefinitely or until other arrangements for birth control are made.

Use of oral contraceptives containing both estrogen and progesterone (combined pills) is generally not recommended during the first several months of nursing. Such contraceptives have been shown to decrease both the volume and the protein content of breast milk in some women. If combined pills are used, nursing should first be well established. In contrast, progestin-only pills (minipills) do not substantially affect breast milk. The minipill and nursing, with its own contraceptive effect, make a very effective *combination* in preventing pregnancy. Minipills can be started right after the baby's birth.

Family Crises

Interactions of physical and psychological factors can precipitate genuine family crises in the days and weeks following a baby's birth. Examples of tough situations are a sluggish baby who won't nurse, whose mother has sore nipples and painfully engorged breasts and is exhausted; an inconsolable baby, with well-meaning, but intrusive and undermining, grandparents who are interacting with parents who feel frazzled and incompetent; and the superwoman who has older children and, thinking she can do it all, refuses to stop waiting on everyone else long enough to care for herself. In such circumstances, the mother is a prime candidate for exhaustion and for having problems with the baby.

Situations such as these, which in the extreme can be nightmarish, call for active involvement by the doctor, midwife, friends and others in the family's support network. Phone contact with the doctor or midwife is helpful, for he or she can assess the family's needs, provide support and offer concrete suggestions. An exhausted mother should be encouraged to get into bed and take her baby with her. She needs to focus on herself and the baby and put everything else on hold. Relatives, friends and members of a couple's prenatal class (the extended family) can be mobilized to bring cooked food, do laundry and shopping and care for other children while the parents focus on themselves and the baby.

For women whose high-level commitment to neatness is a barrier to relaxation, the postpartum period offers an opportunity to learn that people can take priority over things. A family besieged by well-wishers should consider limited, brief visiting hours and turning off the phone during periods of rest. A voice-mail announcement or personal web site can be used to keep friends and relatives posted. Public-health and Visiting Nurse Association nurses, supervised home-health aides and commercial homemakers can also provide support. Women can ask the physician or the hospital or birthing center about such resources.

Other support groups for the postpartum period include independent counseling services and childbirth-preparation organizations, such as the local affiliate of ICEA and La Leche League. Some doulas specialize in postpartum care. Chat lines on the Internet are also playing an increasingly important role.

6

Organ Harvesting Techniques

Introduction

The number of organ donors has, from 1989 to 1991, stayed at approximately 4,000 in the United States. Another study delineates the needs of Americans as follows: 15,000 could benefit from a heart transplant, 22,500 from a kidney transplant and 5,000 each from a liver or pancreas transplant. Interestingly, the most ready market source for harvesting, and thus meeting these needs in the United States, is to be seen in the automobile accident pool that yields approximately 60,000 cadavers each year with some 12,000 to 27,000 of them maintained sufficiently long enough after the accidents to die in hospitals. At a minimum, these statistics suggest something along the lines of 12,000 hearts and livers and 24,000 kidneys are a potential market source for transplantation.

Meeting Market Demands

Whatever statistical profile is used, it can be seen easily that the demand for transplant organs clearly exceeds the supply. The market base for obtaining organs becomes even more fragile and volatile when it is realized that the shortage of cadaveric organs is tied to the very suitability of the cadavers themselves. Thus, to be a suitable cadaveric candidate, the cadaver must have died as a result of either a cerebral hemorrhage or injury to the head and be maintained with respirator and ventilator assistance before its relatively healthy major organs are harvested. The central task, then, is to design a scheme or develop a market mechanism that promotes greater opportunities for obtaining transplantable organs yet at the same time is not antithetical to present ethical values.

Surely, as a society, Americans need to enter into a full dialogue regarding all approaches to saving lives and not dismiss any viable suggestion before it is debated fully (and even tested). This chapter initiates such a dialogue and demonstrates that as things stand at present altruistically induced organ donations at death are not as comprehensive a mechanism for providing a supply of transplantable organs as the demands of modern society require. New market strategies will have to be examined and eventually utilized if a premium is to continue to be placed on restoring health and sustaining life. At this state in the development of an agenda for a national debate, the payment of a standard death benefit as an inducement for organ donations appears to be the most attractive market mechanism to develop.

American Responses and Fears

A 1985 Gallup Poll found 75 percent of all Americans approved of organ donation and transplantation, yet only 27 percent expressed a willingness to donate their own organs in the event of their death, and of that percentage only 17 percent indicated they had signed organ donor cards to effect this commitment. A more recent Gallup Poll in 1993 determined that while 85 percent of Americans now support organ donation, 42 percent acknowledge they have decided to donate their own organs. These figures take on a greater relevance as market indicators of future organ sources when it is realized that approximately 80 percent of all Americans die without a will and thereby lose their opportunity to become donors.

For those queried regarding their reluctance to become organ donors, three common reasons are given for this position: a central unwillingness to consider personal mortality, aesthetic fears or religious beliefs forbidding dismemberment, and an abiding fear that death will be hastened if previous consent to organ donation is given. Meeting, and thereby seeking to resolve, these fears will take time and years of education. Even then, it will be extremely difficult to allay the fears that form the basis of these reasons for inaction.

Common Law Approach

The common law, as interpreted in 1765 by Blackstone *COMMENTARIES*, was clear: no one could have property rights in a human corpse. Since the law of theft operated only to protect rights of property and ownership, a corpse was incapable of being stolen. Thus, body snatchers worked regularly to obtain cadavers for anatomists for subsequent use in medical schools. Interestingly, however, property rights could be held in coffins or shrouds and their theft was an imprisonable act.

While stealing a corpse was a mere indecency, not a felony, consecrated burial grounds were protected and disruption of them carried a penalty as a misdemeanor. This was used as a basis by the common law judges to develop eventually new criminal laws prohibiting the disinternment of corpses without authority. At first, these new criminal offenses applied to body snatchers instead of to their customers. Executors and close family members could assert a right of burial but could still not assert ownership of a corpse. Accordingly, in cases where cadavers were discovered being used in anatomy or surgical dissection classes, there was no clear way of forcing their surrender unless they could be first identified (which, depending on the extent of the dissection, could be difficult) and then made the subject of a legal claim by the family or the descendent's executor. The only right possessed by the family was to have the body retrieved for burial and nothing more.

In 1828, with parliamentary study being undertaken of this area, the courts seized the initiative and expanded the criminal law of body snatchers as applied to cemeteries to reach to the points of common delivery: the medical school anatomy classes. And, in 1832, Parliament passed the Anatomy Act which destroyed the trade of body snatchers altogether by essentially introducing a strict licensing procedure on anatomy schools as well as on instructors and students themselves who wished to perform anatomical examinations. Government inspection, fines and imprisonment were set in place for violations of the act.

Contemporary Legislative Initiatives and isappointments

With the promulgation of the Uniform Anatomical Gift Act (UAGA) in 1968 and its subsequent adoption in some form by the fifty states and the District of Columbia in 1973, a statutory right was conferred on all individuals allowing them, prior to death, to designate either their complete bodies or organs from them for donated transplants. When a descendant's wishes are not communicated prior to death, the act provides a right of disposition to the next of kin allowing him the right to decide whether to donate his relative's organs. The UAGA was silent on the subject of sales. Thus the common law position was largely controlling here and provided no one was acknowledged as having a definitive property interest or right in a human corpse. This meant no one was granted any form of authority to enter into a sale or to make a gift of a cadaver or any of its parts. It is important to note that this did not mean sales or gifts of this were illegal; rather, only contracts for sales or deeds of gifts were, at law, not enforceable.

National Organ Transplant Act

To redirect national thinking from a purely voluntary behavior basis *vis-a-vis* organ donation, the UAGA was built on a principle of encouraged voluntarism. To advance this principle, the whole process of consent was simplified. This was accomplished by the introduction of donor cards designed to allow individuals, carrying them as such, to indicate their consent to donate their organs upon death. Wishing, if possible, to enhance the voluntary principle of altruism implicit in the UAGA for transplantable organs, yet facing the realities of the failure of UAGA's "encouraged voluntarism" to produce enough donors, the U.S. Congress acted in 1984 by passing the National Organ Transplant Act (NOTA). In addition to underwriting financial support for the development and maintenance of local nonprofit organ procurement organizations and additionally the National Organ Procurement and Transplantation Network to assist in matching organ donors with those needing transplants; the act criminalizes the intestate acquisition, receipt or transfer of all transplant tissue (e.g., organs) with the exception of blood. Since the legislation is directed toward imposing a prohibition on sales affecting interstate commerce, some doubt has been raised about the validity of suppression of intrastate organ sales. Interestingly, NOTA has been strengthened specifically on this issue of intrastate sales by the enactment of specific statutes prohibiting either the purchase or the sale of human organs. Again, in a national effort to both educate the public to the communal values associated with organ transplantation and thereby encourage and hopefully, enhance opportunities for more organ harvesting, in 1986 a provision was added to the Omnibus Budget Reconciliation Act that was passed into law in 1987, mandating all Medicare-and-Medicaid- affiliated hospitals to establish "written protocols for the identification of potential organ donors". This means that requests be made for organs and tissues whenever a death occurs in a hospital setting. Options to donate organs are to be presented in a discreet and sensitive manner to all families of potential donors enrolled as Medicare or Medicaid patients.

Hospital compliance with required request provisions of the federal law or complementary state-enacted legislative schemes is very uneven, characterized in fact as poor to grudging in some states. It is said that a number of physicians view the law here as an intrusion into their professional autonomy. Still others are angered over perceived inequities in the distribution of the organs and tissues. These attitudes translate into a lukewarm enthusiasm, if that, as the physicians seek to comply with required request provisions by phrasing their requests for permission to harvest the organs of a family member "in a way that encourages a positive response and does not impose distress on the survivors".

With no set of rules designed to achieve this delicate balance, how can such a legal requirement as this be met? As one organ transplant coordinator observed, "The consent rate when someone asks who does not want to ask, or does not know how to ask, is zero". Thus, the reality of the situation is that unless negative incentives can be structured and then imposed on doctors or hospitals the net enforcement effect of required request laws will be viewed as little more than excessive hortatory language typical of so many congressional enactments.

Living Donors

Since World War II, in the United States live donors have been used as sources for organ and tissue transplantation running the gamut from blood and bone marrow to kidneys. Interestingly, while no adult can be forced without giving a mature, informed consent to donate any organ, a minor, mental incompetent or prisoner has traditionally not been accorded this option. The case law in the

United States, although lacking in any unified rationale, does evidence three bases for testing the validity of the application for a compulsory, nonconsensual donation.

Under one test, the court inquires whether the donation would be in the best interests of the donor, with no relevance being given to any measure of sympathy for the proposed recipient of the family. The second test is one of substituted judgment, where the court speculates how the minor (if mature or competent) would decide relative to the request to donate. But this act of speculation is not flippant or inconsequential; rather, the court seeks to make a decision utilizing the same motive and considerations as would move the incompetent himself. In this regard, then, the test of substituted judgment does not deviate from adherence to the ethical principle of respect for persons. Indeed, it has been suggested that this very principle recognizes that one's welfare, rightly understood, may well depend on an act that helps others. An absolutist approach to this principle of respect, however, would allow for no compromise of any nature. The third test utilizes a judicial review of whatever parental decision has been made here, with the court accepting in principle the importance of the parental position yet, without accepting any correlative duty to the donor, weighing the entire family dilemma, making an ultimate decision based on achieving a balance of family interests.

Ethical Concerns

Some argue ethically and morally that all intrafamilial donations should be prohibited simply because of the coercive forces operating within the family unit which, hypothetically, could justify the need for requiring an incompetent healthy sibling to make a forced organ donation to a competent, unhealthy brother or sister. If such a scenario were in fact to be written, no destructive harm to the particular family unit would occur. Indeed, just the opposite would happen, for the unit would be preserved and strengthened by such a donation. At a minimum, the factors that constitute a valid consent should be defined with as much precision as possible, recognizing as such that there is an enormous factual difference between a family member authorizing tissue removal from the body of a deceased relative and, on the other hand, from a living relative.

There are other ethical and social considerations raised regarding organ transplants from living donors. One simply finds such actions to be inherently immoral. This idea builds on the belief that the general ethical principle that life should always be preserved and that one should never seek his own destruction nor endanger in any way his own life except as an expression of love for another. Commerce in human body parts, it is maintained, also acts to restrict free will and individual autonomy. This, in turn, is buttressed by the view that in harming oneself by deliberately undergoing tissue removal, one may well indeed harm society by later becoming sick or enfeebled and thus a burden on it. Abstract moral principles and concerns of this nature must give way to the realities and the needs of contemporary society and not stand as roadblocks to the maintenance of actual life.

Utilitarian Reality

The counterutilitarian argument to these moral-ethical concerns states that any absolute prohibition on the use of organs from minors or incompetents is unjustified this in light of the fact that donations from such classes restore health and renew life to others and they do this without jeopardizing or ending the lives of the donors. Where the risks from the donation to the minor, incompetent or incarcerated prisoner are minimal or even if substantial—yet much less than the harm that would occur to an individual donee deprived of the benefits of sustained living organ transplantations should be undertaken.

Additional Schemes and Procedures

The prevailing system for organ donation is one of presumed non consent; in other words, one is presumed "unwilling" to be an organ donor at death unless her or his family gives permission. As noted, this scheme is failing to generate sufficient resources for transplantation; thus new approaches must be evaluated and then implemented.

Postmortem Examinations

One such approach was first proposed in 1968 and simply calls for compulsory postmortem examinations to determine the salvageability of cadaveric organs. As such, autopsies would be done routinely, not, as now, performed only when requested by the decedent's family or as a consequence of violent death under suspicious circumstances. The postmortem examinations and autopsies would be carried out in all cases as long as they did not interfere with homicide investigations, and the dying person or his next of kin would be allowed to object to such procedures and give contra instructions thereby opting out.

Right of First Refusal

A more contemporaneous suggestion has been to design and implement a system wherein persons who object to forced donations of this type could refuse to participate in a manner wholly consistent with individual patient and/or family sensitivities yet is both efficient and cost-effective and also meets the plethora of religious, ethical and legal requirements of informed consent. This suggestion, as engrafted on to the basic approach, is very sensitive and seeks to balance personal attitudes with the demands of a market society. Perhaps, in fact, the suggestion is too broad in its focus and seeks too wide an accommodation of personal interests. In any event, considerable more research must be undertaken to test its practical feasibility.

Escheatage

A more expanded version of the compulsory postmortem examination and autopsy retrieval approach is seen in escheatage. Although viewed as immoral by some authorities in the United States, as a system promoting recognition of the state's inherent right of ownership in the bodies of all its citizens unless otherwise specified by the citizen or its family, escheatage is being utilized by some fourteen European countries as a means of combatting the shortage of donor organs. In practice, the state simply delegates its ownership rights to licensed physicians who are thereby authorized to harvest and allocate salvageable organs to compatible donees. Here is an example of utilitarianism at its highest order. Yet the practice has been analogized to both slavery and totalitarianism!

The social policy against escheatage in America is found rather simply in a recognition of the sacredness of the body in life and death and not regarding it as a form of collective personal property disposable at will by the state upon death. But, as dead bodies are recognized more and more as valuable sources of life, through the harvesting of their organs for the living, perhaps with time a definition of their status as property will of necessity be forced on all sophisticated societies in the world community. Yet, even in countries where escheatage is in place, there is a natural reluctance among medical personnel to dismember their former patients' bodies whom they heretofore have worked to sustain life without an actual consent from next of kin; this, even though the state, through escheatage, has adopted a policy of presumed consent. This attitude then, together with the high level of emotionalism rather than rationalism being exhibited on this issue in the United States, means that it is doubtful whether the system would have a real potential for successful adoption.

Additional Mechanisms

Two other mechanisms are also available for consideration: the development of a futures market and a standard death benefit payment. The two central obstacles to implementation of these mechanisms are the need to (1) either repeal or amend present state and federal legislation that prohibits the sale or purchase of human organs and (2) overcome the pervasive reluctance among physicians to seize the initiative at the appropriate moment and make timely inquiries regarding consent to undertake harvesting. To resolve this second obstacle, it has been suggested that tort law be reshaped in such a way as to acknowledge a new standard of care with regards to a patient's body. Accordingly, should physicians fail to determine whether a patient has signified an organ sales contract, to preserve a cadaver for subsequent harvesting, or to inform the proper organ procurement agency of its status, liability would be imposed on the physicians to the estate of the deceased for the value of his organs.

Under a futures market, an individual would enter into a prospective contingent sale of his own organs. Proposed as such, a futures market would be only a small modification of the current system of contingent organ donation. Accordingly, individuals could be presented with an opportunity to execute a contract for the sale of their organs when they received a driver's license, bought insurance, answered a specific solicitation for organ donation through the mail or for that matter, stood on a street corner. The main difference with this proposal from the present system would be that the seller-donor would be promised remuneration, primarily at death. Functioning along the lines of the National Organ Procurement and Transplantation Network, pertinent donor information, including any limitations imposed on which organs were harvestable, would be fed into a computer and accessed by telephone.

Organ Sales Contracts

While payment at death for those organs harvested successfully would be the most efficient, two other payment systems would be available: under one, at the time of execution of the organ sales contract, a vendor could be paid a fee for all of his organs made available at death; or under another scheme, an executory contract could be entered into by both vendor and vendee, specifying that the vendor's estate or designated person would be paid a set fee for the cadaver whether or not upon examination at death the organs were determined harvestable. Of central concern regarding the second scheme payment at the time of contracting would be the necessity to develop a monitoring system whereby individual sellers were not able to enter into multiple contracts for the sale of their body parts. It has been suggested that the donor fee could be set at $5,000 for each major organ (e.g., liver, kidney, heart), with lower amounts for blood, skin bone marrow, corneas, and pituitary glands. If, for example, married male donors could be educated to the fact that the contract for the sale of their organs at death had the effect of being a form of supplemental life insurance policy with a payoff as high as $30,000, it is thought many such men would sign on as donors.

Death Benefit Payments

The final economic mechanism for obtaining organs for transplantation has been a standard death benefit payment of $1,000. This would be paid by presently operating organ procurement organizations to the families of the organ donors; ideally it would not be viewed as coercive in any way but rather only motivational. The amount and the source of the benefit would be controlled strictly by law thereby hopefully continuing the prohibition on bartering for organs. Under this proposal, any organ obtained, regardless of whether the donor family accepted the death benefit payment, would enter the national organ allocation system where all donee-recipients are registered and treated alike and where allocations are made, in turn, on matching medical need and period of time waiting.

Of course for this proposal to be adopted without any real or implied complications, as with the futures market itself, the illegality of such payments presently set forth in the NOTA and the Uniform Anatomical Gift Act of 1987 would have to be amended to allow administration of this one-time death benefit to a donor family. Since these present laws allow reasonable payments to be made to those who participate in the actual harvesting of the human organs for transplantation (e.g., surgeons, hospital staff involved in donor care) why, it may be asked, should not a similar reasonable payment be allowed to the family members of the donor, who, next to the donor himself are the most important participants in the process of harvesting and transplantation.

Clinical Options

Brain-dead patients, termed "heart-beating cadaver donors" (HBCDs), exhibit no brain function, but their hearts are kept beating in order to maintain perfusion of their vital organs. These donors are typically victims of automobile accidents or gunshot wounds to the head. Ironically, as the demand for transplantable organs increases, the pool of HBCDs are decreasing as a result of the implementation of strict automobile safety and gun control legislation. As the availability of organs from HBCDs dwindles, physicians have begun to look to other groups for the needed organs.

In an attempt to satisfy the growing demand for donor organs, or at least contain the growing crisis, the University of Pittsburgh Medical Center approved a protocol which allows patients who would not otherwise qualify as HBCDs because they have some brain function, to nevertheless donate their organs if they or their surrogates so choose. These patients, known as non-heart-beating cadaver donors (NHBCDs), are taken off life-support equipment at a predetermined time in an operating room. The donors are declared dead at the "irreversible cessation of cardiopulmonary function", and after two minutes their organs are then immediately harvested.

The protocol is applicable where the prospective donors cannot otherwise qualify as organ donors by the now traditional neurological criteria. These patients range from those who have full use of their mental faculties but suffer from various degenerative neurological or cardiopulmonary diseases that leave them respirator dependent to others who are terminally brain injured but nevertheless have sufficient neurological function to disqualify them as HBCD candidates. After the patients or their surrogates (who are entrusted to act in the best interest of the patient) make known their desire to forego further life-sustaining treatment, and their desire to donate their organs, the attending physician may discuss the possibility of withdrawing treatment within the controlled environment of an operating room. Two minutes after the heart stops beating, the patient is declared dead and the organs are harvested. NHBCD organs acquired in this manner are without perfusion for only a short period of time. Warm ischemia time is greatly reduced, and the available evidence indicates that organs thus obtained are as viable as those from HBCDs.

A fundamental question in determining whether the Pittsburgh protocol may be maintained as an ethical means of increasing the pool of organ donors is whether the patients or their surrogates knowingly submitted to the procedure. Was consent given as part of an informed decision-making process, or was it obtained through coercion or the withholding of necessary information? The protocol provides numerous measures to ensure patient autonomy. Foremost is that the physician cannot initiate discussion about the removal of lifesustaining equipment. He may only discuss the steps outlined in the protocol after the patient manifests a desire to be free of artificial life support in conjunction with desire to become an organ donor. Moreover, the protocol provides that decisions involving patient management are to be made prior to and separate from discussion of the procedure.

The protocol mandates full disclosure of all information regarding the decision to forego artificial life support. The physician must inform all involved parties regarding the procedures for removing life sustaining therapies and specifically the organ procurement process for NHBDs' acknowledge that organs will not be harvested until the patient is pronounced dead, and further advise the concerned parties that consent for the procedure itself may be withdrawn at any time.

Furthermore, the Pittsburgh protocol minimizes the perception that patients may have been coerced in their decision by providing that the physician responsible for the withdrawal of life support cannot be involved in the harvesting or transplant procedure. Similarly, physicians involved with the transplant procedure may not be involved in patient management prior to the death of the donor. Finally, in addition to the conceptual separation of patient management from the transplant procedure, the protocol goes so far as to recommend the physical separation of the treating physician from the transplant team and that the transplant surgeon not be present in the operating room until after the patient is declared dead. The personal interests of the physicians, as well as any institutional bias resulting from a perceived need to maintain a reputation or increase revenue, are thus effectively nullified.

Loyola Protocol

Under a protocol approved by the Loyola University Medical Center, as well as several other hospitals, physicians are allowed, at death, to infuse the cadaver with a preservative fluid without obtaining consent from the family of the dead person. The fluid preserves the vital organs for an adequate period of time long enough to allow discussion with the family and formal consent for organ donation. Interestingly, to date, no organs obtained from this protocol have been actually transplanted. Rather, the protocol was designed to test the feasibility of harvesting under these specific circumstances and the manner in which families would respond.

Criticism of both the Pittsburgh and Loyola protocols as "rationalized cannibalism" are nothing but appeals to unrestrained emotionalism and neglect totally the immense practical value of these rational and ethically balanced approaches to problem solving. These two protocols are not definitive solutions to a grave societal problem. Rather, they should be viewed as but prisms through which the complex issue of the procurement of organs for transplant may be analyzed further.

Ethical, Moral and Religious Concerns

As might be expected, various ethical, moral and religious concerns have been raised to these market mechanisms designed to increase the supply of harvestable organs for purposes of transplantation. Chief and foremost has been the financial vulnerability of the poor to being pressured into becoming "forced" donors, forced by their own circumstances and coerced by enticement of affluent buyers. Other concerns are whether a commercial market would enhance opportunities for suicides and murders and promote harvesting of the organs of anencephalic infants before actual death. Those religious views and traditions that regard the body as a gift of God and man's rights in it as merely those of a steward with no correlative rights of ownership would include a prohibition on the sale of body parts and would thus be in direct conflict with these market mechanisms.

These fears are understandable. However, while it is recognized that commercial profit making with nonrelated donors may have a tendency to promote an exploitation of those who are financially vulnerable, and may lead to progressive abuses and self-degradations, it is argued here that death payments benefits cannot be properly viewed as morally objectionable. This is simply because the verifiable benefits of sustained life that accrue to participating donees of noncommercial organ sales outweigh the moral fears or costs of using this mechanism as an inducement for stimulating the market for transplantable organs.

Utilitarian *vs.* Egalitarian Allocative Standards

The search for rational and principled standards of apportionment of scarce resources is and will remain a vexatious problem for decades to come. Informal "rules of thumb" cannot be countenanced. Of course, one way to avoid totally the problem of distribution is to avoid using the scarce medical resource altogether. But this would mean certain death to the countless thousands of transplant hopefuls.

Both in the formation of the transplantation waiting list and the actual distribution of donated organs, there is, however, a consensus that the primary criterion operable at both stages should be medical: that is, medical need and probability of success. Intense debate focuses rather on whether these medical criteria should be defined broadly or narrowly (i.e., the relevance of factors such as age, lifestyle and probability of success measured by a qualitative survival). Rehabilitation or salvageability, consistent with basic principles of triage, is also of relevance.

Since the law provides at present no uniformly agreed-upon principles that may be applied in order to regulate the allocation of scarce medical resources (e.g., cadaveric and human organs), current medical practice draws upon a structure for decision making evolved as such from a number of philosophical and ethical constructs. There are five utilitarian principles of application that are operative in the hierarchy of triage: the principles of medical success, immediate usefulness, conservation, parental role and general social value.

Decisional Operatives

Translated as such into decisional operatives, there emerges a recognition that priority of selection for use of a scarce medical resource should be accorded to those for whom treatment has the highest probability of medical success or would be most useful under the immediate circumstances, that is, to those candidates for use who require proportionally smaller amounts of particular resource or to those having the largest responsibilities to dependents or to those believed to have the greater actual or potential general social worth. The utilitarian goal is, simply stated, to achieve the highest possible amount of some good or resource. Thus, utilitarian principles are also commonly referred to as "good maximizing strategies".

Egalitarian alternatives, on the contrary, seek either a basic maintenance or a restoration of equality for persons in need of a particular scarce resource. There are five basic principles utilized here: (1) the principle of saving no one; thus priority is given to no one because, simply, none should be saved if not all can be saved; (2) the principle of medical neediness under which priority is accorded to those determined to be the medically neediest; (3) the principle of general neediness which allows priority to be given to the most helpless or generally neediest; (4) the principle of queuing, where priority is given to those individuals who arrive first; and

(5) the principles of random selection, where priority of selection is given to those selected by pure chance.

To the utilitarian, maximizing utility and hence what is diffusely referred to as the "general welfare" are both the primary ground and subject of all judgments. That which is required in order to maximize utility overall may thus infringe upon an individual's own entitlement of rights to particular goods. Accordingly, moral rights are either rejected generally or recognized as certainly not absolute.

Philosophy and religion may well provide us all with the necessary balance and direction for life and allow us to develop an ethic for daily living and a faith as to the future. The basic challenge of modern medicine should be, simply, to seek, promote, and maintain a level of real and, when the case may indicate, potential achievement for its user-patients which allows for full and purposeful living. Indeed, man himself should seek to pursue decision-making responsibilities and exercise autonomy in a rational manner and guided by a spirit of humanism. He should seek, further, to minimize human suffering and maximize the social good. Defining the extent and application of the social good will vary obviously with each case.

Summary

Thus far, it has been seen that voluntary donations of cadaveric organs have been an ineffective means of tackling the crisis in organ transplantation, and the same is true of the required request provisions of the federal legislation in 1987. Under current federal and state legislative directives, sale of human organs is prohibited. Compulsory postmortem examinations and retrievals bear a close resemblance to recognizing a new collective property right by the government, through escheatage, in all the dead bodies of its citizens. Strong antigovernment sentiments against intrusiveness into issues of privacy and autonomy, when combined with equally strong moral, religious and ethical attitudes about the sacredness of the body, will preclude these two mechanisms from ever being adopted successfully in America.

The development of a futures market, although fraught with two major obstacles, as observed, nonetheless bears further study and testing. Perhaps the most attractive of all the suggested mechanisms is the standard death benefit simply because of its noncommercial focus. But, as with the futures market option, present laws in the United States would surely have to be re-written or amended regarding present prohibitions against the sale of organs to make certain such one-time death benefit payments would be allowed. As well, harvesting physicians will have to be educated to the needs allowed. As well, harvesting physicians will have to be educated to the needs (or legal "rights") of their living patients to "prosper" from dead ones. Education on a massive scale in both public and private sectors is called for here.

Instead of trying to develop new and innovative approaches to organ retrieval, it has been suggested that more emphasis be placed on promoting voluntary, altruistic donations and ensuring the access to transplants is fair and the process for assisting transplant recipients to pay for their new organs is equitable. Indeed, the suggestion is even carried further urging public funding of transplants for the poor as well as establishing specific reimbursements policies for not only the costs of pretransplant evaluation, food, baby-sitters, travel, and housing for prospective patients but all economic assistance for those who are unable to work posttransplant.

These are noble sentiments and set a broadly defined philosophical goal to total equality of opportunity. Yet these concerns are but one facet of the most central problem here: developing a reliable (market) mechanism for assuring a ready supply of cadaveric organs for ready transplantation. Once this mechanism is set, remedial problems can be tackled. Some type of informed consensus must soon be reached in any event that develops a new mechanism for retrieving organs if, that is, the preservation of human life is to be advanced and not paralyzed by social taboos. Stated otherwise, "If human lives are to be saved, the agony of hard choices cannot be avoided". In the final analysis, then, a price economic, social, legal, ethical, moral, or religious *must* be set in determining the allocative process for organ retrieval and transplantation and market mechanisms would appear to be the most functional and objective tool for achieving this. Forced altruism, nurtured as such through the pursuit of lofty educational goals, does not have a practical history for dealing with the problems of the day. Perhaps the words from the book of Deuteronomy provide both a contemporary and useful ethic to utilize here: "I have set before you life and death, blessing and curse; therefore choose life, that you and your descendants may live."

7

Healthy Pregnancy and Its Delivery

Introduction

Your general medical history will include a review of any drugs (prescribed or over-the-counter) you regularly take; any chronic illnesses that might affect or be affected by the pregnancy, such as recurrent herpes infection, heart disease, phenylketonuria, AIDS or HIV infection, hepatitis, phlebitis or diabetes; and past surgical procedures, such as appendectomy, that could be important in evaluating symptoms that may arise, such as abdominal pain.

Your health practices with regard to diet, exposure to cats, exercise, dental care, alcohol, tobacco, drugs and seat-belt use will all have a bearing on the pregnancy and should be reviewed. Ideally, women taking drugs for chronic illnesses will have a preliminary discussion about the safety of these drugs before they become pregnant.

Your menstrual history, including menarche (age of first period), the interval between periods and the date of your last period or of ovulation, if known, is useful in dating the pregnancy.

Information on past pregnancies, including the gestational age of the baby, complications, the type of delivery (vaginal or C-section), the use of episiotomy and oxytocin, the weight and condition of the baby at birth and his or her current health, abortions, any difficulties becoming pregnant and your experiences with care providers during the pregnancy and birth, including relations with doctors, midwives, hospitals and birthing centers, are important data to share with your current care provider.

It will be useful for your doctor or midwife to know whether you and your partner planned to have a baby at this time and what impact the timing of this pregnancy has on your lives. Do you need professional assistance in resolving ambivalence about the pregnancy or in making the decision to continue or terminate it? Do the answers to these questions relate to the quality of your relationship in any way? Would you benefit from couples counselling or further discussion with your partner?

The family history takes on even greater significance in this era of rapidly improving prenatal diagnosis and treatment. Increased risk factors for a genetic disease may include age, racial and ethnic background, history of having produced a genetically abnormal child or a child with mental retardation (or such a history in either partner's family), recurrent abortions and birth of a child with a major malformation or chronic illness. Family history also affects the risks for the woman during pregnancy. For example, a history of phlebitis and thromboembolus in family members raises the question of a hereditary abnormality in a blood-clotting protein for which the woman should be checked. Identification of this disorder allows for evaluation for preventive treatment.

It's also helpful to construct a family tree for each partner. The bottom of the tree has the children of the partners' generation, including those of their siblings. The tree flows upward through the partners and their siblings, their parents, grandparents, and so forth. List under each person's name any chronic illnesses, including mental retardation and deaths with their causes if known.

Pregnancy Tests

A hormone indicating pregnancy can be detected in the blood of the pregnant woman as early as three days following fertilization and in the urine within one week. This hormone, known as human chorionic gonadotropin (HCG), is produced by the placenta (or, more precisely, by the trophoblast, the placenta's earlier form). Current tests for HCG done in medical laboratories or physicians' offices are over 98 percent accurate. Over-the-counter urine-pregnancy-test kits are somewhat less accurate, giving correct readings 85 to 95 percent of the time.

The level of HCG rises rapidly during early pregnancy, doubling every two days. The level peaks at ten weeks, then gradually declines to about one-half of peak levels, where it tends to remain. After an abortion or miscarriage the level falls off over the course of one week. Occasionally, if trophoblastic tissue has been left behind in the uterus, the hormone may be detectable for as long as several weeks. The level of HCG is markedly increased in hydatidiform mole.

Measurement of HCG can be helpful when a miscarriage or an ectopic pregnancy is suspected early on, before ultrasound can indicate the presence or viability of the embryo. The predicted rise in hormone level does not occur in pregnancies that are failing; the level may plateau or actually decline.

Physical Examination

The physical examination is an opportunity for the woman to learn a great deal about her body. If a woman chooses to include her partner, they both can learn more about her body. The exam Female reproductive organs: (a) ovaries, (b) fallopian tubes, (c) uterus, (d) cervix, (e) vagina is also an opportunity for a woman and her doctor or midwife to build up mutual trust. The examination is clearly more than a simple checkup. You can add to the value of this experience in the following ways:

1. Read something about the female body and reproductive organs beforehand. Ask the doctor if he or she can supply any charts or other informational materials.
2. Ask questions if you do not understand something. Good, open communication is essential throughout the childbirth experience. Speak up if you feel pain.
3. Relax and participate in the examination. For the doctor or other attendant to feel the uterus and ovaries properly, the abdominal muscles must be relaxed. The examiner's hands, one in the vagina and the other on the lower abdomen, move toward each other to feel the structures in between. If the abdominal muscles are tense, the examination is hindered. You are an active participant in the examination. To help relax the abdominal and vaginal muscles you might try

breathing in and out twice deeply, bearing down as though to push out a baby, then letting go of the buildup of muscle tension.

4. Ask for a mirror to see the cervix and other intravaginal structures. Many women have never seen a cervix and this is an opportunity to understand its structure.
5. Bring your husband partner or a friend who will be of support later. If you plan to have your partner or a friend present at the delivery, this is a chance to involve that person from the start. Make clear to the doctor, nurse or midwife that this person is an important member of the labor and delivery team.

Although the initial physical examination during pregnancy is a complete physical, from head to toe, its focus is on the reproductive system. The pelvic examination includes inspecting the labia; determining perineal muscle tone; inspecting the vagina and the cervix; taking cultures of the cervix for gonorrhea, chlamydia and herpesvirus in women considered at increased risk for these infections; taking a Pap test of the cervix and feeling the uterus and ovaries.

The size of the uterus reflects the *gestational age* (the length of time the embryo or foetus is carried in the womb) and is recorded during early pregnancy in terms of weeks; for example, six to eight weeks' size (the uterus can first be felt to be enlarged at about six weeks' gestation). Later in pregnancy the size of the uterus is measured with a tape measure.

Perineal Muscles

One part of the examination that requires collaboration between the examiner and the pregnant woman is the assessment of the perineal muscles. The perineum is the portion of the female body between the lower junction of the labia and the anus. These muscles are used in childbirth, during intercourse and in the stopping of urination. Since many women are unaware of the workings of these muscles and relatively few exercise them regularly, their tone is apt to be weak. The examiner assesses the muscle tone by placing the fingers of the gloved hand onto the perineum just inside the entrance of the vagina and pressing down. The woman is then asked to tighten the muscles. The experienced examiner can determine whether tone is nonexistent, weak, average or good. If your doctor or midwife does not check these muscles, you can do it yourself, using two fingers and pressing toward

External female genitals: (a) clitoris, (b) urethra, (c) vagina, (d) perineum, (e) rectum the spine. If your perineal tone is nonexistent, weak or average, you should exercise these muscles. (My suggestion is to tighten and relax in units of five contractions, each lasting ten seconds and to repeat the process ten times a day whether or not you are pregnant.)

Toning these muscles can help prevent tearing during birth and minimizes the need for an episiotomy. Good perineal tone can also enhance the sexual satisfaction of both partners in intercourse; women can increase their chances for and control over orgasm and many men appreciate the gripping sensation they experience when the perineal muscles are tensed. Strong perineal muscles also prevent bladder sagging as women age (particularly if they have had children) and stress incontinence, the involuntary passage of urine during sneezing, coughing, laughing or lifting. Perineal exercises, also known as *Kegel exercises* (after Arnold Kegel, the physician who first described them), have traditionally been a part of female hygiene in many preindustrial societies, passed on from mother to daughter as part of folk knowledge. The effect on childbirth of having well-conditioned perineal muscles during childbirth has not been critically evaluated, although common sense would suggest its value.

Blood Pressure and Testing for Preeclampsia

Blood pressure is measured at each prenatal visit. An inflatable cuff is secured over the upper arm just above the elbow. A stethoscope is placed on the artery that passes under the crease at the elbow. The cuff is inflated to stop the pulse below the cuff and gradually deflated. The upper reading of the blood pressure, called the *systolic pressure* (*systole* refers to the contraction of the heart when blood is ejected with maximum force into the blood vessels), is the reading on the gauge when the pulse sounds first become audible. The lower reading or *diastolic pressure* (*diastole* refers to the filling, noncontracted phase of the heart cycle), is the gauge reading when the pulse is no longer audible. The gauges are calibrated in millimeters of mercury. Thus, a pressure of 120 means that the pressure will balance or support a column of mercury 120 millimeters (about five inches) high in a thin tube. The systolic and diastolic readings are expressed as a fraction: the numerator is the systolic pressure and the denominator is the diastolic pressure.

A pressure reading of 140/90 is regarded as the upper limit of normal. If either figure is higher, the blood pressure is considered too high (hypertension). Blood pressure varies in a predictable way during pregnancy. There is a normal dip of about five millimeters in the systolic and diastolic pressures during the first and second trimesters.

Blood-pressure determination is one of the most important serial measurements made in pregnancy. A blood-pressure reading over 140/90 occurring with protein in the urine after the twentieth week defines preeclampsia, a relatively common disorder with important risks for the woman and the foetus. Blood-pressure readings are also essential in monitoring women who are being treated for established hypertension whether or not it is complicated by preeclampsia.

Dating the Pregnancy

Many decisions about the growth of the foetus and the timing of delivery of a baby depend on accurate dating of the pregnancy. Every effort must be made to determine gestational age by twenty weeks, beyond which dating becomes progressively less accurate.

Growth of the uterus. Unbroken curve in middle is size of uterus at twenty-four weeks. Dotted line shows position of uterus after baby's head engages in the pelvis.

The date of the last menstrual period is the primary way of estimating when conception occurred (at roughly fourteen days before the next menstrual period is anticipated). Even better is the last date of ovulation, as determined by basal body temperature. Another milestone, but not a very accurate one, is the *quickening*, the moment when the woman first feels the foetus move, sometime between sixteen and twenty weeks. A woman's recognition of this sensation will vary, depending in part on whether she has had other pregnancies and is familiar with the sensation. Measurement of the size and the height of the uterus is a good dating method, particularly in first pregnancies. Between eighteen and thirty weeks, the height of the uterus, measured in centimeters, correlates fairly well with the number of weeks of gestation, especially in first pregnancies. The foetus's heart can first be heard with a stethoscope between sixteen and nineteen weeks after conception and by *Doppler ultrasound* by twelve weeks.

With ultrasound, fetal heart movements can be visualized by six to seven weeks. The gestational sac is visible as early as five to six weeks. Between eight and twelve weeks, the distance between the head and buttocks of the fetus, the crown-rump distance, dates the gestational age very precisely. Between sixteen and twenty-six weeks, measurement of the diameter of the baby's head can date the pregnancy to within one and a half weeks of the gestational age with 95 percent confidence, a strong argument for routinely doing ultrasounds in pregnancy. Ultrasound researchers have also found that the length of the femur (thigh bone) of the fetus, measured during the second trimester, is 95 percent accurate to within six days of the fetal age. Other physical measurements are being studied for their correlation with gestational age.

Growth of the Fetus

The First Week

Egg and sperm cells meet during fertilization to form one cell with forty-six chromosomes. From this one cell, through cell growth, division and differentiation, the fetus and placenta will eventually develop.

After fertilization, rapid cell division produces a hollow sphere with a blob of fifteen to twenty cells, the *blastocyst*. Most of these cells will differentiate into the tissues and organs of the body and placenta. Some will remain as genetically unchanged copies of the fertilized egg and form the future egg or sperm cells of the fetus, preserved for the life of the individual. After passing through the fallopian tube and reaching the uterus, the blastocyst continues to enlarge. In another three or four days it attaches to the surface of the uterus's lining in a process called *nidation* (meaning "nesting"). For recent research breakthroughs in the growing of pluripotent cells removed from leftover embryos obtained by in vitro fertilization while in the blastocyst stage, and the opportunities for treating human diseases that may result.

After seven days, the blastocyst, now composed of several hundred cells, invades the now-prepared lining of the uterus, known as the *decidua* and gains a firm attachment to the woman. In the process, the sphere collapses like a cooling popover. The cells from the inside of the sphere form the germinal disk from which the fetus will develop. The rest of the cells compose the invading *trophoblast*, or primitive placenta. The trophoblast is unique, because it is the only human tissue that interphases with another immunologically separate individual, the woman and escapes graft-host type rejection. Some cells from the trophoblast cross into the woman's blood and through special techniques can be identified as such. Because the trophoblast has the same genetic characteristics as the fetus, it is potentially useful in prenatal diagnosis.

The Second Week

Once the blastocyst is implanted, its trophoblast grows at an astounding rate, sending out fingerlike projections into the surrounding decidua. These projections become honeycombed, with walls and spaces. When the embryo is about two weeks old, maternal tissues are eroded to such an extent that the maternal blood vessels allow the woman's blood to rush into these trophoblastic spaces. Placental circulation is thus established and the woman's blood begins to nourish the developing embryo.

The trophoblast also produces HCG, without which the entire lining of the womb, including the developing blastocyst, would be cast off. Tests used to detect pregnancy measure HCG in the woman's blood and urine.

The embryonic disk at this point is a double-layered plate, resembling an empty sandwich. The upper outer layer is called the *ectoderm*; from it the skin, hair, nails and the entire nervous system will develop. The lower layer is the *endoderm*, which gives rise to the digestive tract, the respiratory system and many of their accessory glands.

Between these two layers a third layer, the *mesoderm*, soon develops. The muscles and tissues lining the abdominal and pleural cavities derive from the mesoderm. Scattered between these three germinal layers are loose cells, called the *mesenchyme*. The mesenchyme does not belong to a single layer, but acts as a sort of loose packing tissue between layers. The mesenchyme gives rise to the heart, blood vessels, bones, and cartilage.

The Third Week

During the third week the oval germinal disk becomes pear-shaped and then takes on the form of a violin. It also bends in the middle, so that it is no longer flat. Down the center of the ectodermal surface, which will become the baby's back, two parallel ridges form. A groove, or trench, between them, known as the *neural groove*, will form the central nervous system. The heart and blood vessels also begin to develop during the third week of embryonic life.

The Fourth Week

Very rapid changes take place within the body of the embryo during the fourth week. Shortly after the laying of foundations for the nervous and circulatory systems, the *gut*, or early digestive system, begins to form. By a process similar to the formation of the neural groove, the endoderm gives rise to the foregut in front and the hindgut in the tail region. A blind pouch in front pushes gradually forward, soon breaking through the undersurface of the head to form the mouth.

At four weeks and one-quarter-inch long, the embryo does not yet look like a fetus. It has a head and a tail, which can be distinguished readily. The neural groove has sealed over completely, and formation of the brain is progressing rapidly. In the head, the beginnings of the eye and ear can be seen. A growing area called the mandibular process is beginning to form the face. The heart is now a large bulge on the underside of the embryo, already beating rhythmically.

Two Months

By two months the fetus, over an inch long, has assumed a reconizable human form. It has eyes, ears and a nose. The hands have fingers and the feet have toes. The head still looks too big for the body, which is potbellied because the liver is too large for the abdominal cavity. The sexual organs have begun to form.

Three Months

In the third month of development many different organs become more specialized. In the mouth, series of ten tooth buds appear in the upper and lower jaws. The most dramatic changes of the third month are seen in the sexual organs, especially those of males. Differentiation is more rapid in males than in females and by the end of the third month, close inspection of the fetus will reveal whether it is male or female.

Four and Five Months

The changes occurring during the rest of pregnancy are much more subtle. Development is largely a matter of simple enlargement and maturation of the various organs. The four-month-old fetus, though tiny, looks like a baby in every respect, although the head is still relatively large and the legs relatively short. The skin is thin, red and wrinkled.

From Six Months to Birth

By six months' gestational age, specialized structures in the fetus's skin are formed. On the head and sometimes over the back and shoulders there is a fine growth of hair, the color of which is unrelated to the color of the hair the child will have. Fingernails and toenails appear and grow slowly. At the time of birth they will project slightly at the tips of the fingers and they will have to be trimmed in the first few days of life to keep the infant from scratching himself or herself. Oil glands appear in the skin and manufacture a greasy, sticky substance known as the vernix caseosa, which is like a salve or ointment coating the skin. By the end of the sixth month the fetus is fully developed; it needs only to grow in length, weight and strength to face the demands of the world outside.

Through research we continue to learn about the complex and wonderful aspects of fetal behavior. We now know, for example, that fetuses go through sleep-wake cycles (appreciated by women as periods of quiet and movement); they yawn and suck their thumbs; they are responsive to both light and sound. After birth, infants pay preferential attention to their own mothers' voices and to musical selections to which they were exposed in utero. Fetuses have a keen sense of hearing and need to be protected from noisy environments, as evidence now suggests that noise can stress them. Fetal sensitivity to sound is used in the nonstress test, a late-pregnancy measure of fetal well-being. A good source of information about the world of the fetus is the book Your Amazing Newborn by Marshall Klaus and Phyllis H. Klaus.

The Placenta

The *placenta,* or afterbirth, plays a central role in pregnancy. It is a flat, circular structure about seven to eight inches in diameter and an inch in thickness and weighs roughly one pound. It is composed of millions of fingerlike projections, called chorionic villi, which are part of the fetal blood-vessel system and connect with the rest of the fetal blood vessels by way of the large umbilical veins and artery in the umbilical cord. In the body of the placenta, the villi are suspended in maternal blood and only a thin layer of cells covering the villi separates the maternal from the fetal circulations. Nutrients and oxygen pass from the woman to the fetus across this layer and waste products from the fetus, including carbon dioxide, are returned to the woman's circulation for elimination.

Fetal cells, usually in small numbers, also cross this fetal-maternal interphase in the placenta. These migrated cells, of various types, are important in several ways. Fetal red blood cells, (most commonly, Rh D-positive cells) can sensitize the pregnant woman who has a different blood type (most commonly, Rh D negative) to produce antibodies that bind to and destroy the fetal cells in both the woman's and the fetus's circulations). A similar process can occur with the fetus's platelets (the cells involved in blood clotting) if the type differs from that of the woman.

Trophoblasts from within the placenta and of fetal origin are found in the woman's blood and can be analyzed for genetic characteristics. This process, still in the development stage, offers a way to obtain genetic information about the fetus without having to do the riskier procedures of chorionic-villus sampling or amniocentesis. A procedure already in clinical use is the extraction of DNA from fetal cells in the woman's circulation to identify the Rh D blood type of the fetus. Fetal DNA obtained in this way will probably have widespread use. Fetal DNA has been isolated from the skin lesions of a common rash of the third trimester, opening up a whole new area of research. Intriguingly, there is now evidence that some kinds of fetal cells can persist in the woman indefinitely, either without known ill effects or, as research now suggests, as a contributor to the development of autoimmune diseases, such as systemic sclerosis. (In autoimmune diseases lupus erythematosis is the best-known example the person produces antibodies against her or his own organs.)

Membranes, known as the *amniotic membranes*, which are thin, semitransparent sheets of tissue, attach to the rim of the placenta and form a baglike, round dome that adheres to and conforms with the shape of the inner lining of the uterus. Tethered at the end of the umbilical cord, the fetus is suspended throughout pregnancy in the amniotic fluid within this rounded dome of membranes. Because of this fluid, it is practically impossible for the fetus to sustain injury from the outside.

The production of hormones is another important function of the placenta. Pregnancy places unique demands on the entire maternal organism; its special requirements must be met by adaptations that involve almost every organ system in the body. The size of the uterus and breasts and the volume of blood in the body must increase tremendously. To some extent, the pelvic joints loosen. Smooth muscles relax in the intestines and urinary tract and may contribute to such problems as constipation heartburn and urinary tract infection. These and many other adaptations are largely brought about by the action of the placental hormones on the woman's body. The placental hormones are also thought to be important in maintaining pregnancy and in initiating labor.

Physical Changes

Weight Gain and Growth of the Uterus

The most dramatic and obvious physical changes that occur with pregnancy are those related to the woman's shape and weight. A woman with an average pregnancy, who is carrying one fetus, has an overall pregnancy-related weight gain of 25 to 30 pounds. The fetus accounts for 7.5 pounds; the placenta and membranes, 1.4 pounds; the amniotic fluid, 1.8 pounds; increase in size of the uterus, 2.1 pounds; increase in maternal blood volume, 2.8 pounds; increase in breast size, 0.9 pounds; fluid in the skin and other tissues, 3.7 pounds; and maternal reserves, 7.4 pounds.

During pregnancy the capacity of the uterus increases 500 to 1,000 fold. Its muscle cells stretch and thicken and the elastic and fibrous tissues increase markedly, adding to the strength of the uterine wall. Its blood supply also increases. For the first few weeks of pregnancy, the normal pear shape of the uterus is maintained. As the fetus grows, the uterus becomes more globelike and by the third month, spherical. Then it elongates more than it widens to assume an ovoid shape. After the third month the uterus is too large to be confined in the pelvis, so it rises into the abdomen. As it grows further, it comes in contact with the front wall of the abdomen, pushing the intestines to the side and eventually it reaches almost to the level of the liver.

Weight gain in pregnancy begins slowly and picks up steadily later on. It is obviously correlated with the size of the uterus. About two pounds are gained during the first trimester; the other twenty-five or so pounds are gained during the second and third trimesters, with some levelling off during the last few weeks.

The growth in size of the uterus can be represented on a graph as a straight line that is directly proportional to the fetus's gestational age. This relationship holds primarily in first pregnancies and less so in later ones; it is especially accurate between the eighteenth and thirtieth weeks of gestation, again, more so in first pregnancies. A rule of thumb is that the number of weeks' gestational age equals the number of centimeters of uterine height. Uterine size is a good indicator of fetal growth.

Any abnormalities in the growth of the uterus need to be investigated. Smaller-than-predicted uterine growth over several months could be a result of *intrauterine growth disturbance*, *oligohydramnios*, the relatively uncommon condition of insufficient amniotic fluid, or both. Apparent excessive uterine growth could be explained by errors in dating the fetus (that is, the fetus is older than was thought); *hydramnios*, an excess of amniotic fluid; multiple pregnancies; *hydatidiform mole*; or, simply, a large fetus.

From the beginning of the second trimester the uterus contracts irregularly. Toward the end of pregnancy, women are able to perceive these contractions and report that they feel like menstrual cramps. During the last two weeks of pregnancy Braxton Hicks contractions (named for the physician who first described them) can occur as often as every ten to twenty minutes. They may be quite uncomfortable and account for false labor, or uterine contractions that are not accompanied by progressive dilatation of the cervix.

In some women a distinct bulge can be seen and felt in the midline of the abdomen between the two rectus muscles that run from the lower rib cage to the pubic bone. This bulge results from a spreading apart of these muscles, which deprives the midabdominal wall of one of its major supports. The gap between the muscles is bridged primarily by skin and *fascia*, which stretch relatively easily in response to the enlarging uterus. Treatment of this separation of the recti (also called a *diastasis recti*) is discussed in the section on prenatal exercise.

Cervix and Vagina

The number of its mucous glands and of the mucous glands in the vagina, markedly increases, as does the production of secretions. These glandular secretions account for the thick, white vaginal discharge that is common during pregnancy. Soon after conception the cervical canal is filled with a clump of thick mucus the *mucous plug* which is expelled during or shortly before labor. The mucous plug also serves as a barrier to the invasion of germs from the vagina.

The vaginal wall characteristically becomes duskier, softer, thicker, moister and more elastic, all in preparation for the stretching it will undergo during delivery. The labia enlarge and turn a dusky blue.

Abdomen and Skin

By the third trimester, in about 50 percent of women, reddish, slightly depressed skin markings, called *striae gravidarum* ("lines of pregnancy"), are present on the skin of the abdomen and sometimes on the breasts and thighs. Their cause is unknown. After delivery these markings gradually change to silvery lines that shrink as the contracting abdominal and breast skin firms up. They are permanent *stretch marks* of pregnancy. There is no way to prevent or eliminate these scars; creams and ointments sold for this purpose are ineffective.

In many women, particularly women with dark hair and complexions, the skin of the midline of the abdomen becomes pigmented from the pubic bone to close to the tip of the breastbone. The dark line curves around the umbilicus. Neither the cause nor the significance of this line is known, and it rapidly disappears after delivery.

It is quite common in pregnancy for brown patches to appear on the woman's face and neck. These are known as chloasma, or the "mask of pregnancy," and usually disappear after the birth.

In white women in particular, tiny red spots commonly appear on the face, the neck, the upper chest and arms. Each red dot consists of several tiny blood vessels branching from a central feeder, which can be seen with a magnifying glass. If pressure is gently applied to the center, for example, with the point of a pencil, the entire network is deprived of its blood supply and blanches. These spider hemangiomas, as they are sometimes called, are believed to be related to increased estrogen levels during pregnancy. Why some women have these spots and others do not is not understood and their significance is not known. They disappear after giving birth. Another transient skin change is redness of the palms. Like the spiders, this redness is believed to be related to estrogen levels. Again, its significance is unknown, and the phenomenon vanishes after delivery.

Breasts and Preparation for Breast-Feeding

Women commonly experience tenderness and tingling of the breasts as one of the earliest signs of pregnancy. The breasts increase in size, often dramatically and become lumpier as the milk-producing glands enlarge. Delicate blue veins appear beneath the skin and reflect the increased blood flow. The nipples enlarge and darken and are more erectile. Scattered through the areola (the dark circle around the nipple) are small bumps, which are enlarged sebaceous (oil) glands (also known as the glands of Montgomery). After the first few months, if the nipple is squeezed, colostrum, the thick, yellow fluid that comes in before the milk, will come out.

A woman who plans to breast-feed her baby should wear a nursing bra large enough to support her breasts during the last few months of pregnancy and during nursing. The bra can be worn day and night if her breasts are heavy or if she feels uncomfortable.

An inverted nipple can be identified by pressing the areola between the thumb and the forefinger. A normal nipple, or one that is simply flat, will protrude, whereas an inverted nipple will retract. Inverted nipples are uncommon, since most nipples that appear to be inverted are merely flat and will pose no difficulty for breast-feeding. Inverted nipples are best treated with breast shells (milk cups) during the days after birth. The cups can be worn under the bra between feedings and a breast pump can be used to draw out the nipple before nursing. Breast shells must fit so that the nipples fit completely into the holes and the base of the cups does not irritate the skin. With the exception of treating inverted nipples, there is no evidence to support measures to toughen nipples by massage or application of creams.

Circulatory System

In pregnancy, blood volume increases about 45 percent. The two major components of the blood the red cells and the plasma do not contribute equally to this increase. The red blood cells increase by about 25 percent, whereas the plasma expands by 40 percent. As a result of this disproportionate increase, the hematocrit (the percentage of the blood made up of red blood cells) actually falls, since there are fewer red cells per unit volume of blood during pregnancy. Thus, the standards for defining anemia based on the hematocrit differ for pregnant and nonpregnant women. The predictable fall of the hematocrit begins between the sixth and eighth weeks of gestation.

During pregnancy the pulse rate at rest increases an average of ten to fifteen beats per minute. The volume of blood pumped by the heart increases significantly during the first trimester and even slightly more during the second and third trimesters. *Heart murmurs,* which reflect increased blood flow within the heart, are common in pregnancy. These flow murmurs must be distinguished from those related to heart valve disorders, for which antibiotics against infection of the valves may be indicated during labor.

Respiratory System

Late in pregnancy many women experience some breathlessness, a result of compression of the lungs by the expanding uterus. Breathing becomes easier if the baby moves down into the birth canal before the onset of labor.

Urinary System

During pregnancy more blood flows through the kidneys. Even in women who are not pregnant, a small amount of protein and glucose is passed from the blood to the urine. As the amount of blood filtered increases, the amount of protein and glucose passed in the urine also increases, accounting for the common occurrence of measurable protein and glucose in the urine of pregnant women.

The urine-collecting system undergoes dilatation during pregnancy. The ureters, the muscular tubes that transport urine from the kidneys to the bladder, are relatively lax and dilated, in part a result of hormonal influences and in part a result of partial blockage of the lower ends of the ureters by pressure from the expanding uterus. The right ureter is subjected to further compression by the enlarging veins from the right ovary (which lie directly over the lower end of the right ureter) and by the weight of the uterus, which is usually rotated to the right. The dilatation of the ureters and relative stagnation of urine flow through them is believed to be a factor in the increased susceptibility of pregnant women to urinary tract infection.

Gums and Teeth

Gums soften and thicken during pregnancy, probably in response to increased blood flow. Even with the mild irritation of toothbrushing, they may bleed very easily. A lump of thickened gum tissue (called a *pregnancy epulis*) may bleed vigorously when touched. Both the normal swelling of the gums and the pregnancy epulis disappear after delivery.

The increase in the size of the gums predisposes pregnant women to gingivitis, a gum inflammation that can weaken the supports of the teeth. For this reason, daily brushing, flossing and regular dental cleanings and checkups are especially important for pregnant women. Contrary to folk belief, pregnancy creates no more long-term dental problems than those encountered in nonpregnant women, as long as the woman pays careful attention to diet and dental hygiene. However, dental health before and during pregnancy is taking on added importance as evidence mounts that periodontal (gum) disease may play a significant role in causing premature labor.

Psychological Issues

T. Berry Brazelton and Bertrand G. Cramer, in their book *The Earliest Relationship*, describe the emotional ups and downs, the mixed feelings and the opportunities for growth provided by pregnancy. They describe the work of pregnancy as divided into three separate tasks, each associated with a stage in the development of the fetus.

In the first stage, parents adjust to the news of pregnancy, which is accompanied by changes in the woman's body but not yet by evidence of the existence of the fetus. In the second stage, the parents begin to recognize the fetus as a being who will eventually be separate from the woman. This recognition is confirmed at the moment of quickening, when the fetus first announces its physical presence. In the third and last stage, parents begin to experience the coming child as an individual, as the fetus contributes to its own *individuation* by distinctive motions, rhythms and levels of activity.

In a book entitled *On Becoming a Family*, Brazelton writes about "a predictable kind of turmoil" in the last half of pregnancy, reflected in a series of questions parents-to-be ask of themselves: "Will I ever get to be a parent?" "Will I make it as a parent, or will I ruin my baby?" "If I get to be a parent, will I have to be like my parent? I certainly don't want to be like that!" As parents question themselves they wonder, "Have we made a mistake? Do we really want this baby?" And if there are such doubts, the question that follows is, "Could we already have damaged the baby by our being ambivalent?" Brazelton and his colleagues also found that parents-to-be rehearse for a damaged infant and as new parents are prepared to blame themselves if the baby is impaired in any way. This confusing swirl of emotions and mixed feelings is best understood as normal and represents a mobilization of energy to deal with the unprecedented challenge that lies ahead. At birth and thereafter this energy will flow into bonding with the baby.

Other psychological hurdles are more matter-of-fact. For some couples the change in the woman's body size and shape raises certain anxieties. For one, it is a public announcement of their sexual relationship, the only one allowed by society for an essentially private act. Some couples may feel embarrassed about publicizing what they have been up to.

Another anxiety has to do with a woman's self-image in light of accepted standards of beauty. The mass media decry obesity and portray slimness in the extreme as the only real kind of beauty. Being pregnant is often confused in many people's minds with being fat or unattractive. Because of the intense concern of women with weight and figure, the growing abdominal girth may touch a sensitive nerve. A woman may be concerned that she is no longer attractive to her partner, whereas a man may worry about whether he can still see his partner as beautiful.

Weight gain and increase in size are not the only factors in creating a sense of decreased attractiveness. Other bodily changes, such as large, sagging breasts, puffiness of the skin, stretch marks, swelling of the vulva, increased vaginal secretions, and tan spots on the face may contribute to a sense of loss of physical appeal.

Birth itself involves distortions of the female anatomy (bulging of the vulva, bleeding, stretching of tissues and so on), which can be seen as inconsistent with views of a woman as a sexually attractive being. "How would a man ever want to sleep with a woman he's seen giving birth?" a question asked by men and women alike reflects this concern. Couples can use such fears and reservations about pregnancy as opportunities to acknowledge their concerns to each other, drawing closer through considering them together. The deep emotions of pride and joy in being pregnant and in anticipation of having the baby generally override concerns that negatively affect the woman's self-image.

Common Problems

Morning Sickness

The queasiness very commonly experienced by women during early pregnancy, usually between four and fourteen weeks, may extend beyond the morning hours. The cause of this loss of appetite, nausea and sometimes vomiting during the first trimester is not fully understood. Hormonal influences are believed to play a major role. There is no evidence to indicate that the decreased food intake associated with morning sickness is harmful to the fetus.

Measures that have proved helpful, more by experience than by systematic research, in relieving nausea are eating small, frequent meals, such as six per day; separating ingestion of liquids and solids by one-half hour; and eating a dry, unsalted cracker or biscuit before getting out of bed in the morning. The drug Bendectin, a combination of vitamin B6 and doxylamine, effectively treats nausea in pregnancy. Although the drug was approved by the U.S. Food and Drug Administration (FDA), after a rash of lawsuits, all unfounded, in the 1980s alleging that it caused birth defects, it was withdrawn by the manufacturer from the U.S. market. Bendectin is available in other countries, including Canada. Vitamin B6, which is available over-the-counter, has also been proved effective. The usual dose is 50 milligrams twice a day with a maximum daily dose of 200 milligrams. Also available without a prescription is Emetrol, taken in doses of one to two tablespoons on arising and repeated every three to four hours as needed. Several effective prescription drugs are also available.

Severe nausea and vomiting in early pregnancy suggest a hydatidiform mole. Causes unrelated to pregnancy also need to be considered. If other known causes of severe vomiting have been ruled out, the diagnosis of *hyperemesis gravidarum* may be considered. With this serious, though uncommon, disorder hospitalization is usually required to prevent sometimes life-threatening maternal illness. The cause is unknown, although psychological factors have been suggested, and hypnosis as a treatment has been effective in some cases. A 1991 controlled study involving fifty-nine women with severe nausea and vomiting, reported in the journal Obstetrics and Gynecology, showed that vitamin B6 taken by mouth effectively reduced and shortened symptoms.

Frequency of Urination

Among several causes of increased urination in pregnancy, the most important is decreased bladder capacity resulting from compression of the bladder by the growing uterus. Another factor that contributes to increased output of urine is the consumption of extra fluids, whether they are intended to relieve constipation or to assist in treating urinary tract infections. Frequency of urination may in itself reflect a urinary tract infection and should be watched. When there is doubt, a urine culture should be obtained.

Urinary Tract Infection

Urinary tract infection can be frequent and bothersome during pregnancy. The relative slowing of urine flow from the kidneys to the bladder during pregnancy is a factor that both predisposes a woman to urinary infection and interferes with its treatment.

Infection can involve the lower urinary tract (bladder and urethra), the upper tract (ureters and kidneys), or both. Upper-tract involvement is suggested by such symptoms as fever, chills, nausea, vomiting and abdominal or flank pain. The signs of lower-tract infection (*cystitis*) are urgency and frequency of urination along with pain or burning (*dysuria*).

Symptoms and signs of upper urinary tract infection present the more serious problem. The evaluation of urinary complaints requires a urinalysis and urine culture. The presence of the typical symptoms described here and the presence of white blood cells along with bacteria in the urine argue for the diagnosis of urinary tract infection and the initiation of treatment.

The cornerstone of treatment for urinary tract infection is antibiotics, usually administered for ten days. Several-day, short-course antibiotic therapy for lower-tract urinary infections is effective for nonpregnant women and in asymptomatic infections during pregnancy. It has not been sufficiently studied with symptomatic bladder infections in pregnancy to be recommended yet. The treatment with antibiotics by mouth customarily recommended for lower-tract infections may not be adequate to treat upper-tract infections and intravenous treatment may be needed, at least initially.

Silent urinary tract infection (*asymptomatic bacteriuria*) predisposes pregnant women to symptomatic infection. For this reason, urine cultures are part of routine prenatal testing. Positive results are treated with antibiotics. Both asymptomatic and symptomatic urinary tract infections may increase the risk for premature birth.

Pain in the Lower Abdomen and Thighs

Pain in the lower corners of the abdomen, especially on the right, is common in pregnancy and is believed to result from stretching of the uterine supports, especially the round ligaments. This pain, sometimes known as round ligament syndrome, usually occurs at about twenty weeks and must be distinguished from pain arising from appendicitis, cholecystitis (inflammation of the gallbladder), kidney stones, urinary tract infection, hernia and other disorders. Pain that arises in the supporting structures of the uterus is related to position. It usually improves when a woman lies down, especially when she turns to the painful side. It is not normally associated with fever, loss of appetite, nausea, vomiting, diarrhea, or urinary symptoms. On physical examination, there are no signs of tenderness from pressure over the painful area, a response that is more common in the other conditions mentioned. Most women are able to accept stretching pain as long as they know it does not represent a threat to themselves or to the fetus.

Numbness or pain in the upper front thigh is believed to result from pressure of the uterus on the nerve that loops toward the thigh over the brim of the pelvic bone. The resulting discomfort is similar to that experienced when the "funny bone" in the arm is hit (also related to pressure on a nerve, in this case the ulnar nerve, which can be subjected to pressure as it crosses the inner part of the elbow). Numbness in the thigh can often be relieved by lying on the back or side, especially on the numb or painful side. This symptom does not usually persist after delivery.

Recognizing appendicitis in pregnancy can be tricky. First, loss of appetite, nausea and vomiting are common in pregnancy, as they are in appendicitis. Second, the enlarging uterus can displace the appendix upward out of its usual position in the right lower part of the abdomen, confusing diagnosis. Third, some degree of elevation of the white blood cell count is common in pregnancy, as it is in appendicitis. A physician who suspects appendicitis must act decisively to make a diagnosis before the appendix ruptures. The safest approach is to err on the side of early operation if appendicitis is suspected.

Pain in the pelvic girdle late in pregnancy and a feeling of coming apart are related to the softening of the ligaments that hold the bones together, which allows the pelvis to give during birth. It is a counterpart to the molding of the baby's head, made possible by its open cranial sutures. There is no specific treatment other than avoiding activities that can intensify the strain. Very rarely, the pubic bones actually do separate and require strapping for support.

Pain in the Upper Abdomen

Pain in the upper abdomen warrants a call to the doctor. There are several possible causes that need to be sorted out, including gallstones, heartburn and preeclampsia.

Fibroids

Fibroids are benign (noncancerous) tumors of the uterus that become more common as a woman gets older. If present, fibroids commonly increase in size during pregnancy. Although they usually cause no symptoms, they can occasionally be mildly annoying or confuse a diagnosis. For example, a fibroid may suddenly increase in size and cause pain, usually because of bleeding within it. This complication resolves with time.

Fibroids may make the uterus appear larger than it is, leading to a mistake in estimating gestational age. A fibroid that impinges on the cavity of the uterus may be a factor in miscarriage. Fibroids that are strategically situated in the lower portion of the uterus may obstruct labor, but this is very rare. Generally, fibroids shrink markedly after delivery. During pregnancy they can be identified by ultrasound.

Hair Loss

Hair loss, which results from premature cessation of growth in the hair follicles, is one of the more distressing developments of pregnancy, occurring after the birth. Fortunately, even though it may persist for up to one year, it is temporary. This conversion of the follicles from the growing (anagen) to the resting (telogen) state resembles normal hair follicle behavior at the end of a normal growth cycle. Giving birth is one of the causes of a widespread premature conversion of hair follicles from the growing to the resting state. Diffuse hair shedding during combing may occur for three months after delivery. Should there be any question of this diagnosis, the shedding phenomenon can be duplicated by stroking the hair with a gentle tugging action. The hairs removed can be examined under a microscope, and, in the usual case, the follicles will be seen to be in a resting stage.

Constipation

Less frequent, harder stools that are difficult to pass are common in pregnancy. Factors involved include relaxation of the muscles of the intestine because of pregnancy hormones, pressure on and displacement of the large bowel by the expanding uterus, relaxation and stretching of the muscles of the abdominal wall and the constipating effects of iron supplements. Hemorrhoids may intensify and be intensified by constipation.

Constipation can be corrected through increased fluid intake, increased fiber intake (raw fruit and vegetables, bran, psyllium seeds, and so on), and exercise. Stool softeners, such as dioctyl sodium sulfosuccinate, can also help. If necessary, gentle laxatives can be used, for example, senna concentrate (Senekot), in a dose of one to four tablets at bedtime, or milk of magnesia, in a dose of two to four tablespoons followed by a glass of water.

Varicose Veins and Hemorrhoids

Varicose veins of the legs, rectum (hemorrhoids) and vulva are common in pregnancy, particularly in women whose relatives also have or had them, suggesting a familial susceptibility. The pressure of the pregnant uterus on the large vein (vena cava) that drains blood back from the pelvis and legs is a major factor in varicose veins in pregnancy.

Although some women complain of aching, the significance of varicosities of the legs is primarily cosmetic. They can be relieved by elevating the legs (keeping the legs outstretched in a horizontal position) and wearing elastic (support) stockings.

Hemorrhoids can bleed and form painful fissures. They are ameliorated by measures to prevent constipation (see previous discussion), sitz baths in warm water, lubricating creams, suppositories (witch hazel, Anusol) and avoidance of straining (having what the English sometimes call an unhurried motion). Thrombosis (clotting) of an external hemorrhoid can be very painful. The clot can be removed under local anesthesia. If bleeding persists, if the hemorrhoids cannot be pushed back into the rectum, or if they become infected, hemorrhoidectomy (surgical removal of the hemorrhoids) may be required, although this procedure is very unusual in pregnancy. Tying off the hemorrhoids or injecting them with chemicals that collapse and scar them are preferred to surgery.

Varicosities of the vulva may be contained and relieved with counterpressure by a foam-rubber pad held in place by a belt. Although women can expect relief from varicosities of all kinds following delivery, hemorrhoids may be more pronounced in labor and the immediate postpartum period. Because improvement normally occurs after delivery, surgical correction of varicosities, if considered at all, should be delayed if at all possible until the necessity for it becomes clear.

Dizziness (Light-headedness)

Light-headedness, especially when the woman stands up quickly after lying down for a while, is common during pregnancy. It results when not enough blood reaches the brain because the heart does not receive enough blood to pump. During pregnancy, when a woman stands, blood tends to pool in her legs and thus is less available to the heart. Given the time to adjust, the heart and arteries accommodate this redistribution of blood. The time needed varies. When light-headedness is a problem, it is a good idea to stand up slowly; if dizziness occurs, bending forward or sitting down will relieve it. Dizziness that occurs while the woman is lying down is usually caused by pressure of the uterus on the great vein (inferior vena cava) that returns blood from the legs, pelvis and abdomen to the heart. Lying on the left side usually alleviates the problem.

Leg Cramps

Painful spasms of the calf muscles, particularly at night, affect about half of pregnant women. The cause is not known. Physical measures to relieve a cramp include massage and stretching maneuvers to bend the foot upward at the ankle. When lying in bed, the woman should avoid pointing her toes straight down or under. Although often recommended, dietary change or calcium supplements have not been proven effective.

Backache

As pregnancy progresses, women compensate for the weight carried in the abdomen by hollowing out the lower (lumbar) spine so they can maintain the normal upright position of the upper torso. This forward bend of the lower spine, know as *lordosis*, stresses the muscles and ligaments of the lumbar back, a setup for backache. Wearing high heels further increases the lumbar curve. Preventive measures include wearing low-heeled or flat shoes, taking rest periods during the day, strengthening the abdominal muscles through pelvic tilting and curl-ups, and maintaining general body fitness.

Measures to treat backache include applying ice (in the acute stage), stretching toward the feet as far as is comfortable while sitting in a warm bath with legs outstretched, practicing relaxation techniques, resting more, placing pillows under the knees when in bed and least desirable, analgesic drug therapy with acetaminophen or, in the first and second trimesters only, aspirin and nonsteroidal anti-inflammatory drugs (NSAIDs), such as ibuprofen and naproxen. If these steps do not work or if the backache is incapacitating or associated with any combination of leg pain, weakness and numbness, the health-care provider should be consulted.

Lightening

Lightening is the normal sensation women experience, particularly in first pregnancies, as the fetus (now almost a baby) drops during the latter weeks of pregnancy. Less stretching of the abdomen makes a woman feel lighter, hence the name. Lightening is accompanied by less shortness of breath, decreased pressure in the stomach, the feeling that the baby has dropped, increased pressure in the pelvis, increased backache and more frequent urination. Descent of the fetus may also contribute to constipation, the initial appearance or aggravation of hemorrhoids and varicose veins of the legs and swelling of the legs and feet. Nothing much can be done about lightening except to recognize what it represents and to bear with its associated, but temporary, discomforts.

Heartburn

Heartburn is a common problem in pregnancy and represents the backing up (reflux) of the acid contents of the stomach into the esophagus (food tube). Factors that contribute to heartburn are compression of the abdominal organs, including the stomach, by the enlarging uterus; the elevation of the stomach above the uterus; alterations in the action of the valve between the esophagus and the stomach; and hormone-induced loss of muscle tone in the esophagus and stomach.

Heartburn can be relieved by eating smaller quantities at a time, by avoiding lying down immediately after eating, and, if these measures fail, by using antacids at the end of each meal. If the symptoms come on when a woman lies down, the head of the bed can be raised six to eight inches by blocks beneath the bedposts to allow gravity to work against reflux.

Edema

Edema, or fluid accumulation in the tissues, is indicated by visible swelling and is normal in pregnancy. Edema of the feet and legs is very common in the third trimester and is related to hormonal effects on blood vessels and to increased venous pressure in the lower extremities from pressure of the uterus on the large collecting vein in the abdomen (inferior vena cava). When the uterus presses on the large veins that drain blood from the legs, backup of blood and the passage of proteinrich fluid from the vessels into the skin result. When the woman sits or stands in an upright position, the force of gravity also contributes to this phenomenon. Many women report that late in the day their rings are tight and their faces are puffy, showing fluid retention in the upper part of the body. Neither edema nor weight gain alone during the third trimester is predictive of increased fetal or maternal problems.

If edema is annoying, raising the legs will help. The best treatment is to lie down one or two times a day on the left side (to tip the uterus off the vena cava). In addition, the woman should avoid salty foods and eat more complex carbohydrates and proteins (fresh fruits and vegetables) and lean meats. Fluid, especially water, intake should be increased to eight to twelve glasses a day. Elastic hose will help reduce the swelling, but some women find these stockings too uncomfortable to be worth the bother. When edema is associated with *preeclampsia*, protein is present in the urine and the blood pressure is elevated.

Vaginal Infection

Vaginal infection is common in pregnancy and Candida albicans (a yeast) is the major culprit, causing an infection called moniliasis, or monilia. Symptoms of infection are itching, burning, and vaginal discharge. Examination of the vagina with a speculum reveals a yeast infection resembling cottage cheese. Microscopic study of a sample shows the characteristic branching structure of the budding yeast. Several effective antifungal drugs are used for local treatment. Candida in the vagina can be picked up by the baby during birth and infect his or her mouth, producing the condition known as thrush.

Two other causes of vaginitis and vaginal discharge in pregnant (as well as nonpregnant) women are Trichomonas, a one-celled amoeba-like organism, and bacteria. Anaerobic (not requiring oxygen) bacterial infections are commonly referred to as bacterial vaginosis (BV). These vaginal infections may cause no symptoms and are diagnosed by microscopic examination and culture. Both are treated with metronidazole (common trade name, Flagyl), which is considered safe for the fetus after the first trimester.

Bacterial vaginosis has recently attracted attention because of its association with premature rupture of the membranes and premature labor. It is now recommended that women with a history of premature rupture of the membranes be checked for BV in subsequent pregnancies and treated if positive. A large study of treating BV in women without symptoms after sixteen weeks, which was reported in 2000, showed no decrease in premature labors.

Itching

Itching (pruritus) of the body, especially of the arms and legs, is a common and sometimes annoying symptom of the third trimester. It may be related to a rash. When a rash is not present, the most common cause of itching is a partial blockage in the liver of the excretion of bile into the biliary system, including the gallbladder. Bile salts in greater quantities than usual spill into the blood and circulate throughout the body. In the skin these salts cause itching and mild jaundice, a yellow color that may also be seen subtly in the whites of the eyes. Over-the-counter anti-itch preparations can relieve mild symptoms. These include colloidal oatmeal for baths (Aveeno), cooling lotions (Sarno), and antihistamines (Benadryl, Chlor-Trimeton). If these measures are ineffective, a doctor can recommend various prescription medicines. This type of itching quickly resolves after birth.

Skin Rashes

Several rashes that appear in the third trimester are unique to pregnancy. One in about 200 women develops itchy, sometimes blotchy, red bumps or blisters on the abdomen, thighs, arms and buttocks, which disappear after the baby is born. This rash is known as the *polymorphic eruption of pregnancy,* or PEP. There is no known treatment other than measures to lessen the itching. In 1998, Selim Aractingi and his colleagues in the United Kingdom reported the isolation of fetal DNA in the skin lesions of PEP. The role of this DNA is unclear, but its presence is further suggestive evidence for the immediate and long-term impact of the fetus on the woman, a connection that appears ripe for further inquiry.

Another rash, less common than PEP and also very itchy is called prurigo gestationis. It consists of small bumps, often distorted by scratching, located on the forearms and trunk. Its cause and treatment are unknown.

Fatigue

Even in the most physically fit women, fatigue is a common feature of pregnancy. Although psychological factors may play a role, it is likely that weariness has a still-unexplained physical basis. Pregnant women tire easily and need to rest and sleep. There is no treatment for this problem other than rest, especially rest that is not associated with guilt about being tired or shirking responsibilities. Most women experience fatigue more during some periods of the pregnancy than during others. Some women are tired throughout their pregnancies, but others report having more energy than ever and experiencing no fatigue at all.

Headache

Headaches, whether resulting from migraine, tense scalp and neck muscles, or a mixture of both, can be treated much the same in pregnant women as in nonpregnant women. For pregnant women the emphasis is on nondrug treatments, such as massage, ice, avoidance of migraine triggers, and relaxation. A helpful technique is to stretch the neck while seated under a hot shower with the head and neck loosely dropping forward, hands clasped behind the head to allow the weight of the arms to pull the head gently down as it is turned from side to side to bring the tense neck muscles into the line of pull.

When a woman has a headache that for her is unusual in its intensity or other characteristics, she should consult her health-care provider. Headaches are one of the symptoms of preeclampsia.

Insomnia

Difficulty in falling asleep and interrupted sleep are common in pregnancy, particularly in the third trimester. Known causes include kicking by the fetus, heartburn, frequent need to urinate, shortness of breath, difficulty in finding a position of comfort and worry. For some of these factors there is not a lot that can be done but to grin and bear it. A pillow under the uterus for support can make a side position workable; a waterbed allows sleeping on the abdomen. For excessive worry, anxiety, or depression, all of which can disturb sleep, the pregnant woman should seek professional help.

A pregnant woman having trouble falling asleep can try the same measures used by nonpregnant women: eliminating caffeine-containing beverages; avoiding use of alcohol; not eating before bedtime; taking a warm shower; drinking a glass of warm milk. Relaxation techniques can also help. If the woman doesn't fall asleep within about ten minutes, she should stop trying, get up and leave the bedroom. TV is out (too stimulating), but reading a (preferably boring) book, with the lights turned low, is in. When drowsiness sets in, it is time to return to bed. If all else fails, a sedating antihistamine, such as diphenhydramine, is an option, after checking with the health-care provider about the dose.

Nosebleed

Nosebleeds appear to be more common in women who are pregnant than in those who are not. The best explanation offered is that the already very vascular inner lining of the nose (mucosa) becomes even more full of blood in pregnancy, presumably an effect of hormones. The vast majority of nosebleeds can be controlled by finger pressure along the outside of the nose sustained for five to ten minutes. For bleeding that won't stop, the woman should see her health-care provider or go to the nearest emergency room while continuing to maintain pressure.

Emotional Sensitivity

Many women report wide mood swings, forgetfulness and unusual sensitivity to the surrounding emotional climate during pregnancy. For no apparent reason, or with only the slightest provocation, an otherwise well-composed woman will burst into tears. This heightened reactivity is no reason to avoid stress or to be treated with kid gloves. Knowing that emotionality is a normal feature of pregnancy should promote understanding by the woman and those around her that outbursts and withdrawals are normal and need not be taken too seriously.

Later Prenatal Visits

The prenatal visits build on the important earlier steps of taking the initial history and performing the first physical examination and laboratory tests. These later visits offer expectant couples an opportunity to take a more active role if their professional attendants agree. Women can weigh themselves, for example and can check their own urine for protein and glucose. Couples can learn to listen to the fetal heart with the fetoscope and feel the various parts of the fetus through the abdominal wall. They can keep their own records, plotting the growth of the uterus and the increase in weight over the course of the pregnancy. A woman can pay particular attention to the first feeling of fetal movement, recording the time and date and she can note changes, especially decreases, in kicking, allowing for sleep periods toward the end of pregnancy. Decreases should be reported promptly to the nurse or doctor. Couples can come to the prenatal visits together and can even include their children. They can share their observations, fears and pleasures with the doctor or midwife and can insist on fully understanding what is happening and what choices they have throughout the pregnancy.

It is possible for couples to lay claim to their own prenatal care just as they do to labor and delivery. The doctor or midwife then becomes a ready resource and a support, not merely a director of the birth. Obviously, parents-to-be need to decide if they want this kind of relationship and will accept the responsibilities it implies. Many people elect a less active role for themselves or are in health-care settings in which no other option is available.

In uncomplicated pregnancies, after the initial examination, visits are traditionally scheduled every four weeks until the thirty-second week, then at thirty-four and thirty-six weeks, and weekly thereafter until birth usually thirteen visits in all. A recent U.S. Public Health Service expert panel has recommended reducing this number for healthy women to nine for first pregnancies and seven for later ones.

The content of the visits depends on the stage of the pregnancy. Weighing in, checking the urine for protein and glucose and measuring blood pressure are standard procedures. Maneuvers having to do with the uterus and baby obviously depend on the size of the uterus, which by the second trimester (twelfth week) has risen out of the pelvis into the abdomen. The height of the uterus is determined by stretching the measuring tape from the pubic bone up and over the uterus to its top.

By sixteen to twenty weeks it is possible to hear the fetus's heartbeat with a stethoscope. Since the fetal heart sound transmits best through the fetus's back, the location of the loudest sounds indicates the position of the back. In normal, head-down (vertex) presentations, the heart tones are generally heard best below the woman's umbilicus; in breech presentations they are heard best above it. When the fetus's back is pointing forward, the tones are best heard in front of the abdomen.

When the fetus's back is pointed toward the woman's back (called the posterior position), its heart tones are apt to be loudest in the woman's flanks. It is possible to hear the heartbeat by placing an ear directly on the abdomen. An extra-long tubing attached to the stethoscope will allow the pregnant woman to listen. An inexpensive, wooden listening device, shaped like a megaphone, may also be used. With an ear against its tip, the examiner places its base directly on the abdomen. These devices are available through the International Childbirth Education Association and its affiliates (see Appendix) and sometimes from doctors or midwives.

By normal adult standards, the heartbeat of the fetus is very fast, ranging from 120 to 150 beats per minute. It is sometimes faint and hard to hear, but this does not mean there is anything wrong. Since the sounds have to travel a variable distance through amniotic fluid, the wall of the uterus, and the fat, muscle and skin of the woman's abdominal wall, it is easy for them to be muted.

With Doppler ultrasound, the fetal heartbeat can be detected as early as the twelfth week. The sounds heard through the ultrasound monitor are not those of the heart itself, but are machine made sounds triggered by the movements of the heart, as sensed by the monitor from echoes of sound waves pulsed to the heart. The visual detection of fetal-heart movement by ultrasound imaging can occur as early as the sixth or seventh week of fetal life.

During the last trimester the examiner can feel the fetus through the abdominal and uterine walls. The firm pressure required to outline the fetus will not harm it. The woman can assist the examiner by letting her abdominal muscles relax completely; blowing air out and then letting go helps relax the abdomen. By feeling the location of the fetus's head and buttocks, the examiner can tell whether the fetus is head down (vertex), breech, or transverse (lying horizontally). Each position has implications for subsequent care in pregnancy. Palpation is also a reasonably good guide to the number of fetuses present. The fetus's size can be estimated as average, large, or small, a judgment useful in predicting its fit to the birth canal.

Physical examination can reveal whether the fetal head has descended into the pelvis. The examiner feels whether his or her fingers can get around the bottom of the head and come toward each other. If the fingers surround the head, it is still high in the abdomen; if not, it has descended into the pelvis. By differentiating between the lumpy hands and feet and the smooth back and by the location of the heartbeat, the examiner can conclude whether the back is facing left, right, front, or back.

Schedule and Contents of Prenatal Visits

Here I present as representative of current practice the contents and timing of routine prenatal visits as we now conduct them at our branch of Kaiser Permanente. There may be variations in other settings. Further, some tests not regularly done at Kaiser might be done routinely in other populations because of the prevalence of certain diseases in those groups.

As soon as you know you are pregnant: meet with a trained health education professional for orientation to prenatal care and to issues such as common problems, nutrition and drugs in pregnancy.

Blood pressure and weight are determined at all visits, as is the size (height) of the uterus once it can be felt.

Twelve weeks: first individual medical visit, pelvic exam, Pap test, cervical culture for gonorrhea and chlamydia; schedule expanded AFP test for fifteen to twenty (ideally sixteen to seventeen) weeks.

Eighteen weeks: review results of expanded AFP and next step if any; check fetus's growth and heartbeat (done at all subsequent visits); determine whether more specialized attention may be needed because of risk factors.

Twenty to twenty-four weeks: arrange for ultrasound and tests for anemia, diabetes and Rh D factor.

Twenty-eight to thirty-two weeks: review results of ultrasound and lab tests and take indicated action if any. Review and revise if necessary the estimated delivery date; Review record of fetal heart kicks.

Thirty-six to forty weeks: review record of fetal heart kicks; pelvic exam may be done to check on fetal position and status of cervix; discuss labor signs and when to go to the hospital or birthing center.

Nutrition and Weight Gain

A good diet is a cornerstone of a healthy pregnancy, necessary to create a healthy baby and to sustain the woman through pregnancy, delivery, and nursing. Nutritional needs of women increase during pregnancy and nursing because the woman is really eating for two. The best available advice on diet can be summarized as follows:

1. Follow the guidelines and consider the recommendations based on the new food groups described later in this chapter.
2. Gain a minimum of twenty-five pounds (unless you are overweight to start), but do not allow yourself to become overweight.
3. Gain weight gradually and steadily.
4. Do not attempt to lose weight during pregnancy (even obese women should gain weight).
5. Do not restrict your intake of salt (sodium); use iodized salt to optimize thyroid function.

The best recommendation based on the evidence available at this time is that underweight women should gain twenty-six to thirty-five pounds normal-weight women between thirty and thirty-seven pounds and overweight women no more than fifteen pounds. A pregnancy is safer for the woman and the fetus when the woman's weight going into pregnancy is normal, a fact worth considering when you are planning a pregnancy. Another point is that women will weigh, on average, six pounds more after the postpartum period than they did when they first became pregnant. Many women do not return to their prepregnancy weight unless they make a special effort. For a large number of women, pregnancy is the first step in a pattern of weight gain, which increases with subsequent pregnancies. Be aware of this risk and watch your weight, diet and exercise during and after pregnancy. Extra pounds gained are hard to lose. Notice during prenatal visits where your weight plots out from month to month on the graph of weight gain that is a part of many prenatal charts. If your pattern of weight gain starts to move up and off the normal curve, stop and ask why. If it is important to you to return to your prepregnancy weight after your baby is born, eat carefully and exercise so that you will return to your desired weight within weeks. The Daily Food Guide is adapted by me from the one recommended in our practice at Kaiser Permanente.

Table 7.1. Daily Food Guide

What Is a Serving?	Recommended Servings You Need Every Day	Write in the Number of Servings You Ate Today
Bread, pasta, rice tortillas, cereal, oatmeal	7 or more	
1 slice bread		
1 tortilla		
3/4 cup dry cereal		
1/2 cup hot cereal,		
cooked rice, noodles, pasta		
6 crackers		
Vegetables	3 or more	
1 cup raw or 1/2 cup cooked vegetables		
1 cup green salad		
3/4 cup vegetable juice		

What Is a Serving?	Recommended Servings You Need Every Day	Write in the Number of Servings You Ate Today
Fruits	2 or more	
1 medium piece fresh fruit		
1/2 cup chopped, canned, or cooked fruit		
3/4 cup orange or other fruit juice		
Milk, yogurt, or cheese	3 or more	
1 cup low-fat or nonfat milk or yogurt		
1 cup of low-fat or nonfat frozen milk or frozen yogurt		
1 1/2 oz. of low-fat cheese		
2 cups cottage cheese		
Meat, turkey, chicken, fish, eggs, dry beans	2 or more	
3 oz. lean meat, fish, or poultry		
1 cup cooked beans, lentils, or tofu		
2 eggs		
4 Tbs. peanut or almond butter (nonhardened, nonhydrogenated)		
Choose High-Vitamin Foods: You can get the extra calcium, iron, and folate that you and your baby need to be healthy if you eat some of these foods every day.		
Calcium-rich foods		
• Dairy products (milk, cheese, yogurt)		
• tofu (calcium fortified)		
• canned fish with bones (salmon, sardines)		
• almonds		
• broccoli		
• green leafy vegetables (spinach, bok choy; mustard, turnip, beet and dandelion greens; collards, kale, chard)		
• corn tortillas		
• orange juice fortified with calcium		
Iron-rich foods: Try to eat iron-rich foods in combination with foods or juices high in vitamin C such as oranges, pineapple, broccoli, or strawberries. Vitamin C helps your body absorb the iron.		

• beef, chicken, or turkey
• liver or other organ meets
• oysters
• tofu
• green leafy vegetables (spinach, bok choy; mustard, turnip, beet and dandelion greens; collards, kale, chard)
• dry beans
• iron-fortified cereals
• raisins and dried fruits
Folate-rich foods
• dark green, leafy vegetables (like spinach or greens)
• broccoli
• asparagus
• liver
• fortified breakfast cereals
• oranges and orange juice
• peanuts and almonds

Fats

Fats are important in the diet and should supply between 20 and 30 percent of calories. Although fats do contain more calories, gram per gram, than other food components, reducing fat in the diet to the vanishing point with reduced-fat foods in an attempt to control weight, a major public preoccupation, can backfire often people consume even more calories to achieve satiety. No matter what anyone tells you, it's *the calories that count*. Marked restriction of fat in the diet has paradoxically contributed to obesity.

The type of fat consumed is as important to health as is the overall amount. Foods containing trans fats should be limited. Trans fats result when liquid vegetable oils are hydrogenated to harden them. They are present in margarines and in many packaged, prepared foods, such as refrigerated biscuit dough, ready-to-eat cake frosting, cheese crackers, chocolate chip cookies, doughnuts, french fries, graham crackers, microwave popcorn, pound cake, snack crackers, and taco shells. Read the labels. You will probably not see the term *trans fat* as such (regrettably, not a food-labeling requirement), but you may see the word *hydrogenated* in such phrases as "partially hydrogenated soybean oil". Or, when you subtract individual fats (saturated, polyunsaturated and monounsaturated) listed on a label from the total amount of fat given, there may be some quantity of fat unaccounted for. Many fast foods, such as doughnuts and french fries, which contain high levels of trans fats, are exempt from labeling requirements and can be advertised as cholesterol free and cooked in vegetable oil. Trans fats are worse than saturated fats in negative effects on the blood-fat profile (cholesterol level, etc.) and as contributors to coronary artery disease. A promising exception in margarine products, although data on safety in pregnancy are lacking, is Benecol, popular in Finland since 1995; its key ingredient, sitostanol, derived from pine trees, appears to reduce blood-cholesterol levels. A similar product derived from soybeans is Take Control. Whether these margarines have an effect on reducing coronary artery disease is not known. Also not yet known are the long-term effects, positive or negative, of the plant fats (sterols) contained in these products.

A healthy diet should emphasize fats that are oils at room temperature, including canola, safflower, olive and corn oils. The diet should include fish at least twice a week (salmon-deep-sea is healthiest and mackerel are among the most beneficial because they contain high levels of omega-3 fatty acids, which have a positive effect on body fats) and should minimize saturated fats found in red meats. Recent data show that eating one egg a day, or an egg several times a week, is not harmful.

A gram of fat has the same number of calories whether it comes from peanuts, meat, or olive oil. Gram for gram, fat has the most calories of all food components, so quantity of fat as well as quality is important.

Sugar

Sugar is added to many foods, and average consumption is increasing, a factor in obesity. It is difficult to tell from labeling, which lists total sugar, how much is from the food itself, how much is added, and how the total compares to recommendations. Clues to added sugar are mention of corn syrup and fructose in the list of ingredients. Also, don't be fooled by the claim of "all-natural sweeteners".

Grains

A healthy diet during pregnancy should emphasize whole grains. Most of us eat very refined products most of the time. Studies suggest that eating whole grains can reduce the risk for heart disease, minimize the chances of developing the most common type of diabetes and prevent several types of intestinal disorders. A whole cereal kernel including oats, rye, barley and wheat contains all three parts of the kernel, including the *bran*, which is rich in fiber (a good preventive for constipation) and B vitamins; the carbohydrate- (and calory) rich *core*, or *endosperm*; and the *germ* (as in *wheat germ*), also rich in B vitamins and other important nutrients. To find whole-grain products, look for the word *whole* as part of the first ingredient on the label. A product that lists enriched or wheat flour is a refined product, missing some of the key elements found in whole grains. If you're not used to whole-grain breads and cereals, add them to your diet gradually, as they can cause intestinal cramps and constipation at first.

Virtues of Soy

Tofu and other soy preparations (including soy milk) may be as close to perfect foods as any. They are complete proteins, containing all the amino acids the body needs but cannot manufacture itself. Like other legumes (members of the bean family), they have no cholesterol, contain healthy forms of fat (mono and polyunsaturated fats and omega-3 fatty acids) and are rich in fiber. Soy has the additional advantage of being rich in naturally occurring chemicals called isoflavones, which, in conjunction with other components of soy, lower blood cholesterol. Isoflavones may also help prevent the damage that narrows blood vessels in the process of atherosclerosis, may hinder the clotting of blood that leads to heart attacks and may even play a role in preventing breast cancer. Apparently isoflavones are beneficial only when consumed as part of soy, not as purified supplements. Processing greatly affects the amount of isoflavones present in a soy product. For example, one ounce of soy isolate contains sixty milligrams of isoflavones; one-half cup of soy flour, fifty milligrams; one cup of soy milk, thirty to forty milligrams; and soy sauce and oil, none.

A note of caution comes from a recent study in the United Kingdom, which showed that boys whose mothers ate an exclusively soy-based vegetarian diet during pregnancy were five times as likely as others to have hypospadius, an abnormality of the penis in which the opening occurs on the lower shaft instead of on the tip. So, pending further studies, it's best to use soy to meet just *part* of protein needs.

Folic Acid

The vitamin folic acid deserves special mention. A daily intake of 0.4 milligrams taken from the time of conception through the first three months protects against fetal neural tube defects and possibly against certain heart defects, cleft palate and prematurity. If a fetus in a previous pregnancy has had a neural tube defect, the recommended daily dose of folic acid is ten times greater, 4.0 milligrams. Because women do not usually know for several weeks that they are pregnant, this vitamin should be taken at the protective dose when pregnancy is being planned in order to gain the full benefit from it.

The average diet supplies 0.05 to 0.5 milligrams of folate, the salt form of folic acid, daily, mainly from meat and dark green, leafy vegetables. Since January 1998 all enriched cereal grains sold in the United States must by law contain 0.14 milligrams of folate per 100 grams of cereal. Considering that dietary folate is only about one-half as bioavailable (usable by the body) as supplementary folic acid, it is easy to see why a supplement is required to reach 400 milligrams a day.

Vitamin Supplement

With the exception of folic acid, other nutrients for the fetus can be obtained by eating a well-balanced diet as described. The extra folic acid can be obtained from a supplement containing this vitamin alone or in combination with other vitamins, even though a combination is excessive. Taking quantities of vitamins greater than the daily requirements for pregnancy and lactation serves no purpose and should not be done. Megadoses (much more than the recommended daily amount) of some vitamins have been reported to damage the fetus.

Inadequate dietary iodine has recently received attention as a cause of underfunctioning of the woman's thyroid gland, resulting in less maternal thyroid hormone available for the fetus and greater risk for impaired fetal-brain development. Factors in decreased iodine intake include reduced use of iodized salt and reduced fortification of animal feeds and bread with iodine. Corrective measures include, in addition to reversing these trends, adding iodine to prenatal vitamins and other foods. Whether testing pregnant women for thyroid hormone would be useful is not yet known.

Iron Supplement

The question of whether iron supplements are necessary in pregnancy has not been evaluated with a randomized control study. Despite the lack of evidence in favor of iron supplements, it is common practice to include iron in the prenatal vitamins recommended in pregnancy. My opinion is that this practice is unnecessary.

Herbs in Pregnancy

Food Preparation

To prevent infection of yourself and the fetus by food-borne bacteria, follow these rules:

1. Fully cook meat, poultry and seafood. Eat cooked food immediately. Avoid undercooked foods. Avoid cold, ready-to-eat seafood and cold leftovers. Do not eat pate and raw egg dishes. Heat processed meats (bologna, hot dogs, salami, sausages) to steaming.
2. Use only pasteurized milk and avoid soft cheeses (for example, camembert, brie, feta cheese, and blue cheese).
3. Thoroughly wash fresh fruits and raw vegetables.

Pregnancy and a Plant-Based Diet

Pregnancy is an excellent time to consider in a fresh and thoughtful way what you eat. There is mounting evidence that a grain-based diet, with less animal (meat, fish, dairy, eggs and poultry) protein and fat will help prevent heart and blood-vessel disease, high blood pressure, kidney disease, osteoporosis, obesity and even some cancers. Although recognizing that the U.S. government has recently revised its dietary recommendations based on this new evidence, many experts on nutrition believe that the government is too strongly influenced by the meat and dairy industries and that these changes do not go far enough. Reducing the fat in hamburgers in our kitchens and in fast-food restaurants a step in the right direction taken several years ago and regrettably, reversed still doesn't get at the crux of the problem, namely, the hamburger itself.

Apart from the considerable direct health benefits for individuals, a shift toward a diet that includes less meat and more reduced-fat dairy products will have highly beneficial ecological and economic effects. For example, a meat-based diet requires the continual creation of new farmland, raising of more cattle, clearing of forests, costly and inefficient use of crops and water and heavier use of fossil fuels in food production and processing. Environmental effects, although counteracted in some instances by new farming methods, range from increased soil erosion and water pollution to increased levels of greenhouse gases in the atmosphere. The Physicians Committee for Responsible Medicine, a national, nonprofit organization of physicians and consumers, has been actively addressing these problems and has promoted a new four food groups.

The new four food groups are (1) whole grains, (2) legumes, (3) fruits and (4) vegetables. A healthy diet meeting dietary needs for calcium, protein, iron and vitamins includes a variety of foods from each of these groups. Other foods, including nuts, sweets, dairy products, meats and oils, are options; it isn't necessary to include them in the diet. If you do consume them, use small quantities and select those with the healthiest kinds of fats. During pregnancy, be sure to include a moderate amount of non-plant-based proteins.

Exercise and Relaxation

Pregnancy offers a wonderful opportunity to develop habits that will work for a lifetime. The purpose of prenatal exercise is to improve muscle strength and stretch tight muscles, since muscles are frequently tensed and shortened, as well as weak. Many common discomforts of pregnancy backache, varicose veins, cramps, constipation, breathlessness, heartburn, postural discomfort may be prevented or alleviated through a balanced program of exercise and relaxation. Also, a woman in good physical condition can withstand the rigors of a long or hard labor, as well as the exertion needed to care for the new baby, better than a woman who is out of shape. But conditioning takes time to develop, and the sooner a pregnant woman begins exercising, the better.

In addition to strengthening and stretching muscles, prenatal exercise provides several benefits that may enhance the birth experience. Women who exercise regularly throughout pregnancy claim heightened body awareness, confidence in their physiological functions and knowledge of how these functions are affected by the changes brought on by pregnancy. A woman who learns to trust her body can better trust her uterus and let go during labor and will feel comfortable enough after birth to bond with her baby. After delivery, the physical fitness skills learned during pregnancy should be continued as an integral part of a healthy lifestyle. The exercises described here can be done in an exercise class or on your own. Don't feel guilty if, for whatever reason, you can't participate in an exercise program. Look on exercise as an enhancement, but not a crucial aspect of the care you give yourself.

Choosing an Exercise Class

Although the obstetrics and gynecology section of the American Physical Therapy Association has an increasing number of registered physical therapists who are trained to support women in achieving good musculoskeletal care during the childbearing years, in many communities there are no such therapists. Often, no exercise classes are available, either. Health spas, fitness centers, yoga classes and dance schools offer prenatal or postpartum exercises, but these vary greatly in quality. Unfortunately, many of these programs neglect the muscles of the pelvic floor and reflect little understanding of the physiological changes of pregnancy. However, as long as a woman listens to her body and does nothing that causes strain or pain, she can usually reap the benefits and avoid the hazards of any reasonably good exercise program. With increasing consumer demand, more quality exercise classes should become available, so women should make their preferences known. If no classes are available, the exercises that follow should be of help.

Exercise classes for pregnant women and their partners may be held separately or as part of general childbirth-education classes. In either case, they provide contact with other childbearing couples. In addition to gaining group support, couples in these classes can learn about other resources early in their pregnancies, when they may still be open to making choices and changes in their birth arrangements.

The ideal exercise class has a small number of participants who can be individually evaluated and supervised, rather than trained as a group to follow the leader. The instructor explains the rationale for each position and movement, along with the role of the muscles in pregnancy, birth and afterward. The best classes present the exercises in a broad context, coordinated with breathing, relaxation and psychological preparation for birth.

General Principles

A suggested exercise session lasts for one and one-half hours and consists of roughly equal proportions of calisthenics, stretching and relaxation. Aerobic exercises, such as walking, swimming, dancing and cycling, can be done for recreation. The exercises here need be done only a few times each session to be beneficial, but they must be performed slowly and properly. Jerking and straining should be avoided. The goal is increased body awareness and comfort, not training for the Olympics. Quivering muscles or sudden jerky movements that bypass a weak muscle group indicate that the exercise is too difficult and should be modified. Once an exercise is mastered and is no longer taxing, it is advisable to make it more challenging by changing the position of the body or the leverage of the limbs, instead of merely doing it more times.

Breathing must be coordinated at all times with exercise movement. A good rule of thumb is to exhale during exertion. Another is to breathe in through your nose and out through your mouth (with your lips slightly parted). For example, when doing a curl-up for strengthening the abdominal muscles (to be discussed), fill your lungs by inhaling through your nose while your head, neck and upper back are flat on the surface (floor or mat). As soon as your lungs are full, immediately begin exhaling through your pursed lips while elevating your head, neck and upper chest. Then inhale again. When you reach the curled-up position and as soon as your lungs are full, exhale as you lower yourself back to the surface. To increase the time in the curled-position, lengthen the time of your breathing in and out. Straining while holding the breath in the throat has an undesirable effect on the circulation of blood, especially in pregnant women. It limits the return of blood to the heart; hence, less blood is pumped from the heart to the lungs to receive oxygen and then out into the body. Since less oxygenated blood can reach the woman's tissues, including the placenta, less oxygen is available to the fetus. Exhaling during exertion not only prevents such negative cardiovascular effects, but also avoids strain on the pelvic-floor and abdominal muscles. In fact, exhaling during exertion actually improves the return of blood to the heart, as positive pressure is maintained in the abdomen relative to that in the chest. This principle is even more important during the pushing stage of labor.

A woman should become conscious of the natural expansion of the chest and abdomen during inspiration and their contraction during exhalation. Strange as it may seem, not everyone breathes in the most efficient way. Many people contract their abdominal muscles during inspiration and expand them during expiration rather than the reverse and this needs to be pointed out to them. Tightening the abdominal muscles on exhalation is a good preliminary exercise that demonstrates the role of these muscles in forced exhalation; the abdominal muscles can be strengthened only during exhalation.

It is important to focus on the muscles most stressed in childbearing the muscles of the abdomen and the pelvic floor. In most woman, both are weak. Typically, the abdominal muscles are rarely exercised, although they are quite visible and most women sit or stand and rarely use the perineal muscles by squatting. During pregnancy, these muscles must meet the demands of increased weight gain, changes in the center of gravity and support for the enlarging uterus, as well as meet the challenge of the expulsive phase of labor.

Abdominal and Back Muscle Exercise

The muscles of the abdominal wall provide much of the support for the spine and thus play an important role in the health of the back. Together with the *gluteus maximus* muscles the major muscles of the buttocks the abdominals control the angle of the pelvis in relation to the spine, which affects stability and stress of the lower back. The common view is that backache is due to weakness of the back muscles, but back muscles are more likely to be too tight than too weak. Thus, it is the abdominal muscles that need emphasis in back-care programs.The abdominal muscles run from the lower edge of the ribs in front and on the sides to the rim of the pelvis. You can feel them if you lie on your back, knees bent and raise your head and shoulders. Move your hand around over your abdomen from your ribs to your pelvis and feel the firmness over the entire area. The abdominals actually consist of several sets of muscles arranged in layers:

The recti, which run straight down the center of the abdomen and consist of two bundles about three inches in width, one on each side of the midline, separated by about an inch and a half of tough, fibrous tissue.

The obliques, two layers of muscles that run diagonally, one on each side of the body, from the ribs to the pelvis, crisscrossing in opposite directions.

The transversus, which is wrapped around horizontally.

During pregnancy the growing uterus stretches the abdominals from a straight line between the pelvis and ribs to an expanding curve between upper and lower attachments. Therefore, it makes sense to begin abdominal strengthening exercises as early as possible.The curl-up is the basic exercise for the abdominal muscles. A curl up is a modified sit-up, done to a maximum of forty-five degrees off the surface, with knees bent and the back of the waist flat on the surface used. To exercise all abdominal muscles adequately, curl-ups should be done in both straight and diagonal directions.For a diagonal curl-up, twist one shoulder toward the opposite knee, alternating shoulders on successive curl-ups. Lie flat after each curl-up. Repeat the exercise up to fifty times, but stop if it starts to hurt.The work of the abdominals can be progressively increased by changing the position of the arms as follows:

1. In the initial position, the arms reach toward the knees, assisting the movement (60 percent abdominal-muscle effort).
2. The next progression involves a neutral position, with arms folded across the chest (80 percent effort).

3. Finally, the arms are clasped behind the head to increase the leverage (100 percent effort).

Each woman begins at the appropriate level and progresses at her own pace. The physical changes that occur in later pregnancy make the more advanced curl-ups (2 and 3) too difficult.

It is important to check regularly through pregnancy for any separation of the rectus muscles from the stretching of the fibrous band that unites them like a central seam. Such a separation is called a *diastasis* recti. This condition is usually observed after the fifth month, but may be seen earlier in women who have retained it from a previous pregnancy. Many women notice the bulging in the midline of the abdominal wall as they get up off the floor after exercising or as they get out of bed or the bath. Although diastasis recti is painless, it may lead to postural backache because of abdominal wall weakness.

To check for diastasis, lie on your back with knees bent. Raise your head (which activates the rectus muscles), allowing your hands to reach toward your knees. You or your exercise coach can then check the width of the soft area between the tense rectus-muscle bundles. If three or more fingers can be placed between the contracted rectus muscles, diastasis recti is present. With this degree of separation, the bulging can usually be seen as well as felt.

A woman with a diastasis should avoid strenuous work with the abdominal muscles, as in double leg-raising exercises on the back (described later) and heavy lifting or straining. She should also be careful, when arising from the floor or bed, first to roll on one side and then push herself into a sitting position with her arms. It is usually not possible to close the gap of a diastasis during pregnancy because of the progressive and continuous stretching of the abdominal wall by the enlarging uterus. However, couples can be reassured that it is possible to bring these muscles together again with exercises after birth. The presence of diastasis recti requires that a woman's exercise program be modified only with regard to curl-ups; the other essential exercises are still suitable. If the rectus muscles cannot stay parallel when the head only is raised, it makes no sense to increase the load by bringing the shoulders off the floor as well. Furthermore, the oblique abdominal muscles contract when the shoulders curl forward. Because they attach to the sheath covering the rectus muscles, their action will lead to further strain and muscle imbalance, which can increase the diastasis.

To perform the modified curl-up, the woman with diastasis recti lies on her back with knees bent and hands crossed at the area of the gap to support the muscles. She performs head raises only, taking care that the abdominal wall is pulled *in* as the breath is exhaled, in order not to increase the bulging. She should do the exercises frequently for a short time, following the same program postpartum. After a few days postpartum, the woman can evaluate the gap while performing a modified curl-up without hand support. If the diastasis persists, she should continue the modified curl-ups. If the muscles are parallel at the midline, she can slowly increase the curling up by bringing the shoulders off the floor, but only little by little. Too rapid progression can lead to reseparation.

Note the difference between curl-ups and sit-ups. Sit-ups involve lying flat on the floor with legs extended and straight and then sitting up. With curl-ups, the knees are bent to stabilize the lower back (lumbar spine). The movement is limited to the abdominals and is never more than about forty-five-degrees forward flexion off the surface. A sit-up, which involves a ninety-degree movement, is performed primarily by the hip flexor muscles, which run from the front of the upper thigh bones to the lower spine and pelvis. When these muscles contract, they pull the spine and the thighs closer together and hollow the spine just the effect that should be avoided. The abdominal muscles, on the other hand, roll the body forward as the ribs approach the pelvis without straining the lower spine. In the early part of a sit-up, the abdominals do most of the work; the second half of a sit-up hardly exercises the abdominals at all and may actually conceal weak abdominal muscles, as is typically seen in a person who jerks quickly through the first phase of the movement. Keeping the legs straight and, as is sometimes done in sit-ups, fixing the feet with external force (as, for example, by tucking them under a horizontal bar) further encourages use of the hip flexor muscles and thus increases lumbar strain. *Avoid sit-ups at all times.* Conversely, bending the knees minimizes use of the hip flexors and brings the abdominals into full play. The American College of Obstetricians and Gynecologists guidelines recommend against the supine (on-the-back) position for resting or sleeping after the fourth month. Not all experts agree.

Pelvic Tilting and Bridging

Pelvic-tilting movements focus on the lower part of the abdominal wall and can be done in many positions. The action is to decrease the curve of the lower spine (the small of the back) by squeezing the buttocks tightly together and pulling in the abdominal muscles, thus rotating the pelvis to the back (posteriorly). Like curl-ups, pelvic-tilting exercises can be done progressively in three different positions while lying on the back.

1. The knees are bent, the feet flat on the floor.
2. With heels sliding along the floor, the legs are extended as far as possible while the pelvic tilt is maintained. With practice and increasing muscle strength and control, the tilt will be possible with the legs fully extended.
3. Finally, with the tilt maintained, the legs and thighs are bent and brought over the waist. Then the thighs and legs are simultaneously and gradually lowered and extended to the point at which the pelvic tilt is maximally stressed, yet maintained. Usually this point occurs before the thighs are lowered forty-five degrees. Many women will be able to lower the legs as far as forty-five degrees only after considerable practice. In late pregnancy this maneuver is difficult for many women. Do not perform this exercise if diastasis recti is present.

There is a difference between leg lowering as described and double leg raising, with which it is often confused. In double leg raising, the woman lies on her back with her legs outstretched and perfectly straight. She then lifts the stiffened legs together from the surface upward. The problem with double leg raising is that during the most difficult initial part of the movement, the pelvic tilt is out of control because the hip flexors, not the abdominals, do the work. As with a seesaw, the short lever of the pelvis rises before the longer lever of the outstretched legs. This exercise can cause much discomfort and aggravation of back pain. The point is not simply to raise or lower the legs. You must be able to maintain the pelvic tilt and protect the lumbar spine while the muscles that do so are challenged and thereby strengthened. *Double leg raising should be eliminated from any exercise program, especially one designed for pregnant women.*

Basic pelvic tilting can also be done in sitting, standing, kneeling, side-lying and hands-and-knees positions. In the hands-and-knees position, the work of maintaining the pelvic tilt can be increased by extending first one arm, then one leg, then opposite arms and legs together. In this exercise, the abdominal and gluteal muscles hold the pelvis in line with the spine against gravity and the leverage of the different arm and leg positions. This is also a good position for the woman with a diastasis who cannot do curl-ups. The hands-and-knees position relieves backache and pressure from the uterus, and the progressive exercises mentioned improve balance and strengthen the arms and shoulders.

Bridging is the act of raising the buttocks off the floor. It helps improve the pelvic tilt by strengthening the gluteal muscles, which pull the pelvis down in conjunction with the upward movement of the abdominals. Bridging is done lying on the back, preferably with the legs straight at the knees and with the heels resting on a low table or foot stool. The buttocks are lifted from the floor to form a bridge with the body. If this exercise is done with the knees bent, the woman must be taught to feel the difference between gluteal contractions and the leverage exerted by the hamstrings, which run from below the knee to the sitting bones of the pelvis. The closer the heels are to the buttocks, the more substitution occurs with the hamstrings, which can extend the hips when the knees are bent and thereby reduce the value of the exercise. Bridging should be done with the pelvis tilted back and buttocks held as firm as possible. A further progression is to straighten alternate knees while in the bridge, and then to move the extended leg from side to side, keeping the thighs parallel throughout.

Pelvic-Floor Exercises

The importance of the muscular and fascial layers that make up the pelvic floor cannot be overemphasized. Particularly important is the *pubococcygeus* muscle, which runs from the coccyx (tailbone, or tip of the spine), encircles the vagina and rectum, and attaches to the pubic bones at their point of joining. In Western cultures, the muscles of the pelvic floor are typically not exercised, and many women are unaware of them. The three main functions of the pelvic floor are:

1. To support the pelvic abdominal organs and the increasing weight of the uterus in pregnancy
2. To provide sphincter control of the anus and urethra
3. To enhance sexual response, since healthy muscles grip and massage the penis during intercourse and vigorously contract during orgasm to provide increased satisfaction to the woman and her partner

Structural changes in the pelvic floor, such as laxity and various degrees of sagging of the uterus, bladder, or rectum, are common in Western society, particularly in women who have borne children. Functional changes, such as urinary-stress incontinence (the leakage of urine with coughing, sneezing, or straining), lack of sexual satisfaction for either partner and incomplete emptying of bowels or bladder, are also very common. Many women believe that stress incontinence and falling-out feelings are normal consequences of pregnancy, since many of their friends have the same symptoms. Smoking, obesity and chronic chest conditions, which all cause increases in intra-abdominal pressure, aggravate pelvic-floor dysfunction. Although softening of tissues related to hormonal and blood-supply changes and some descent of the pelvic floor are normal during pregnancy, adequate urinary control can be expected to be maintained throughout.

Healthy pelvic-floor muscles can help facilitate the safe progress of the baby during the second stage of labor. Well-exercised muscles with an enhanced blood supply can better withstand stretching before their fibers become underoxygenated or stretched to the point of tearing. Arnold Kegel, a pioneer in studying the pelvic floor, has shown that during the crowning of the baby's head, a strong pubococcygeus muscle remains protected by the pubic bones, whereas a thin, fibrous, unexercised muscle is dragged down with the fetal head and is more likely to be injured.

There are problems in learning to contract the pubococcygeus, because the action is internal and out of sight and no bones are involved in the movement. Many women are unaware of the pubococcygeus and cannot contract it in isolation from other muscle groups. Typically, when asked to tighten this muscle, women contract other muscles, such as the muscles of the buttocks or inner thighs. Since vaginal examinations are not performed during exercise or childbirth classes, it is essential for the woman, perhaps with the aid of illustrations, to locate this muscle herself.

A woman can become aware of this muscle while urinating simply by stopping in midstream several times and paying attention to the muscles used to do so. A woman who cannot do this will need to reeducate this muscle. The muscle can also be identified and evaluated during the prenatal physical examination. Inserting one or more fingers into the vagina, while at the same time trying to squeeze, is another way for a woman to identify this muscle.

Once a woman has identified the correct muscle, she tightens the anal and vaginal sphincters, thereby also raising the perineum (the region between the lower end of the vagina and the anus). Useful analogies to this action are the rising of an elevator and the drawing up of a hammock. The muscular contractions must be done slowly enough to recruit as many muscle fibers as possible. Contract-relax exercises (also known as Kegeling) can be done at any time. In particular, the pelvic floor should be braced during such exertions as sneezing, coughing, or lifting.

Research has shown that the pelvic floor readily fatigues with exercise and that the average woman cannot make more than a few contractions of consistent strength. Similarly, holding a contraction for more than ten seconds is beyond the ability of most unconditioned women. The exercise should be done little and often—just three or four contractions in a series, followed by a rest interval. A total of about fifty should be done daily before, during, and after pregnancy. Sexual intercourse is another opportunity for the practice and improvement of pelvic-floor control and has the advantage of feedback from the woman's partner. Pelvic-floor exercises can be done anywhere, anytime. They should become as routine as brushing the teeth.

In societies in which squatting is common, the pelvic floor is always being strengthened because it must support all the internal organs when in the squatting position. Squatting also strengthens the muscles of the thighs and promotes safe lifting habits by avoiding bending at the waist. Squatting is a useful exercise in pregnancy, and the squatting position is also recognized as useful during childbirth both in terms of effective pushing and in maximizing the space in the birth canal.

Stretching Exercises

The muscle groups that are tight are typically the hamstrings, calf muscles, inner thighs, hip flexors (muscles that bend the thigh toward the abdomen) and back extensors (muscles that straighten out the back, as in a position of attention). Yoga exercises are particularly suited to enhance flexibility.

The hamstrings can be stretched by standing with one leg elevated on a chair or table, by long sitting (knees straight, legs outstretched) and by lying on the back and lifting *one* straight leg at a time. (Avoid double leg raising, as described previously.) In pregnancy these positions are preferable to bending forward, which usually involves rounding of the back and excessive pressure on the spinal disks (the structures that act as shock absorbers between the individual vertebrae). In stretching the hamstrings it is important to bend at the hips rather than to bend the spine.

Calf stretching can be done kneeling on one knee (runner's stretch) with the foot of the forward leg firmly applied to the floor as weight is shifted progressively forward; or by standing with one foot in front of the other, keeping the knee of the rear leg straight with its foot planted squarely on the floor as the forward knee is bent. The hip flexors can also be stretched in the half-kneeling position (the position runners assume at the starting line), one foot in front of the other, with the weight transferred onto the forward foot until a pull is felt in the opposite groin.

The back can be stretched in a tailor-sitting position (knees bent, ankles crossed and legs allowed to fall apart). The trunk is then bent forward to bring the head toward the floor. A modified back stretch can also be done in a half-tailor-sitting position (one leg outstretched and one leg bent) with the trunk bent to either side. Sitting with the legs extended (long sit) and holding the back at a ninety-degree angle (without leaning on the arms) is an excellent stretch and postural exercise. The lower back can also be buttressed against a wall and the exercise made more difficult by raising the arms while keeping contact with the wall.

The adductor muscles (which pull the thighs inward toward each other and contract to hold an object between the knees) can be stretched while sitting on the floor with the soles of the feet together, allowing the force of gravity to let the thighs fall apart. The pelvic clock exercise, arching the pelvis around like the hands of a clock, of Moshe Feldenkrais can also be done in this position and increases pelvic awareness. This maneuver involves sitting on the floor with the soles of the feet together and rotating the pelvis round and round, first clockwise, then counterclockwise.

Aerobic Exercise

Aerobic exercise refers to activities that increase the pumping of blood by the heart and the movement of air in and out of the lungs and includes any combination of walking, skipping, jumping, jogging and dancing, using backward, forward and sideways directions for variety. Other aerobic activities are running, cross-country skiing, brisk walking and non-weight-bearing activities such as swimming and cycling. Warming up and cooling down, including stretching before and after aerobic exercise, are particularly important to prevent injury and are often overlooked. Women can continue with their favorite sports, listening to their bodies for signs about what to do and how much, as the pregnancy progresses and after delivery. Table 7.2 contains guidelines for planning appropriate aerobic activities.

Relaxation

An ability to relax is a great asset during childbirth, when actively being is as important as doing. For one thing, relaxation during labor allows the woman to conserve energy. Giving birth involves using the forces that push the baby down the birth canal as well as reducing the forces that oppose this descent. Tightening up increases resistance; opening up decreases it. In a sense, a pregnant woman allows her baby to be born simply by yielding to the forces pushing the baby out. Letting go through increased awareness of the body is a skill that can be learned and practiced.

Sheila Kitzinger, noted British childbirth educator, has described the "puppet-string" approach to relaxation. In a comfortable lying position, with plenty of pillows, the woman imagines various parts of her body attached to strings operated by a puppeteer. The puppeteer can pull the strings straight up or at various angles and can pull them in any combination; for example, the right shoulder and the right index finger can move together, or the right shoulder can move with the left knee and so forth.

Table 7.2. Exercise Guidelines for Pregnancy and Following Birth

1. Regular exercise (at least three times per week) is preferable to intermittent activity.
2. Avoid vigorous exercise in hot, humid weather. Stay well hydrated before, during, and after exercise. Wear light clothing that "breathes".
3. Ballistic movements (jerky, bouncy motions) should be avoided. Exercise on a wooden floor or a tightly carpeted surface to reduce shock and provide a sure footing.
4. Avoid deep flexion or extension of joints because they are looser in pregnancy and more vulnerable to trauma. For the same reason, avoid jumping, jarring motions or rapid changes in direction.
5. Vigorous exercise should be preceded by a 5-minute period of muscle warm-up. This can be accomplished by slow walking or stationary cycling with low resistance.
6. Follow vigorous exercise with a period of gradually declining activity that includes gentle, stationary stretching. Because connective-tissue laxity increases the risk of joint injury, stretches should not be pushed to the point of maximum resistance.
7. Measure heart rate at times of peak activity. Do not exceed 140-150 beats per minute unless in consultation with your physician.
8. Take care to rise from the floor gradually to avoid orthostatic hypotension. Continue some form of activity involving the legs for a brief period.
9. Drink liquids liberally before and after exercise to prevent dehydration. If necessary, activity should be interrupted to replenish fluids.
10. Women who have led sedentary lifestyles should begin with physical activity of very low intensity and advance activity levels very gradually.
11. Stop activity if any unusual symptoms appear. Consult your physician.

Pregnancy Only

1. Do not let your heart rate exceed 140-150 beats per minute.
2. Do not exercise strenuously for more than 15 minutes. Limit total time to 45 minutes and stop before you're worn out. You should be able to carry on a conversation at all times.
3. Avoid contact sports, scuba diving and high altitude exercise (unless you are specially conditioned for thin air). Otherwise,

(Contd.)

there are no restrictions on what you can do safely, but take it easier than when not pregnant.

4. Strength training with light weights and frequent repetitions are okay.
5. After the fourth month don't do exercises while lying flat on your back.
6. Avoid exercises that require holding your breath and bearing down (thereby markedly increasing pressure in the abdomen.)
7. In the second half of pregnancy, swimming is by far the ideal exercise. It takes the weight off you while you work out.
8. Limit your use of saunas and whirlpools to a few minutes at a time.

A woman can activate the strings herself, or she can ask her partner to do so and to let her know which strings are being pulled. After an imaginary string has been pulled, the woman allows the muscle to relax and the body part involved to sink back into a resting state.

The method of relaxation based on Stanislavsky acting techniques uses imagined activities. In a relaxed sitting or lying position, with eyes closed, the woman gets in touch with various parts of her body by imagining them engaged in activities such as chewing sticky taffy, walking barefoot on sharp pebbles at the beach, kneading dough, following an airplane overhead to the distant horizon, tasting a sour lemon and so forth. She does not actually make these movements, but does them in her mind.

Although there are many relaxation techniques, relaxation cannot really be taught. People learn how to relax *indirectly*. Childbirth classes often include training for conscious release, yet the receptors that control muscle tension do not reach a conscious level in the brain, so conscious release is not physiologically possible. The most effective body-work approach to relaxing a muscle is to tighten the muscle that has the opposite action. Examples of this approach include dragging down the shoulders for tense and elevated shoulder muscles; fingers long, to extend overactive finger flexors; and dragging down the jaw, for tension in the face. As you do these exercises, note which muscles are tense and which are relaxed. Then let go of the tense muscles to permit maximum movement in the intended direction. In actively dropping your jaw you can become aware of relaxation in the muscles of your cheeks.

Mental relaxation must be encouraged along with physical release. These skills form the basis of yoga and meditation programs. Focusing on the natural rhythms of breathing will quiet the mind and facilitate relaxation of the body. Controlling the breath, on the other hand, requires effort, diminishes awareness of the body and impairs relaxation. Couples can experience these phenomena for themselves by alternating controlling breathing with simple observation of it.

The passive state of mental relaxation can also be obtained by repeating the number "one" or any other word silently, or by using a mantra, as in meditation. The procedure, adapted from Herbert Benson's *Relaxation Response, is as follows (note that this exercise does not work well after a heavy meal):*

1. On an empty stomach, in a quiet environment, select a comfortable chair, sit in a relaxed position and close your eyes. Place your feet comfortably on the floor and rest your head against the wall or back of the chair.
2. Deeply relax all your muscles, from your feet to your face-toes, ankles, calves, thighs, lower torso, chest, shoulders, neck, head. If this is hard, try tensing each part and then relaxing it. Squeeze your fists and arm muscles. Then let them relax and hang loosely at your side, on the arms of the chair, or in your lap. Repeat with your feet and legs, squeezing them first and then letting them loose.
3. Breathe normally through your nose. Pay attention to your breathing and to the air moving through your nose. Do not overbreathe. As you breathe out, say "one" or another word silently to yourself. Rather than focusing on breathing, some people find it easier to imagine a pleasant scene.
4. When other thoughts and feelings float into your mind, just let them be. Do not push them away, but do not pay attention to them either. Be indifferent; adopt an "oh, well" attitude. If a reminder (to do something, for example) comes into your mind, open your eyes, get up, write it down, sit back down and start again from the beginning.
5. Continue for ten to twenty minutes. Open your eyes to check the time, but do not use an alarm. If you have done the exercise for too short a time, close your eyes and go back to

it. Then sit quietly for several minutes, at first with your eyes closed and then with them open.

6. Do this exercise daily. Do not expect immediate results and do not expect any results unless you do the exercise on a regular basis. Some people prefer doing the relaxation exercise at the beginning of the day, others at the end of the day. Some do it at both the beginning and the end of each day. Once you have practiced the exercise and feel comfortable with it, you can also use it at times of particular stress.

Breathing in Labor

As part of a changing emphasis in childbirth education, many practitioners are reevaluating traditional psychoprophylactic breathing techniques, such as the Lamaze and Bradley methods. This rethinking recognizes that each woman's labor is different and that women, left to themselves and encouraged to experiment, are capable of finding the laboring position and breathing patterns that work best for them.

Increasingly, controlled patterns of breathing are coming to be considered excessively rigid. This view in no way minimizes their historical importance as a reaction to the totally anesthetized childbirth practiced in the early twentieth century, nor does it deny the continuing appeal of these methods to women who want consciously to control pain in childbirth. All too often, however, women become preoccupied with fixed patterns of breathing that do not respond to the needs of the body. Breathing normally and in response to internal cues, may be more beneficial. The purposeful alteration of breathing, with the goal of pain control through distraction, consumes energy and limits feeling and awareness. Women who have had a normal childbirth often report that lack of energy, rather than unbearable pain, is their most common difficulty during labor. This lack of energy may result from anxiety and tension and may be exacerbated, rather than helped, by the distraction techniques and breathing interventions that have been taught by childbirth educators.

Shallow chest breathing does not permit sufficient fresh air to enter or sufficient stale air to leave the lungs for adequate gas exchange to occur in the tiny air sacs. If this type of breathing becomes rapid, dizziness and light-headedness (symptoms of hyperventilation) may occur as the woman accelerates her breathing to stay on top of her intensifying contractions. Hyperventilation also leads to chemical changes in the blood that decrease its oxygen-carrying capacity and change its acidity. Both effects are undesirable for the fetus.

Although women are commonly taught to achieve an inverse relationship between the speed and depth of respiration (the slower, the deeper; the faster, the more shallow), research has shown that as the breathing rate increases, women in labor do not naturally decrease the amount of air they breathe in and out with each breath. The rate of breathing is the only practical guide for couples. It should not exceed twenty breaths per minute and to stay within optimum limits, it should be much less.

Traditionally, women have been told after full cervical dilatation to "breathe in, hold your breath, and push!" an effort that results in a forced expulsive effort against a closed glottis. This approach is now being reconsidered. The closed-pressure system formed after even five seconds of forced breath retention leads to increased pressure inside the chest, reduced return of blood to the heart and lungs and a reduction of the amount of blood pumped by the heart through the body, including the placenta. Thus, blood flow to the fetus can be impaired. Holding the breath also results in reflex tensing of the pelvic floor, which increases resistance to the baby's descent just the opposite of what is desired.

A more beneficial approach, according to recent thinking, is to push with lips pursed to let air out gently during bearing down in effect, to breathe the baby out. Furthermore, women need to bear down only to the extent that such pushing brings a feeling of relief.

The birthing center at Pithiviers, France, directed by renowned obstetrician Michel Odent, works on the assumption that women know how to give birth if left alone. No formal prenatal instruction is given. Instead, women come to the center about a week before their due date and learn what they need from other women who have just given birth. They spend much time singing around the piano. When they go into labor, they are free to assume any comfortable position, and many labor and give birth in a warm pool. The reported results are excellent.

My opinion is that preparation for labor and delivery, including breathing techniques, should be kept simple, with emphasis on natural events and normal physiology. If childbirth can be seen as an involuntary process that needs only to be allowed to unfold, rather than to be controlled, the laboring woman will be better able to direct her energy within, instead of dissipating it by attempting to put her mind outside her body. Each woman should strive to find her own way, fully recognizing that women already know how to have babies if left to themselves.

Guidelines for Work

Sex during Pregnancy

Sexual feelings during pregnancy may fluctuate widely, from intense passion to no interest whatsoever. For example, in early pregnancy, a woman experiencing morning sickness is not likely to be interested in intercourse with her partner. Several studies indicate a decrease in desire in the third trimester as well. Yet at certain times during pregnancy, some women experience an increased desire for genital sex.

The dramatic changes in a woman's body that are part of a normal pregnancy run counter to some of society's most cherished ideals of beauty. In American society, which tends not to acknowledge and respect the sexuality of the pregnant woman, these changes are thought of as anything but sexual turn-ons. Couples would do well to concentrate on their own positive feelings toward each other, deemphasizing any stereotyped negative feelings toward sexuality, pregnancy and sex and pregnancy.

Intercourse is perfectly permissible during pregnancy, although adjustments in position and penetration will have to be made to accommodate the woman's expanding abdomen. The man-on-top position is too uncomfortable for late pregnancy; a side-by-side or sitting position is preferable. After the baby has dropped, rear-entry positions are particularly comfortable, with the woman kneeling, crouching, or lying. Lots of pillows can be used for support, to keep weight off the abdomen. Pillows and more pillows are to intercourse during pregnancy what a rocking chair is to breast-feeding.

Kitzinger has pointed out that in advanced pregnancy, it may be better for the man to ejaculate and withdraw just before a woman comes to orgasm. An erect penis in a heavily pregnant woman may prevent her from making the kind of pelvic movements that will bring on orgasm. In pregnancy, as at other times, the man should be aware that the clitoris can be overstimulated. A good general rule is that, once the clitoris has become swollen, the man should ask the woman when she wants penetration.

Table 7.3. When to Terminate Various Levels of Work During a Normal, Uncomplicated Pregnancy

Job Function	May Work to (weeks)
Secretarial, light clerical, professional, managerial	40
Seated; light tasks (prolonged or intermittent)	40
Standing	
Prolonged (more than 4 hrs)	24
Intermittent (more than 30 min/hr)	32
Intermittent (less than 30 min/hr)	40
Stooping and bending below knee level	
Repetitive (more than 10 times/hr)	20
Intermittent (between 2-10 times/hr)	28
Intermittent (less than 2 times /hr)	40
Climbing Vertical ladders and poles	
Repetitive (more than 4 times/8 hr shift)	28
Intermittent (less than 4 times /8 hr shift)	28
Stairs	
Repetitive (more than 4 times/8 hr shift)	28
Intermittent (less than 4 times /8 hr shift)	40
Lifting	
Repetitive	
More than 50 lbs	20
25 to 50 lbs	24
Less than 25 lbs	40
Intermittent	
More than 50 lbs	30
25 to 50 lbs	40
Less than 25 lbs	40

During pregnancy, many couples prefer to express sexual feelings in ways other than intercourse cuddling, showering together, massage, or caresses that lead to orgasm. The sensitivity of a woman's breasts and nipples often markedly increases in pregnancy. Breasts can become the focus of erotic arousal, but need to be handled gently. Pregnancy offers couples the opportunity to explore new forms of sexual expression, which can be continued after the birth.

Pioneering childbirth researcher Niles Newton identified eleven points of comparison between undisturbed childbirth and sexual excitement:

1. Change in breathing.
2. Tendency to make vocal noises.
3. Facial expression reminiscent of an athlete under great strain.
4. Rhythmic contraction of the upper segment of the uterus.
5. Loosening of the mucous plug from the opening of the cervix
6. Periodic contractions of the uterus.
7. Use of a position in which the woman's legs are drawn up and spread apart (a dated observation, as women do not necessarily give birth or have intercourse in this position) .
8. A tendency to become uninhibited.
9. Unusual muscular strength.
10. A tendency to be unaware of the world, and a sudden return to alert awareness after climax (orgasm) or birth.
11. A feeling of joy and well-being following the orgasm or birth.

The degree to which a couple can experience labor and delivery in such sexual terms will depend on the setting in which birth takes place and how it is conducted. Relaxation and a sense of security are important factors. Common fears regarding intercourse and orgasm during pregnancy relate to precipitation of an abortion (miscarriage), initiation of premature labor and causing harm to the fetus in some way. There is no evidence that intercourse causes miscarriages, although it may be the precipitating factor in a pregnancy that is destined to abort. Although there is some evidence that intercourse and orgasm may trigger the onset of labor, research findings are divided on this question; the consensus is that intercourse is not a factor in premature labor. There is no evidence that intercourse harms the fetus. If certain conditions are present or suspected, intercourse during late pregnancy is best avoided:

1. Broken amniotic sac, allowing communication between the uterus and vagina and thus increasing the chances of infection of both the uterus and the fetus.
2. Premature labor.
3. Placenta previa.
4. Impaired well-being of the fetus for example, if the infant is suspected of having intrauterine growth disturbance.

Born of Baby Later in Life

The number of American women over the age of thirty-five who are having children is steadily increasing as more women postpone parenthood because of career choices. Women over thirty-five and their fetuses do face special problems. However, data from the Royal Victoria Hospital in Canada (reported by Ruth Fretts and her colleagues) show that if serious genetic problems and birth defects are eliminated by genetic testing and therapeutic abortion and if the women are treated properly for chronic illnesses such as diabetes and hypertension, 994 of 1,000 babies will be born alive to older women compared with 997 in 1,000 for younger women, a difference of 3 per 1,000. With modern treatment the difference in maternal mortality based on age, once significant, can be largely eliminated. Thus the news for older pregnant women is very encouraging.

Problems remain, some of them without ready answers. Older pregnant women are more likely to have placenta previa or placental abruption and to require cesarean sections. Fetuses of older women are at increased risk for miscarriage, fetal defects, premature birth, and stillbirth. Because older women are more likely than younger women to have a chronic illness, such as hypertension, that requires treatment, decisions about drugs safest for the fetus will have to be made, preferably before conception.

Children and Birth

There is an increased focus on preparing older children for the birth and arrival of a new sibling. Some parents choose to include an older child during labor and delivery; many do not. In any case, thoughtful preparation of the older child is important.

Many parents who have been through the experience of preparing an older child for the arrival of a sibling emphasize three points:

1. The key to success in preparation is the attitude of the parents; if the child is to be unafraid, enthusiastic and excited about the birth, the parents must be that way, too.
2. The bonding that takes place after birth should occur not only between the parents and the newborn but between the older child and the new sibling as well.
3. Children participate to the degree to which they are comfortable. They should not be forced or pressured to do more than they want to do; and they should be permitted as much or as little involvement as they can comfortably handle.

Conveying the Unfolding of Pregnancy and the Time of Birth

Parents should tell their child about the expected baby as soon as they are sure the woman is pregnant. Many parents say their child needed the nine months to prepare as much as they did. Even though time is a difficult concept for small children, they seem able to grasp it if it is linked to their own experiences. Some parents use the signs of the seasons to convey the passage of time. If, for example, the baby is due in June, a parent may say something like, "First there will be fall, when the leaves turn pretty colors; then winter, when the trees are bare and it is cold and snow is on the ground; then spring, when the crocuses peep above the ground and the willows turn yellow; then the forsythia, then the lilacs and then our baby will be born when the roses bloom." Of course, the age of the child will be a factor in trying to convey time this way; but this pattern can be understood by children as young as two and a half years, who may memorize and repeat the sequence.

One mother said she used pictures showing the month-by-month changes in the uterus and fetus to make up a time line for the wall of her daughter's room. Sources of pictures for such a time line include the illustrated booklets given out by many physicians and midwives, sets of posters available in stores and illustrations copied from picture books on pregnancy (see Appendix). By adding the appropriate picture to the time line each month, the child gets a clear sense of the progression of the pregnancy from the pictures as well as from his or her mother's increasing girth. Another kind of time line is a series of photographs of the mother, perhaps taken by the child, showing the changing configuration of her body throughout the pregnancy.

Another idea that works particularly well for children between ages two and eight is to make a special calendar they can use to count down to the due date, beginning at about thirty-eight weeks. (We suggest having the calendar run at least two weeks beyond the due date in case the baby arrives late.) Each day on the calendar is a small movable door or window that opens to reveal a picture or surprise, preferably related to new life such as a baby animal toy, a toy robin's egg, or seeds.

Family Celebrations and Activities

Family celebrations holidays, birthdays, festivals can be used to convey passage of time before the birth of the baby. Some religious and ethnic groups have holidays with strong associations for children. For Christians, Christmas, with its focus on baby Jesus, is the time to celebrate babies in general, first anticipating their coming, then marveling at their birth, and finally rejoicing in their arrival. Repeating Christmas traditions that center on the birth of a baby (such as the calendar just described, which is similar to an Advent calendar, candles around the house, or familiar music) helps young children get into the spirit of the event and makes it real for them. The same can be achieved with birthday customs already followed in the family cake and candles, presents, singing, and retelling family members' memories of past birthdays. Children of all ages and adults too, love to hear the story of their birth. Retelling and rehearing their own beginnings helps them prepare for another birth in the family.

Many parents have found that focusing attention on a pet helps a child understand that another being needs care and space of its own and has a will of its own and that its needs must be respected. Parents can take their children to visit younger animals in pet shops, in children's zoos, or in the homes of friends to let them experience new lives. With pets, children can learn, over a period of time, that care is a never-ending circle of love and attention. Of course, contact with human babies is even more to the point.

The idea of a nickname may come from the child when he or she refers to the baby during the pregnancy. If not, parents can suggest one, realizing it may not catch on. One eighteen-month-old had a beloved doll she called "Wolly". When she saw her mother's belly growing, she transferred the name to the baby inside. She would talk to "Wolly" and pat her mother's stomach. The nickname did not stick after little sister Katy's birth, but it did help the toddler relate to her new sibling during the pregnancy.

Often it helps to talk about the baby as a special gift to the whole family, to be cared for by everyone, just as the older child was a special gift to the parents. The older child may then more easily appreciate the idea of preparing gifts for when the baby is born (receiving blankets, quilts, decorated T-shirts, mobiles, special songs). Children can participate in making these gifts. Families who enjoy music together can make up or choose a particular song to welcome the new baby. They can rehearse it together before the baby comes so that it becomes a kind of theme song in the home for many days, or even years, after the birth.

Events Surrounding Childbirth

The caregiver and the developmental level and interest of the child, older children may be included in visits to the midwife or doctor. Parents can explain that these people will be present to help with the birth of the baby. As the pregnancy advances, children usually enjoy listening to the heartbeat and feeling the fetus kick and move around. If at all possible, children should be included in visits to the hospital to meet the doctor or to look through the nursery window. If a home birth is planned, parents should explain to an older child that the woman might have to go to the hospital for help.

Parents may want to bring a child to some childbirth classes. Classes that use slides and pictures of births are particularly useful, depending on the interests and age of the child. Birth movies can give a child who will be attending a home birth a real sense of the sights and sounds of birth. Children can meet the midwife, nurse, or labor coach. Class leaders can suggest well-illustrated, informative books on birth and the arrival of a new baby, as can libraries and bookstores.

Visits to friends who have new babies, especially those whose pregnancies the child may have followed, are helpful. Contact with babies gives children a better idea of what newborns are like how tiny and helpless they are and how gentle and loving one must be with them. Children often enjoy watching and imitating the exercises a woman does in preparation for birth, including relaxation and breathing techniques.

Depending on the age and temperament of the child, parents may want to discuss any fears he or she has about the birth, for example, what happens if the baby does not breathe right away. It is important to be alert to the child's questions and observations and to be aware of the deeper meanings they convey. Children at any age can have distorted ideas of birth, and by listening, parents will have a good chance to correct them.

Including a Sibling at the Birth

If you plan to have children present at the actual birth, assuming this is an option at the site you have chosen for labor and delivery, you need to do extra preparation. Talk about the hard work of pushing the baby out and the concentration and patience it takes to have a baby. Show them the different positions you might assume, and let them hear the kinds of sounds you might make. One family played a tape of their first labor to their older child the sounds of his own birth to accustom him to the sounds he would here.

Don't forget to talk about blood the good blood and its purpose and value when the baby is born. Talk about how a baby looks when it first comes out of the mother and about the importance of the placenta to the baby.

Give the child a task. Four- and five-year-olds can give you ice chips and orange juice, for example. Older children can help time contractions, wipe your face with a washcloth, hold your hand, breathe along with you, hold a flashlight (at a home birth) and so forth. Although most children want to feel useful at a birth, expect that they may also need to be out of the room for a while. Make them as aware as possible before the birth that they can choose to be there or not and that whatever they choose is all right with you.

Identify a caretaker for the child. Unless children are well into their teens, most will need someone at the birth who is there solely for them. Explain that while Mommy is having the baby, she won't be able to give him or her the same kind of attention and care that she normally does. For this reason, this other familiar and loved person will be there. The person you choose for the caretaker role should be comfortable with birth in the setting you have chosen. Consider having this person join you at several childbirth classes and show him or her the books about pregnancy and birth that you particularly like. Also, this "birth-sitter" should understand that if the child does not want to be present at the birth, that is fine, and his or her job is to stay with the child.

Define the father's role at the birth. Will he be the caretaker for the child and leave others to support the mother, or does he want to be primarily involved with her? The child should know in advance what role the father will play.

A surprise bag of goodies, suitable to the age of the child, will keep most children interested and peaceful during what might be a long labor. For young children, these small treats are often the most exciting part. Their interest will alternate between the items in the bag and aspects of the labor and delivery.

Parents who have included their older children in a birth say that it does not eliminate sibling rivalry. But, as one parent reported, "There seems to be a deep reservoir of trust and love from the older to the younger," because, as her three-year-old said to the baby, "I saw you born".

One four year-old was overheard describing to a friend of the same age the recent birth at which she was present: "Mommy cried, the baby cried, and there was blood, but it was good blood".

Following the Birth

When the mother first sees her older child at the hospital or at home, she should reassure him or her that she is fine, physically tired, perhaps, but in no way hurt or unrecognizable. She is still the same person, still the child's mother. Birth is such a dramatic happening that a young child, particularly a child under age six, may feel that the world has turned upside down. The child should see his or her mother behaving normally again walking, talking and laughing especially if the child was present at birth and witnessed his or her mother assuming strange positions and making odd, possibly frightening noises.

The mother should make time during the days following birth for some quiet cuddling and spending time with the older child alone, perhaps when her partner or friend is with the baby.

Depending on the child's age and temperament, he or she may ask for a lot of this kind of physical reassurance immediately or may act reserved and reject the mother's attention. Sometimes this diffidence comes from a feeling of awe toward the mother and the new baby, and sometimes from a feeling of anger and a fear of rejection. Such withdrawal is a common reaction, particularly in children aged five to eight.

Children need time to integrate the experience of birth, just as parents do. If parents continue to show that they love and care for the older child as well as for the new baby, then the child can share affection and positive feelings toward his or her mother and the new baby at his or her own pace. Older children, as well as parents, need time to bond with the newborn. They should have as much freedom as possible within the limits of safety for the infant to explore, touch, kiss and handle the new sibling. With a younger child, parents may have to make it very clear from the beginning that they will not allow the baby to be hurt or even pressed too firmly. A parent can demonstrate touch to the child by encouraging him or her to hug the baby gently; touch the baby's hair, hands and feet; and even hold the baby. Each day special playtime for the newborn and the sibling should be set aside.

A festive birthday party for the newborn can be a long-remembered highlight for siblings. Older children can help in the preparations, such as making and decorating the cake. The party is the time for the special song or for a version of "Happy Birthday". If the celebration includes champagne, children can have their own small glasses with juice or soda, so they can join in the toasts. Children love to receive and give gifts and gift giving can express love within the family. Gifts to the older child from the parents, the new baby, and others and gifts from the older child to the new brother or sister are all appropriate. For preschool children, well-chosen books are particularly fitting. For children who like dolls, they are especially appropriate gifts. A special area where the child can care for the doll can be set up with replicas of the equipment used in caring for the real baby changing table, diapers and bottles. Items can be added over time to keep the child's interest.

A big jar filled with packets of nutritious snacks (raisins, nuts, sesame sticks) that are especially for the older sibling can head off difficulties with the older child during nursing times (a La Leche

League suggestion). The child can have his or her own snack at nursing time and sit with mother and baby. The child might enjoy decorating the jar and putting his or her name on it. The jar should be one the child can open and should be kept within reach.

Bath time can be a delightful opportunity to include the older child. Newborns love water and it seems to have a soothing and pleasurable effect on children of all ages, whether they need to be scrubbed or not. With adult supervision, the older child can support the baby in the water and feel very useful and trusted. Time spent touching and caressing during the bath and immediately after can teach lessons in gentleness and care. After the bath, a little warm oil can be massaged into the baby's skin.

A picture sign can teach a small child about the importance of not disturbing a sleeping infant. The sign can depict each member of the family engaged in quiet activity while the baby is sleeping. When the baby needs to sleep, the older child can hang the sign on the baby's door. The child will quickly learn about a baby's need to sleep without being disturbed.

Older children will probably experience jealousy toward the baby and long for the good old days when they had their mother all to themselves. It is important that children understand and eventually accept that the baby is here to stay, but it is equally important that both parents take time to do things individually or together with older children. If there is more than one older child, parents need to make sure that whoever was the baby before does not get dropped by the older siblings in favor of the new arrival. Parents may need to talk about this with the older children before the birth. Even if the father is the primary caretaker for the older child during the few weeks following birth, it is important for the mother to spend time with the child as well. After those first few weeks, even if a woman is busy nursing the baby full time, there will always be some brief periods when the sleeping baby can be left with another adult while the mother takes the older child on one of those favorite trips to the library, park, or ice-cream parlor. There should be special time each day at home for the older child to read, talk, cuddle and play with the mother while the baby sleeps.

8

Artificial Insemination and Assisted Reproductive Technologies

Introduction

The new advances in reproductive technology, or what has been termed "collaborative conception", it is now possible for a child to have up to five "parents": an egg donor, a sperm donor, a surrogate mother who gestates the fetus, and the couple who actually raise the child. From reading the biblical account of Sarah directing her husband, Abraham, to conceive a child with the assistance of her handmaiden, Hagar, it is evident that the practice of surrogate motherhood has existed for years.

For many, infertility, sterility, genetic incompatibilities and/or physical handicaps do not in any way appear to diminish the need for having children in order to have what is regarded as a complete marriage. Adoption is often a long, complicated procedure lasting anywhere from four to six years. For many couples, continuation of the blood line is of central importance. With the assistance of surrogates, such continuation can be achieved anywhere from a year and a half to two years. Married women who share this view have been known to state: "I want my husband's baby even if someone else carries it". 211 It is astonishing and incongruous to realize that, with children in such great demand for some, there presently exists some 400,000 or more unwanted children in foster care arrangements. Tragically, time, circumstances and socioeconomic conditions often change parental attitudes after an infant is added to the family unit with the result being that the sought after and prized child all too often becomes an unwanted liability.

An early 1969 Harris opinion survey of some sixteen hundred adults from throughout the country concerning advances and applications of the new developing biology revealed a fascinating attitudinal profile. Of all interviewed, 19 percent approved of AID, or heterologous, donor insemination, while 56 percent disapproved of the process. Where the sole method to achieve conception is by use of the AID procedure, that is, obtaining semen from a donor and injecting by syringe into the woman's reproductive tract, 35 percent of those interviewed approved of the technique. Forty-nine percent of the men interviewed in the survey agreed in principle with homologous insemination, that is, taking semen from the husband. Sixty-two percent of the women interviewed approved of pregnancies achieved by the artificial injection of their husbands' semen where physical or psychological difficulties precluded fertilization through sexual intercourse.

Another sampling of public opinion occurred in 1978, shortly after the first recorded *in vitro* success of "Baby Louise Brown's" birth in England, when Gallup conducted a poll to determine American attitudes concerning the process of IVF. The poll revealed public approval of the procedure by a two-to-one margin. A majority stated they would be willing to follow this procedure if they were childless and wished to have offspring. Nationwide, 53 percent would undergo this medical intervention and 36 percent would not. While no sophisticated studies have been conducted regarding the public's acceptance or rejection of surrogate motherhood, there is every indication that it will not be universally accepted or rejected. Rather, a case-by-case response will be forthcoming with the reasons for the initial action being carefully scrutinized.

In a 1994 opinion survey by the Roper Center for Public Opinion Research, 71 percent of those 701 individuals polled said it was wrong for a man to sell his sperm for purposes of artificial insemination. Yet, if the sperm were given as a gift, 59 percent said it would be proper and 35 percent said it would be wrong to assist a couple who could not otherwise conceive in this way. When women in the survey were asked if they would consider paying another woman to be artificially inseminated with their husband's sperm and carrying the baby to term because of their own incapacity to achieve this, 76 percent of the respondents would not consider such actions while twenty percent said they would.

Artificial Father

Generally, in dealing with heterologous AID cases, the donor is unknown. The major issues involve whether the putative father (i.e., the husband of the artificially inseminated mother) becomes the legal father of the artificially conceived child and whether the wife has committed adultery by participating in the act with or without her husband's consent.

In 1948 the New York Supreme Court recognized that a woman artificially inseminated by a third-party donor, with her husband's consent, gave birth to a legitimate child. The woman's husband was "entitled to the same rights as that acquired by a foster parent who has formally adopted a child, if not the same rights as those to which a natural parent under the circumstances would be entitled".

With the case of *Gursky v. Gursky* in 1963, however, a New York trial court held that even though a husband consents to his wife's use of AID, the child is nonetheless illegitimate. In 1968 a considerably more enlightened and contemporary California Supreme Court in *People v. Sorensen* rejected the *Gursky* thesis and held that a husband who gives his consent to his wife's use of AID intervention cannot disclaim his lawful fatherhood of the child for the purpose of child support. The court construed a state penal nonsupport statute to incorporate liability of a consenting father of the AID child finding a genetic relationship, as such, unnecessary in order to establish the required father-child relationship.

A considerable degree of sophistication was shown by the New York Supreme Court in 1973 with its holding in *Adoption of Anonymous*. Instead of adhering blindly to *Gursky*, the court found a strong state policy favoring legitimacy. Furthermore, the court acknowledged that a child born of consensual artificial insemination by a donor, accomplished during a valid marriage, was legitimate and thereby entitled to enjoy all rights and privileges of a child who was conceived in a natural way by the same marriage.

Since *Sorensen* and *Anonymous,* a growing number of states have passed legislation making legitimate the offspring of AID when the husband consents to the procedure. Twenty-four states have chosen to enact legislation that refuses to treat the donor as the father of a child conceived from artificial insemination. For the majority of states addressing donor insemination, the provisions of the Uniform Parentage Act are followed thereby providing that the donor sperm used by a married couple does not confer recognition on the donor of legal fatherhood of a child conceived by assisted conception so long as the procedure itself is supervised by a licensed physician.

Where states chose not to define the legal rights of the sperm donor, paternity may still be established if it is pursued by the legitimacy statutes as an issue of fact. Thus, courts confronted with such a matter, would consider not only the intent of the parties as substantiated or modified by the parties subsequent behavior, but the placement of the name of the donor on the certificate of birth, for example, or the declaration by the donor of his paternity. What these judicial and legislative actions indicate clearly, then, is that both these branches of government no longer equate AID with adultery as they once did and may even signal the public's willingness to sanction more startling genetic developments and to legitimate heretofore illegitimate conduct.

In 1977 a New Jersey court held that an unmarried woman, who conceived a child through sperm artificially donated by a friend, was required to allow custodial and visitation rights for the donor despite her wishes but consistent with what was perceived as the best interests of the child. Even though refusing to take a specific position on the propriety of the use of artificial insemination between unmarried persons, the court recognized the donor as the *natural* father and imposed on him the responsibility to support and maintain the child.

Today, with the social and legal recognition of equality of rights for women and of their reproductive autonomy granted by the U.S. Supreme Court in *Roe v. Wade,* the issue of the necessity of a husband's consent for an act to be performed on his wife's body has become less significant. Nonetheless, it is to be hoped that married women who contemplate offering to become surrogate mothers, or submit to AID for their personal benefit or desire to have a child, will do so only after consultation with their husbands. Failure to disclose such acts may be tantamount to deceit.

Donor Confidentiality versus the Right to Know

A rather interesting and far-reaching precedent in the field of adoption law could, if construed broadly, seriously jeopardize donor secrecy in AID cases. A District of Columbia Superior Court Judge ruled that a twenty-two-year-old mother of two living in Takoma Park, Maryland, who was adopted as a child, should be granted permission to see her sealed birth records and thus learn the identities of her natural parents. The plaintiff in this case asserted her "basic right" to know her total historical identity, and also to discover whether hereditary diseases or other health problems were a part of her genetic inheritance.

A comparable argument can obviously be made by the progeny of AID. The argument for disclosure would gain even more persuasiveness in light of dramatic findings presented in the *NEW ENGLAND JOURNAL OF MEDICINE*. Statistics from a 1979 study showed that sperm from one donor had in fact been used to produce fifty children and thus raised the very real danger of accidental incest among offspring who have the same father. The article also recorded the sloppiness of some doctors in failing to screen genetically the donors who participate in AID procedures. A mere 29 percent of the doctors tested the donors of semen—and then primarily for communicable diseases. Most recipients were inseminated twice per cycle. Seventeen percent of the physicians used the same donor for a given recipient and 32 percent used multiple donors within a single cycle. Only 37 percent kept records on children and only 30 percent kept records on donors. The identity of donors usually was carefully guarded to ensure privacy in order to avoid legal complications. Interestingly, most donors have been over time medical students or resident physicians, thus prompting concern by some that eugenic decisions are made by using "superior" genes for donor insemination.

Of 711 physicians likely to perform artificial insemination by donors surveyed to determine their current practices, 471 responded, and 379 reported that they performed this procedure. They accounted for approximately 3,576 births by this means in 1977. In addition to treating infertility, 26 percent of these physicians used the procedure to prevent transmission of a genetic disease and 10 percent used it for single women. Donors of semen were only superficially screened for genetic diseases and were then matched phenotypically to the recipient's husband.

Subsequent studies have shown the very high degree of carelessness if, indeed, not negligence many doctors exhibit in performing AID. Serious legal cases of "wandering sperm" have arisen when women have alleged that due to the negligent actions of sperm banks or physicians or both in administering inseminations, they have been impregnated with wrong sperm. Additional actions growing from such failed undertakings would be for breach of contract if the sperm banks storing the semen failed to maintain its promised viability together with negligence or strict liability for those participating physicians who failed to properly screen the sperm donors and recipients for infectious diseases.

In 1987 a report of the Congressional Office of Technology Assessment found only 10 percent of 1,558 physicians surveyed tested regularly the sperm donations for the HIV virus. The report found an absence of federal regulatory programming in this area and few states with laws screening sperm donations designed, as such, to protect either the female recipients or possible offspring.

Suppose a donor of semen, at age thirty-four, discovers that he is a carrier of the congenital abnormality Huntington's chorea. His bodily movements become involuntary and his mental abilities become progressively disoriented. Death is certain. Realizing that he was a donor of semen at age twenty-one when he was a law school student, he approaches the physician who administered the artificial intervention and advises him of his condition. The physician advises, regrettably, that his records of the insemination are incomplete. Sensing a grave responsibility, he seeks to learn the identity of those children whom he fathered artificially. He wishes to provide some type of financial assistance for his offspring and/or make provision in his estate for them before he dies. *Quaere*: Should a court of law consider a best interest of the child test, an average ordinary donor's wishes under similar circumstances standard, or a best interest of society test, in ruling on a resolution of this dilemma? If a court-ordered investigation discloses the donor's issue, should they be told of the situation without a revelation of their donorfather's identity? Does the donor in such a hypothetical case as this have a right to know the identity of his progeny even though they were conceived artificially? Why should not the same right to know be provided the donor in cases of this nature as the adopted child is being given some jurisdictions to learn the identity of its birth parents? Even without legal validation of the right to know genetic lineage, all too often independent investigatory means are employed and the missing identity established.

Provisions within the Uniform Parentage Act provide that all records involving AID interventions are to be kept "confidential and in a sealed file". Inspection of records is only sanctioned when a court order acknowledges the existence of "good cause". By drawing upon analogous right-to-know parental-identity cases arising in regular adoption areas, "good cause," in order to discern the identity of a donor in artificial insemination cases, could be determined to exist not only for reasons of obtaining complete medical information regarding the child's donor-father but also for such additional reasons such as allowing the AID child to resolve questions of identity and promote social adjustment, establishing a bond of love, promoting a wish to be of genuine assistance and support to a biological family unit and determining if the rules of intestate succession were applicable.

Future of Artificial Insemination

As the courts begin to recognize "a best interest of the child test" in deciding vexatious cases involving artificial insemination, it would surely appear that where genetic heritage is brought into question concerning the health and well-being of an AID child, the confidential files (*if* such are maintained) of a participating physician to an AID intervention, should be examined by a judge *in camera* and, where necessary, with the assistance of a geneticist. Although a strong argument against disclosure of the donor's identity can be made, the exigencies and circumstances of each case should be considered. And, where the utility of the good in maintaining the confidentiality of the donor's identity is outweighed by the gravity of the "harm" that will arise as a consequence of disclosure, then the veil of confidentiality should be pierced.

Greater safeguards must be undertaken in order to preserve the integrity and value of artificial insemination as a medico-legal process. If physicians are not sufficiently careful in their supervision and administration of the AID process, then the state must act in order to guarantee higher standards of professional care and competence. When a physician is negligent in properly screening prospective donors for artificial insemination, and a genetic abnormality thus passes undetected to the issue the physician must always be held liable for the consequences of his error.

In addition to continued judicial activism, legislative implementation should be sought by creating presumptions at law of the legitimacy of issue born of consensual AID and thus clarifying both the legal rights and duties of the husband. To the extent that greater confidentiality of donor records would be strengthened, additional adoptions of the Uniform Parentage Act should be advocated.

Surrogate Mother

The surrogate mother has been regarded correctly as the female counterpart to AID. This concept embraces several processes of surrogate parenthood. One is the embryo implant in which a married woman's eggs are fertilized by her husband's semen *in vitro* and then implanted in specific human female carriers or "incubators". Another process might be the simple use of semen from a married woman's husband and the insertion of that semen into a female donor or surrogate who will, under a bilateral contract for services rendered, carry the issue to term and after birth, release all her rights to the child by allowing adoption by the biological father and putative mother. Additional situations might arise in which maternally carried dominant genetic disorders exist, where a married woman's eggs would not accept fertilization, or where ovarian failures would arise and prevent the woman from conceiving but which would not preclude her from carrying another woman's embryo. Thus, a reverse surrogate mother situation would exist where a married man's semen was used *in vitro* to fertilize another woman's eggs with the embryo then being implanted into the married man's spouse.

The attitudes that prompt a woman to become a surrogate mother have been isolated to three or four. Some women possess either a sentimental or a maternal instinct, or a fascination with having a child. Others feel a sense of altruism which advances a wish to help others experience that which has been a part of the surrogate's life. Still others have cited a need for money as a reason for seeking the status of surrogate motherhood.

Policy Issues—Legality of the Bargain

A number of vexatious policy issues are inherent in any consideration of surrogate motherhood. Some issues may be resolved now, others must await the test of time to be both sharpened and clarified before a resolution will emerge.

If an illegal performance promised bilaterally or unilaterally is regarded as being heinous, criminal, or immoral to a high degree, courts normally will not enforce the promise that accompanies such performance. Before such drastic judicial action is taken, however, the court will give due consideration to the degree of the offense, the extent of public harm involved if the bargain is recognized as valid, and the nature of the moral quality of the conduct of the parties to the bargain in light of current community standards. Obviously, as times change, so too does the public policy relevant to the particular issue under consideration or in controversy. Public policy in this context may be defined simply as a legal principle which declares an act either to be unlawful (i.e., that which promotes corruption or immorality) or which has a "tendency" to be injurious to either the welfare, health, or morality of the public.

State Positions

A number of states make it a crime to pay anything of value to a parent in consideration for obtaining consent to adopt or obtain custody of a child and impose a heavy penalty or imprisonment for violation thereof. In this way, some deterrent exists to prevent extensive "black market" operations in adoptions. Since the legality of a contract is tested by and depends on the place where it is made, a jurisdiction having such a law would hold a contract between a husband and wife with a surrogate mother, in which the latter relinquished her parental rights to an infant born of such a contract for subsequent adoption by the natural father and putative mother, to be illegal and thus invalid. The bargain is an *adoption* contract. Now, if this same contractual relation is viewed as a contract to *bear* a child, less objection and greater acceptance of the contract, itself, should be recognized simply because the purchaser is the natural father of the child. With such a consideration, fears of commercialization become less worrisome as a competing or undermining factor over the interests of the child or the biological mother.

Interestingly, an unmarried man would encounter even less legal entanglement in dealing with a surrogate. Since no wife would be involved, it would be unnecessary for a man to adopt his own child. He would simply pay the surrogate without risk and, as natural father of the child, take custody upon birth without any formal adoption procedure being required.

Perhaps the easiest way in which to avoid the issue of illegality surrounding contracts to adopt a child or to bear one would be to have the contracting parents either make a simple gift, conditional or absolute, or a voluntary declaration of trust to the surrogate mother.

Presumptions of Paternity

The Uniform Parentage Act, although adopted in only eighteen states, presents an initial obstacle to the establishment of paternity in surrogate contract situations. Section 5 of the act controls the use of artificial insemination and provides: "The donor of semen provided to a licensed physician for use in artificial insemination of a married woman other than the donor's wife is treated in law as if he were not the natural father of a child thereby conceived." While it appears rather obvious that this provision was crafted in order to protect anonymous AID donors from all legal responsibility for those children fathered as a consequence of their donations of semen, if the provision is adopted *in toto* this language could well establish a difficulty for the real father under a surrogate contract to establish either paternity or to assert parental rights, such as visitation.

Children born of a validated marital union are presumed to be the legitimate issue of that union. Regardless of their adoption of the Uniform Parentage Act, all of the states have recognized this presumption. Thus, if a surrogate is married, the issue she bears will be presumed, unless rebutted by proof beyond a reasonable doubt, to be the legitimate child or herself and her husband not of the artificial donor of the sperm. If the donor or biological father brought a custody suit and upon proof (again, beyond a reasonable doubt) that he was in fact the biological father, it would then fall to the court to determine which parent or set of parents could better serve the long term interests of the child.

Section four of the Uniform Parentage Act also establishes presumptions of paternity. When, for example, a man, after a child's birth, receives a child under the age of majority into his home and openly holds the child out as his natural child, a presumption arises, which may be rebutted only by clear and convincing evidence, that the man is the natural father of the child. Another provision allows for the establishment of a presumption of paternity when the man purporting to be the natural father acknowledges his paternity of the questioned child by filing a written statement with the appropriate court or administrative agency, informing the biological mother of this public acknowledgment and no dispute of this acknowledgment occurs. Again, this presumption is to be rebutted only by clear and convincing evidence.

A liberal construction of these provisions of the Uniform Parentage Act could modify the rigidity of the provisions regarding issue born of artificial insemination and thereby enable a surrogate contract father to establish his paternity. To avoid confusion in both interpretation and implementation of the Uniform Act, however, it would be wise to modify the act in such a manner so as to provide a specific provision or state a specific presumption establishing a mechanism for the biological father to establish his unquestioned paternity in surrogate contracts.

Additional Policy Issues

The parallel relationship between AID and contracts to bear children is inescapable. Yet, while donor identity is generally assured of confidentiality in heterologous insemination, the identity of a surrogate mother is generally known by the contract couple. Appearance, in fact, is often a major consideration, together with the prospective surrogate's medical history, education level, environment and cultural background, in making a judgment as to the suitability of a surrogate. Because of the increased potential for genetic anomalies in births by women over thirty-five years of age, this age is usually the cutoff for surrogate candidacy. The availability of the pool of candidates is, furthermore, normally limited to women who are presently married or have been divorced. Single, unwed women are regarded generally as not suitable simply because their involvement would not only be regarded in some circles as promoting immorality (and perhaps technically adultery) but as a practical matter, an unproven record of birth successes might also promote a further element of uncertainty for the contracting parties which is undesirable. The right of a single, unmarried woman to control her own physical autonomy is an ever-evolving concept measured in proportion to the degree of state interest in preserving the public welfare and morals. The right of a married woman to act or conduct her marital affairs without the informed consent of her husband, specifically to submit herself to surrogate mother status, remains an open-ended question as well.

Perhaps an even more unsettled issue is the extent of the surrogate's autonomy during the period of the pregnancy versus the extent and nature of the right of control of her and the fetus by the biological husband and his wife. If, for example, after agreeing to abstain from uses of alcoholic beverages during the pregnancy, the surrogate does in fact imbibe on a regular basis, could a court order be obtained to stop such consumption? If so, how could it be enforced? By total restraint (i.e., hospital confinement)? Suppose the surrogate did not reveal her propensity to consume alcohol (or unprescribed drugs) and upon birth, the child is born with a genetic impairment or defect which is determined to be as a direct consequence of the actions of the surrogate. Could the surrogate be sued for negligence? Suppose, further, neither the husband nor his wife wish to raise the defective child as their own, and the surrogate does not wish to either. Should a penalty be assessed against all concerned parties because of this "misdeed"? In such a situation, the infant would likely become a ward of the state, and therefore a responsibility of the taxpayers if and until an adoption could be arranged.

Other issues arise in the area of physician negligence. If a physician is negligent in failing to screen adequately a prospective surrogate mother candidate and upon birth the infant is born with a genetic deficiency, might a suit for malpractice be obtained against the attending physician or the surrogate? Suppose a surrogate decides to keep the contract baby. Could she in turn sue the biological father for child support? As a practical matter, it would appear that in a case where a court decreed the biological surrogate mother had a right to keep her child and assuming the mother had insufficient funds to support herself and the child that financial support by the biological father would be in the best interests of the child and of the state. But, *quaere,* given this hypothetical, would it not be arguably best for all concerned to have the child in a stable economic environment with its biological father and his wife instead of being placed and raised in the possibly impoverished environment of its biological mother alone and no adoptive father? Yet another interesting question is raised in the case where the surrogate suffers mental trauma or a complete breakdown after relinquishing the baby to the biological father and his wife. Would the surrogate be able to sue the contracting parents for damages?

Further unanswered issues may arise with changes in the status of the contracting couple. What if the contracting couple divorced or one or both died before the surrogate gave birth? What would be the status of the infant upon birth? Would the contract be voided for impossibility of performance and the child recognized as illegitimate and a subsequent ward of the state? Obviously, if the biological father died, severe difficulty would be encountered in establishing the paternity of the infant. Assume further that upon the death of the biological father, the surrogate decided that she wished to keep the infant that she bore, but the widow wanted her husband's child. Would Solomonic wisdom be called into play dictating the birth mother win out over a widow who might never be able to have a child?

To anticipate or forestall these complexities and others that might arise, it is imperative that a tightly drawn contract be executed which defines the rights and responsibilities of all parties and establishes a mechanism or procedure for assessing damages for violations thereof. Clarity of terms and specification of duties will go far toward assisting a court to construe the provisions of a contract of this nature and at the same time, to determine the intent of the contracting parties. Absent such a controlling instrument and definitive legislation in the area, it will fall upon the courts to employ a rather traditional equitable balancing test in determining the merits or demerits of each issue in a surrogate contract case; thus, the gravity of the "harm" (economic, social, personal, religious, etc.) of holding one particular way according to the plaintiff's case, will be weighed against the utility of the "good" (economic, social, personal, religious, etc.) in sustaining defendant's case-in-chief. Fluidity and flexibility, then, become the coordinates of action instead of predictability and stability.

Inextricably related to this area of concern are various religious considerations. Indeed, these considerations remain a serious point of contention to a complete understanding, acceptance and advancement of the aspects of the new human genetic technology. Suffice it to state that from the standpoint of maintaining its strengths and efficiency of power, religion must meet change with the same attitude and spirit as does science. Accordingly, while religious principles may be immutable and eternal, the continued expression of those principles require an open, continual development that staves off stagnation.

New Right of Familial Procreation

The courts have slighted or even refused to recognize the mental elements of procreation by acknowledging that the biology of reproduction is controlling over the psychological and indeed, have chosen traditionally to give little consideration to the motivations of initiating parents. Thus, as might be expected, final decisions in surrogation have included neither an accurate assessment of the child's best interest nor an assessment of adequate care for the child. Adequate care should be but a complement to best interests and not a separate standard of application. With this approach, the "mentally conceiving" (or "initiating") parents would be recognized, of necessity, as holding the priority of right to raise the child without extracustodial visitation rights from the birthing mother. Admittedly, before this approach could be validated, a new right of "familial procurement" would have to be structured whereby the judicial protection of the choice to procreate would be recognized as but a logical analogue to "recognition of a fundamental interest in procuring assistance to overcome a personal inability to procreate". Absent the wide acceptance of this new or coordinate right, the best interests test must, however, remain controlling.

Determining Best Interests

How should the best interests of the child test be developed and for that matter, applied? Obviously, the test is fact sensitive and defies a uniform standard of application. Yet, a core set of factors may be employed to test, as between competing family and state interests in a surrogation case, the extent to which the best interests of the disputed child would be advanced and recognized as reasonable.

Ideally, the following factors could be weighed in performing the balancing test of determining which of the opposing parties would provide for or guarantee that the infant's best interests would be assured: the character and extent of harm (economic, physical, mental, social, psychological, ethical) that would either befall or so threaten the infant as to jeopardize its well-being; the specific social value that would be continued or, alternatively, abridged if the child were placed with one set of parents as opposed to the other set; the suitability of the character of the opposing parties; the burden (economic or social) that would be placed on the parties *and* the infant if one course of action were pursued over another (e.g., custodial or visitation rights); and the practicability of the ultimate action (i.e., ease of enforcement if parties are in different jurisdictions).

Maintaining Middle-Class Standards

Middle-class standards should never be considered a handicap or negative value for a court to consider in determining from whom a child can receive the most adequate care that, in turn, will ensure its best interests are advanced. A good education, attractive job and financial security should mean in the normal course of affairs that a child being raised within a family environment of this nature will be afforded a more enhanced opportunity for care and growth than would be the case otherwise. It really is just that simple. If the goal of law is to maximize the welfare or utility of all human beings, a *prima facie* case could be posited for according children some measure of legal protection against their parents or those who would assert custodial rights. Efficiency, emotional stability and security are minimal investments for a child's development.

Evolving Case Law

The judiciary itself had certain broad, inherent powers to shape a response to specific problems within this area. Specifically, as presented by the facts of the *Baby M* case, the court enforced a preconception agreement whereby a biological mother, Mary Beth

Whitehead-Gould, agreed to relinquish her child conceived through artificial insemination and carried to full term. Mrs. Whitehead was married to another person as was the contracting party, Mr. William Stern. For her services, it was agreed further that Mrs. Whitehead would receive $10,000. After Baby M was born, the biological mother changed her mind and decided she would keep and raise "her" daughter.

Even though determined not to be unfit, the trial judge ordered, as a consequence of the contract, that the biological mother's rights were terminated. It was held further that only the consent of the baby's biological father, William Stern, was necessary for him and his own wife to proceed to adopt Baby M.

The Supreme Court of New Jersey determined that the original contract between Mrs. Whitehead-Gould and Mr. Stern was not legally enforceable. Consequently, under existing principles of family law, the court held both biological or "natural" parents were the legal parents. Even though granting that the primary custody of the child was to remain with Mr. Stern, the biological and legal father, the court granted Mrs. Whitehead-Gould visitation rights. The court proceeded to rule that in future cases where a surrogate mother might refuse to relinquish her child, contrary to contractual agreement, the child would nonetheless remain with the biological mother, in nearly all cases, until the custody issue was determined.

Variations on a Theme

Robert Moschetta, a thirty-four-year-old man and his wife of nine years, Cynthia, aged forty, decided to hire a surrogate mother to bear them a child. Elvira Johnson, a divorced mother of three, became artificially inseminated and conceived in November 1989. The surrogacy contract stipulated that she was to be paid $10,000 for her services. Shortly before the child was born in May 1990, Ms. Johnson learned of the plans of the Moschettas to divorce. Robert and Cynthia had decided previously not to divulge their marital difficulties to Ms. Jordan until after the birth, but complications arose toward the end of the pregnancy and necessitated the disclosure. Upon the birth of the female child, Ms. Jordan agreed reluctantly to nonetheless let the Moschettas take the baby home provided they agreed to seek marriage counselling for a least at year and allow her visitation rights, together with full payment of her contract. Six months later, Mr. Moschetta separated from his wife and let her and the surrogate battle for custody of the child, Marissa. Mr. Moschetta asserts Marissa is his legally because he fathered her with his sperm. His wife, Cynthia, maintains the surrogacy contract establishes her rights as the legal mother while the surrogate advances her claim as the biological birth mother.

Ms. Jordan, whom the court initially denied contact with the child, is a native Spanish-speaking woman who admits that she never read the document relinquishing her parental rights before executing it and furthermore states that she would have never signed it if she had understood the focus of the relinquishment and that the child might not be provided with a two-parent environment in which to be raised. A clause in the contract barring a couple from divorcing would have been unenforceable, however.

During the protracted litigation involding this case, Cynthia Moschetta helped raise Marissa by visting with her two days a week and even going so far as to take maternity leave from her regular employment in order to care for and bond with the child when it was born. Additionally, she helped pay for the expenses the surrogate, Ms. Jordan, incurred during the pregnancy itself. Had it been decided that parenting rights are established by raising the child rather than by participating in its birth, a new precedent setting course would have been charted in family law.

As will be remembered, in the *Baby M* case, the New Jersey Supreme Court gave the biological father, William Stern and the surrogate mother, Mary Beth Whitehead, parental rights, but Mrs. Stern, who helped raise the baby, was awarded no legal rights. In 1991 there was no definitive and tested appellate court decisional law in California indicating whether surrogacy contracts were legal, let alone delineating the respective rights of a divorcing couple and a surrogate mother. Heretofore, unless it could be proved otherwise, a strong presumption is made that the biological bonding of gestational mother makes her a better mother. Indeed, she "is the legal mother for all purposes" since, quite simply, she has assumed the majority of the risks during the pregnancy.

In 1994, showing rather predictable judicial confusion and indecisiveness on the issue of surrogation, the California Court of Appeal in dealing with the *Moschetta* case, called for "legislative guidance" in assisting it to develop standards for determining legal rights under both "traditional" surrogacy arrangements and "gestational" surrogacy. The court proceeded to define traditional surrogation as an arrangement whereby a woman is impregnated with the sperm of a married man, with a full understanding prior to the completion of the act that the resulting child is to be recognized legally as the child of the married man and his infertile wife. Contrariwise, in cases of gestational surrogacy, sperm given by a married man is united artifically with the egg of his wife, with the resulting embryo being implanted into another woman's womb. The court stated

Infertile couples who can afford the high tech solution of *in vitro* fertilization and embryo implantation in another woman's womb can be reasonably assured of being judged the legal parents of the child, even if the surrogate reneges on her agreement. Couples who cannot afford *in vitro* fertilization and embryo implantation, or who resort to traditional surrogacy becaue the female does not have eggs suitable for *in vitro* fertilization, have no assurance their intentions will be honored in a court of law. For them and the child, biology is destiny.

Considerable progress in clarifying the "rights" of a gestational surrogate was, however, made by the State Supreme Court in the 1993 California case of *Johnson v. Calvert*.

Gestational Surrogate

Unlike Elvira Johnson or Mary Beth Whitehead, Anna Johnson had no genetic claim to the baby she was carrying as a surrogate. Rather, she contracted for a $10,000 fee to carry the embryo (fetus) derived from the egg and sperm of Cris and Mark Calvert that had been fertilized in a petri dish. Since Cris had had a hysterectomy and was unable to carry a baby., Anna was hired to perform that biological function. Accordingly, the fertilized embryo was implanted in her womb and she thus became a gestational surrogate. This type of surrogation is on the rise with nearly eighty births being attributed to the process over some three years.

The ethics of gestational surrogacy have focused on whether it is but exploitation of poor women by affluent couples with a coordinate fear that the time is approaching when busy professional women who cannot take the time to conceive and carry a fetus will merely rent another woman's uterus in order to achieve motherhood. If a contract for personal services is entered into freely without fear or coercion, it should, in a free, democratic society functioning as such within a freemarket economy, be allowed. The test is, of course, to assure that there be an absence of coercion in the negotiating or bargaining phase of the contract itself.

On October 22, 1990, Judge Richard N. Parslow, Jr., of the Orange County, California, Superior Court refused the claim of parental rights and custody made by Anna Johnson and ruled that she was a "genetic stranger" to the infant and thus had no legal rights to assert parenthood. Again, this was a valid contract and, absent fraud, should be enforced. Emotional changes of mind simply cannot be countenanced as the rule of the day. Subsequently, the California Supreme Court affirmed, finding that not only was there nothing in the record to support an argument that surrogacy contracts tend to exploit and dehumanize poor women and that they violate state public policy or the constitutional rights of gestational mothers. Accordingly, the court found for Cris Calvert, the genetic mother.

Structuring a New Framework

Since surrogate parenting is the biological counterpart of AID with the surrogate herself being thus equivalent to the semen donor it might be hoped that present laws controlling AID would in turn provide a basis for regulating parenthood arrangements in surrogation. Such is not the case, however.

Statutory distinctions exist that allow payment for semen to donors who participate in AID but deny it for surrogate mothers and thus may well be challenged as an unconstitutional denial of equal protection. Further distinction might be found in separating cases involving surrogating practices when there will be no genotypical relationship between the child and the individuals seeking its procreation and those cases in which a womb is "borrowed" to carry a child conceived by persons who will be the biological parents and who propose to integrate fully the child into their family.

In some twenty-three jurisdictions presently, financial compensation (except for certain specific expenses) is prohibited under state adoption laws. While in Michigan payment to a surrogate based on a contract to perform services was held invalid as a contract to sell a baby, the Kentucky Supreme Court reached the opposite conclusion based on constitutional grounds reasoning as such that surrogacy was not baby selling simply because the biological father already had established a legal relationship with the child.

Some commentators have suggested that an unmarried woman's right to AID may derive from a liberal reading of Supreme Court decisions establishing fundamental rights to procreation and privacy. The following discussion summarizes the points of view presented in those cases.

As society evolves and changes, so do many of its values. Autonomy, selfrepresentation, personhood, identity, intimacy and dignity are all essential to privacy. The extent to which these essentials play a role in shaping sexual, procreational autonomy must surely remain flexible; attempting to define them with precision would challenge and erode any efficacy they might enjoy. The right of the state to control and to shape the behavior of both individuals and groups regarding the birth of children is always an area of high emotion and concern.

The majority view on privacy holds that private conduct between consenting adults or, for that matter, personal conduct of any nature, should be regulated only to the extent necessary to prevent harm to others. Thus, conformity is not a priority and is certainly not a value worth pursuing. The opposing view argues that the business of the law is to suppress vice and immorality. Advocates of this view reason that if violations of society's moral structure are indulged and promoted, the whole basis of society would be undermined.

Arguably, under the majority view, the state would be justified in acting to control personal decision making in the areas of artificial insemination and surrogation for unmarried women. The requirement of harm to others is met because society could suffer economic harm by incurring expenses associated with the maintenance and education of a fatherless child born of artificial insemination. Similarly, the prevention of harm theory could be invoked in surrogation where the state, by attempting to prevent such acts, seeks to maintain the dignity and continuity of the traditional family.

Alternative Legal Approaches

In retrospect, it can be seen that three alternative legal approaches or strategies may be developed by states in order to meet the critical challenges of surrogate motherhood. First, specific legislation that outlaws the practice coupled with stringent enforcement codes could be enacted. This would have the obvious effect of forcing a real "black market" to develop, particularly since the process of becoming a surrogate mother is not an exceptionally difficult one to learn. Furthermore, the enforcement of a law forbidding surrogate motherhood in all forms would be difficult as a matter of policy to enforce. For example, it would be rather distasteful to many to exact a penalty for becoming a mother or to impose a prison sentence for promoting its advancement and implementation. Such would be offensive and morally distasteful to the very policy that both favors and recognizes the family as the bulwark of society.

Second, a legislative program designed to license the procedure and the surrogates participating in it as well as to protect the health and well being of the child, together with the safety of the surrogate, could be enacted. Legislation of this order and dimension would include provisions shaping the rights and determining the extent of the liabilities of the contracting parents in the surrogate compete *vis-a-vis* the infant. Consideration would, additionally, be given to shaping the sphere of responsibility for various types of error which intermediaries (doctors, lawyers, or mere friends of the family) might commit in facilitating the whole process. Courses of action to be taken in many of the other specific policy areas discussed previously would be ideally either tackled legislatively or delegated to administrative decision making by a licensing board constituted in order to set, enforce and implement standards considered relevant.

A third and final strategy would be to purposely allow the very concept or principle of surrogate mothers to develop through case-by-case judicial determination. Obviously, this would yield a crazy patchwork quilt similar to those early and disparate cases dealing with artificial insemination. In some jurisdictions, regrettably, this very process concerning artificial insemination in fact still continues. Judicial activity will of necessity be the order of the day if the state legislatures assume their normal passive role in matters of great moment and controversy, but the preferred approach would be a legislative one.

Practical Consequences

If regulated adequately, the "legitimization" of the status of surrogate mothers, involving a legislative or judicial interpretation, and the corresponding validation of contracts to bear a child, present no insuperable problems to society. It is by realizing the vast dimensions of the 21st century and by preparing for them now that the law assumes its rightful posture as a predictive, rather than a resultative vector of force in a scheme of modern living. Any new change or departure in custom and practice in the philosophies and coordinate actions of biological and technological advances as they impact on social life initially elicit a response of horrified negation. Subsequently with time, this shades into a negation of the acts without horror; then comes a slow, yet nonetheless, perceptible type of curiosity, study and devaluation. This evolutionary thinking process concludes with a slow but steady acceptance and establishment of a new norm or construct.

It is evident that artificial insemination is becoming more widely accepted and approved as a means of family development. The parallels and, indeed, linkage between artificial fathering and surrogate mothering are so obvious that it can be but hoped that wise judges and informed legislatures will give official recognition to this method which is also designed to further and promote the basic unit of society the family.

In Vitro Fertilization

An estimated two hundred conception clinics around the United States currently serve two million couples seeking assistance in combatting infertility. These couples expend nearly $1 billion to arrest their condition. Tragically, the national "take home baby rate" from these clinics is between 11 and 14 percent.

From this, the question that becomes uppermost in the hearts and minds of many is whether there is a fundamental or international human right to health assistance in biological reproduction. In recognizing or structuring such a right, would the state be obligated to spend any and all reasonable amounts of money in order to validate the procreative rights of all women regardless of marital status? Consistent with the fundamental constitutional right to life, liberty and the pursuit of happiness, should the state enforce its protective powers *vis-a-vis* infants at the moment of conception or at some point later in their embryonic development?

In 1983 Sir Harry Gibbs, Chief Justice of Australian High Court, ruled "that a foetus has no right of its own until it is born and has a separate existence from its mother". The common law tied the commencement of life to the time when an unborn first moved in the womb or, in other words, when it quickened. Thus, only after the fetus quickened could its destruction be classified as murder. In the United States, the issue of when individuality is established biologically and when the law should, accordingly, protect such individuals, was determined by the Supreme Court in *Roe v. Wade*. In Roe, the Court essentially held that a fetus does not receive the full protection of the law until it is born.

In September 1989 a judge of the Circuit Court for the Fifth Judicial District of Tennessee ruled that life begins at the moment of conception. The court held that seven cryogenically preserved *in vitro* embryos were children, not personal property. Accordingly, the court placed the embryos in the custodial care of the woman who, during marriage, produced eggs subsequently fertilized by her then husband. The only support the court provided for its momentus decision was a reference to the definition of "conception" in *WEBSTER'S NEW COLLEGIATE DICTIONARY*. Apparently, the court was unpersuaded by the authoritative texts and treatises relevant to the field. Instead, it relied primarily on the testimony of eight witnesses, particularly that of Dr. Jerome Lajeune, a member of the Faculty of Medicine of the University of Paris and the Pontifical Academy of Science at the Vatican.

On September 13, 1990, however, the Tennessee Court of Appeals ruled that awarding the seven fertilized ova to the woman would constitute "impermissible state action" by violating the former husband's "constitutionally protected right not to beget a child where no pregnancy has taken place". The court based its opinion on the U.S. Supreme Court recognition that the decision to "bear or beget a child" is one of protected choice by the Constitution.

Consistent also with state law which recognizes legal protections extending only to viable fetuses, the court remanded the case to the trial court directing a new judgment to reflect the appeals court decision, granting both parties joint control and an equal voice in the disposition of the ova. The court thus held that just as it would be repugnant constitutionally to order the woman to implant the fertilized ova against her will, it would be equally repugnant to order her former husband to bear the psychological, if not legal, burdens of forced paternity. In 1992 the Tennessee Supreme Court affirmed the ruling of the Court of Appeals holding that Mr. Davis could not be forced to become a parent against his will and, thus, the frozen embryos were to remain in storage or be destroyed.

The dilemma of frozen embryos presents no clear course of action for easy resolution. Yet, in the state of Victoria, Australia, alone, there are said to be some two thousand embryos cryogenically preserved. Throughout Australia as many as ten thousand such frozen embryos may exist. Fritze Honduis, the Deputy Director of Legal Affairs of the Council of Europe, has suggested that upwards of twenty thousand embryos are frozen throughout Europe.

Lack of Consensus

The fact that no clear consensus is evolving on even how to begin a dialogue about frozen embryos, let alone develop a legal response-mechanism to deal with the situation, does not bode well for clarity and direction in this area. Indeed, "the ethical debate is even less focused than the unending rhetorical battle over abortion". Before the legislature and the courts are called upon to develop a definitive framework for principled decision making, objective "hard thinking" is required of the major cross-disciplinary participants in this unfolding drama.

The new reproductive biology promises untold opportunities for resolving heartbreaking problems of infertility and will expand the meaning of "procreational autonomy" for women. It also presents difficult problems for the physician, lawyer, ethicist, theologian and for that matter, the average person.

The evolving indeed, fluid parameters of the new reproductive biology defy a single definitive response. This analysis is premised on the belief that medical and scientific interventions that minimize human suffering (genetically or otherwise induced) and maximize quality of life should be pursued. Most always, the untold benefits of noncoital reproduction outweigh the costs attendant with its experimentation and use.

Ethics of in Vitro Fertilization

Typically, the IVF and embryo transfer processes begins with drug therapy to produce super ovulation in a woman. Through a procedure called laparoscopy, the resulting eggs are removed from the woman's reproductive tract and then fertilized. An embryo is then implanted in the woman's uterus and, if the implantation is successful, carried to term. The remaining embryos are stored, either for future implantation should the first attempt fail or for use in scientific or medical experiments. Alternatively, IVF may be used without embryo transfer to produce embryos solely for experimental purposes.

Ethical Complexities

Attention is now drawn to what might be termed as the "ethical morality" of IVF, a discussion which explores the benefits and the harms of IVF use. Ethical complexities attend each of the many variations on the basic IVF theme. For example, when artificial insemination is used to fertilize a married woman's egg with the sperm of a man other than her husband because her husband's sperm is defective, a serious ethical issue is posed. Similarly, moral and ethical issues arise when a third-party surrogate carries an embryo to term for a genetic mother or when a single woman seeks to avail herself of IVF procedures. This section of the chapter probes not all of the ethical issues raised by IVF but instead proceeds selectively.

The most obvious benefit of IVF is that it circumvents infertility and allows persons with a strong desire to have children to rear a family. If it is determined conclusively that frozen embryos can be used without damage to resultant children, IVF could enable women who wish to pursue careers to bear children using embryos created some years earlier, thereby reducing their chance of producing a Down's syndrome child. Beyond family expansion, IVF could be used to provide embryos for scientific and medical experiments. Embryos could be used in infertility, genetic and cancer research; as a source of obtaining embryonic tissue used in the treatment of diseases such as diabetes; and to harvest organs for transplant.

There are several major objections to IVF. The first is that separating sex from procreation is inherently wrong. IVF, followed by embryo transfer to the uterus of the married woman, severs the connection between sex and reproduction. The second objection is that IVF is morally wrong because it involves an abnormal risk of harm to the individual subsequently brought into existence. Physical damage or abnormality (although not documented factually) could result from IVF or from the subsequent transfer of the embryo to the woman's womb. Furthermore, psychological harm might inure to an infant born of the total process.

The third objection is that using IVF as a means to produce embryos for experiments or as sources of tissues and organs subjects the embryo to pain. This objection would have considerable merit where experiments were conducted on substantially developed fetuses. When conducting such scientific interventions with embryos in the first several weeks of their development, such embryos probably do not experience pain, owing to the absence of a critical nervous system.

The fourth objection is that although IVF may not be inherently wrong or wrong because of its effects upon those immediately involved, it may be wrong because of the "slippery slope" to which it is likely to lead. IVF together with embryo transfer may lead to unimpeded use of surrogate mothers as substitutes for genetic mothers, cause the dissolution of the family unit when women who do not wish to marry or have sexual relations with a man use this technique, or even lead to the development of artificial wombs, severing the mother-child connection.

The strongest objection to the IVF process is that the unimplanted embryos will eventually be destroyed an action morally akin to abortion. When embryos are not implanted in the woman's uterus they must be used for scientific experimentation, frozen, or destroyed. Generally, antiabortionists view all scientific experimentation using embryos as morally wrong since it necessarily leads to the embryos' destruction. However, at a recent meeting of the American Society of Human Genetics, a new procedure was revealed which might ease the high tension associated with prenatal genetic testing. This procedure is designed to discover genetic defects in the human egg *before* fertilization. Although considered promising, this procedure must itself undergo further testing. Once validated, this could well take the "sting" out of some moral objections to experimentation and use of IVF and embryo implants as assaults on the right to life. Indeed, the General Counsel for the National Right to Life expressed his opinion that the test was proper since it did not involve "the taking of innocent human life".

Moral Dilemmas

The freezing of embryos also poses difficult moral dilemmas. If frozen embryos cannot be thawed successfully, a decision to thaw would lead to the destruction of the embryos. Moreover, even if successful thawing can be accomplished, the decision to experiment, implant, or destroy arises again. Quite clearly, the ethical dilemma involves very real problems. For example, would a woman whose first implantation was successful be required to keep the remaining embryos frozen in perpetuity to avoid their destruction? The only apparent way to resolve the uncertainty about freezing techniques would be to continue with limited experimentation in the field, using lower animal life forms.

Religious Overtones

Religious values have historically played an important part in public policy debates. Indeed, the very "bedrock of moral order is religion". "And as morality's foundation is religion, religion and politics are necessarily related. We need religion as a guide; we need it because we are imperfect."

Faith and religion have played a dynamic role in the political life of the United States. Today's commitment to democratic pluralism is nurtured and sustained as a consequence of recognizing the inviolability of individual conscience. For some, politics and morality become inseparable. To exclude societal values grounded in a religious base from the public arena would pose a serious threat to the very principle of pluralism. What this commitment to pluralism means, however, is that no definitive posture can ever emerge relative to assisted noncoital reproduction.

Regulation in the United States

The extent to which U.S. states may validly regulate IVF procedures and embryo transfers depends on whether these acts are viewed as fundamental rights. Thus, the threshold question is whether they are "rights" guaranteed by the Constitution as part of the "right to marital privacy".

Various Supreme Court decisions seem to grant "the right 'to marry, establish a home and bring up children'" as among those liberties granted by the fourteenth amendment. Based on these cases, it could be argued that any state regulation on IVF and embryo transfers would be an intrusion on the fundamental right to marital privacy. "If the decision to beget a child is a protected area of privacy, presumably the actual method of begetting also would be protected. Thus, any statute affecting this delicate area would have to serve a compelling state interest and must do so by the least restrictive means."

A more conservative analysis of the Supreme Court decisions in this area recognizes, at the threshold, that the right to privacy is not explicitly mentioned in the U.S. Constitution. No right of sexual freedom is found within the gambit of procreative rights recognized by the Supreme Court nor has the Court fashioned a general right of personal privacy which is sufficiently broad based to encompass sex outside marriage.

Legislative Positions among the States

It is doubtful that Congress could ever enact effective legislation on the legal status of an embryo because society is not of a singular mind. Nor is there a consensus as to when "life" should be legally protected. Judicial interpretation of this issue has aroused national debate with the decision in *Roe v. Wade*. Despite the lack of agreement regarding when life begins, those children born of an IVF procedure using either a donor ova or donor sperm should be recognized as children of the family in which they were born. No issue of illegitimacy should be raised nor should the donors be held to any level of financial support of the child. Similarly, the child should have no right of inheritance against the donors. The best interests of the IVF child are served and more important, the strength of the family unit is enhanced and its stability assured by following this course.

After *Roe*, some twenty-five states enacted fetal research laws designed primarily to control research on aborted fetuses. Several statutes extend their protective coverage to research on embryos. If cumbersome safeguards effecting excess embryo preservation are required, the initiation of medical scientific programs utilizing IVF procedures could be discouraged. Moreover, in a number of these states, the very legality of IVF as a medical procedure to overcome infertility is in question.

Only Pennsylvania and Louisiana have statutes regarding IVF. Pennsylvania's law simply monitors IVF by requiring anyone conducting the procedure to file quarterly reports with the state Department of Health fully describing the processes involved. In 1986, the Louisiana legislature decreed that, "a viable *in vitro* fertilized ovum is a juridicial person" that cannot be destroyed and furthermore that such an ovum "cannot be owned by the *in vitro* fertilization patients who owe it a high duty of care and prudent administration". If a renunciation of parental rights by the IVF patients occurs, the "ovum shall be available for adoptive implantation". Sadly, no other state statutes clarify the legal status of IVF children.

Illinois had a statute which prohibited selling or experimenting upon a "fetus produced by the fertilization of a human ovum by a human sperm unless such experimentation is therapeutic to the fetus thereby produced". However, the statute was struck down subsequently as being unconstitutionally vague and restrictive of women's fundamental right to privacy.

U.S. Government's Position

The HHS has the responsibility for regulating human subjects involved in research conducted or funded by HHS or other federal agencies, including research and development relating to IVF. The HHS Ethics Advisory Board reviews every proposal concerning research projects involving fetuses or pregnant women. The board examines the research projects' "acceptability from an ethical standpoint". HHS regulations specifically protect fetuses that are the subject of proposed experimentation and IVF research.

Although limited to research efforts funded in whole or in part by the federal government, these guidelines made a significant distinction with regard to potential legal rights of unimplanted embryos. The distinction is apparent in the definition of "fetus":

"the product of conception from the time of implantation (as evidenced by any of the presumptive signs of pregnancy, such as missed menses, or a medically acceptable pregnancy test)."

As a consequence of this structured definition, research undertaken on fetuses *in utero* and *ex utero* is prohibited unless the purpose of the activity is either to meet the particular health needs of an at-risk fetus or to obtain biomedical knowledge not otherwise obtainable, but then only if the harm posed to the fetus is minimal. Research undertaken on nonviable fetuses *ex utero* is prohibited unless vital function are not maintained artificially, experimental activities that would terminate vital functions are not used, or the research purpose is to obtain otherwise unobtainable significant biomedical knowledge. The effect of these restrictions on embryonic and fetal research is that the scientific pursuit of knowledge is significantly handicapped. Because of this *de facto* moratorium, no federally funded research on IVF has been undertaken since 1975. Private research into the mysteries and the opportunities of the new reproductive biology continues. But without a balanced regulatory scheme and sources for federal research funding, the initiative and the momentum for scientific advancement is curtailed.

Both as a response to Louise Brown's extracorporeal birth in 1978 and to a grant application for IVF research, FISS and its Ethics Advisory Board decided to study the complex ethical, legal, social and scientific issues raised by IVF and embryo transfer. Their report concluded that federal support of research on human IVF, in order to establish both the safety and the effectiveness of IVF procedures, would be permissible ethically so long as certain conditions were met. The report was ultimately "buried in the bureaucracy". Yet, due largely to the leadership of then the Congressman Albert Gore of Tennessee, hearings were conducted in August 1984 on the very issue of embryo transfers and the legal, ethical and medical responses to such procedures. Although no firm or conclusive steps were taken as a result of these hearings, the hearings served to focus attention on the need for continuing dialogue in this area.

Given the oftentimes strident antiabortion mood of a vocal segment of society, strong positive movement will probably not occur at the federal regulatory level. Indeed, on November 2, 1989, the Bush Administration extended the prohibition on support for research involving fetal tissue transplants from induced abortions.

The principal reason for such action was that the positive health benefits generated by this research were outweighed by the accompanying complex moral and ethical problems. Dr. Louis W. Sullivan, Secretary of HHS, stated that permitting human fetal research "will increase the incidence of abortion across the country". What is once again evident is the inextricable relationship between abortion and fetal research and experimentation and, even more importantly, the almost inextricable relationship between politics and morality.

On January 22, 1993, President William Clinton lifted the moratorium on federal funding of research involving transplantation of fetal tissue from induced abortions. With the execution of a presidential memorandum, then, untold opportunities have been created for developing effective treatments not only for Parkinson's disease and Alzheimer's but also for disorders such as diabetes and leukemia.

Human Embryo Research Panel

On September 27, 1994, the Human Embryo Research Panel of the NIH recommended a series of guidelines allowing for a wide range of research on human embryos (developed from test-tube fertilization) with less than fourteen days of developmental age. President Clinton, however, on December 3, 1994, concluded that no federal monies would be expended for research on human embryos. His order did not bar support for studies using fertilized eggs from fertility clinics. Interestingly, when in January 1996 the president signed a continuing resolution to keep the government operating, it incorporated within its provisions a prohibition on the use of federal funds for human embryo research.

The 1994 findings of the Embryo Research Panel were that several areas of scientific research were well within the limits for federal funding and consisted of research involving fertilization, egg activation, maturation and freezing, methods for improving chances of pregnancy, genetic diagnosis before implantation and the development of embryonic stem cells. Sadly, these vital areas of embryonic research have become linked with the issue of abortion and indeed, become a captive of it. The reality here is that abortion is truly a political issue and its resolution is unlikely to be resolved by ethical argumentation.

A disengagement of embryonic research from the continuing abortion debate must be undertaken if scientific progress is to be made in combatting the problem of fertilization and improvement made in structuring the effectiveness of the process of *in vitro* fertilization itself. Two major points overlooked totally are the fact that research on embryos *ex utero* need not involve abortion since no pregnancy is necessary for this type of research and similarly, that a goal of embryonic research is to serve as an aid to increasing the number of pregnancies and thereby reducing the rate of abortion. Put simply, then, ethical research must be shaped by ethical reasoning rather than political vagaries.

Impact and the Promise of Webster v. Reproductive Health Services

In tackling "the most political divisive domestic legal issue of our time", the Supreme Court, on July 3, 1989, upheld the validity of a Missouri statute which significantly restricts a woman's right to obtain an abortion. The preamble to the challenged statute declares human life to begin at conception and defines conception as "the fertilization of the ovum of a female by a sperm of a male" in disregard of standard medical tests which equate conception with uteral implantation occurring about six days after fertilization. Thus the statute not only sought implicitly to regulate previable abortions but common forms of contraception such as the IUD and the morning-after-pill as well. Yet a majority of the Court held the preamble did not actually regulate abortion and therefore the scope of its application would have to await testing until a concrete example restricting the appellees' activities was shown. The majority of the court refused "to decide abstract propositions".

What is relevant to the present analysis is Justice Stevens' opinion in *Webster* concurring in part and dissenting in part. Stevens would find the Missouri statute violated the Establishment Clause because of the legislative ("theological") finding in the statute's preamble that endorses the state interest in preserving the life of an embryo during the first forty or eighty days of pregnancy to be at the same level of protection and scrutiny as after viability. Justice Stevens would also invalidate the statute because it violates the right of contraceptive privacy set forth in *Griswold v. Connecticut*. Before reaching this conclusion, however, he develops a thoughtful inquiry into the issue of male versus female ensoulment articulated in the early writings of St. Thomas Aquinas which have been accepted by the Roman Catholic Church.

What Justice Stevens concludes after analyzing the Aquinas position is most important to a sophisticated understanding of the complex medico-legal-ethical issue of the scope of protection the state should or may extend to research and experimentation of extracorporeal embryos. He states eloquently:

As a secular matter, there is an obvious difference between the state interest in protecting the freshly fertilized egg and the state interest in protecting a 9-month-gestated, fully sentient fetus on the eve of birth. *There can be no interest in protecting the newly fertilized egg from physical pain or mental anguish, because the capacity for such suffering does not yet exist; respecting a developed fetus, however, that interest is valid.* In fact, if one prescinds the theological concept of ensoulment—or one accepts St. Thomas Aquinas' view that ensoulment does not occur for at least 40 days, *a State has no greater secular interest in protecting the potential life of a sperm or an unfertilized ovum.*

The logic of this position is quite compelling and provides much weight to the position that while the embryo does not theologically have an independent moral status, it is regarded by some as worthy of respect as a "symbol of life". While the embryo might well be treated as "an object of respect", it arguably does not consistent with this position gain any type of moral status or recognition until transferred to a uterus. Accordingly, when no transfer occurs, vexatious decisions concerning unused or stored embryos "become occasions to use embryos as a symbol of life or persons generally" are presented. What then must be evaluated is whether the need for preserving such symbols outweighs "the costs to autonomy or future knowledge that symbol-making necessarily involves".

Justice O'Connor, in concurring in part and concurring in the judgment, addressed the concern that the preamble to the challenged statute might prohibit the development and use of IVF by dismissing them as "intimations of unconstitutionality" that were "simply too hypothetical" to address. Regarding the challenge that the statute is violative of *Griswold*, she found nothing in the preamble that would affect a woman's right to practice acts of contraception.

Justice O'Connor stressed that as to the state's interest in protecting potential life, the point of viability was the crucial determination when such interest could be focused by the enactment of regulations designed to achieve that end. "No decision of this Court has held that the State may not directly promote its interest in potential life when viability may differ with each pregnancy." Its "possibility" can thus be determined within a period of testing—as for example here with Missouri's twenty-week period (that was essentially a presumption of viability of twenty weeks—subject to medical rebuttal). As more advanced medical technologies develop, the testing period may commence earlier. Yet, even with an earlier time frame for testing viability, it is well known that fetal lungs do not mature until some thirty-three to thirty-four weeks of gestation. The physician is also aided in the determination of viability by ultra sound examinations that determine gestational age and fetal weight, as well as fetal lung maturity.

The full Court chose not to address the validity of the statute's preamble that recognized life as beginning with human conception. However, the arguments made by Justices Stevens and O'Connor regarding viability and the tone of the other opinions in the case persuasively show that legal protection of personhood under present accepted biological and medical knowledge ought not be extended to unimplanted, extracorporeal embryos. When implanted, as with normal conception, the embryo must develop into a viable fetus before full state protections will be accorded to it.

Congressional Action

With the enactment in 1994 of the Freedom of Access to Clinics Entrance Act, Congress, unlike the Supreme Court, has stated boldly and unequivocally that efforts to threaten, intimidate or interfere with persons obtaining or providing reproductive health services (e.g., abortion) are prohibited with criminal sanctions. Health services are defined as including "medical, surgical, counselling or referral services including services relating to . . . the termination of a pregnancy whether the services are provided in a hospital, clinic, doctor's office or other facility".

American Fertility Society Guidelines

In an effort to update and supplement its 1990 Report on Ethical Considerations of the New Reproductive Technology, the Ethics Committee of the American Fertility Society issued, in 1994, its sixty-page report titled *"Ethical Considerations of Assisted Reproductive Technology"*. Although their conclusions and recommendations are not binding policy, they do reflect the serious thinking of one of the nation's preeminent groups in family planning. Thus, from this standpoint, they are of considerable importance.

The committee, while acknowledging artificial insemination by a husband is acceptable, nonetheless called for the development and regulation of reliable sperm bank facilities and concluded the cryo-preservation of human sperm is both ethically and medically acceptable. Donor insemination, although controversial, was also found to enjoy the same status as husband, or homologous, insemination. Again, calling for uniform standards for the collection and preservation of sperm in banks, the committee urged donors to be subject to genetic and health screening and suggested cyro-preserved donor sperm be used over fresh sperm because of the opportunity for more extensive screening and testing. Further, it was recommended that no payment be made to semen donors other than for their time and expenses involved and that the same donor not be used for more than *ten* offspring. This latter point, taken together with the conclusion that single, unmarried women should be entitled to donor insemination, shows a very sad and tragic societal direction for traditional families. Indeed, both recommendations regarding multiple donor use and the availability of donor insemination for single women if accepted popularly and acted on would destroy the very notion of the nuclear family and glorify the motto of popular feminism: "My Body, My Choice!"

IVF was found to be not only safe for both mother and child but was also an extension and thus, not a radical separation of procreation and sexual intimacy. If whatever risks involved with the procedure are found acceptable by the participating couple, then its use should be permitted. While recognizing the ethical difficulty with the process which allows the selection of some pre-embryos for transfer and the discarding of others not used, the committee concluded that there was no ethical objection to the discarding of those pre-embryos. which were clearly degenerate or abnormal. In order to lessen the rate of discard, adjunctive cryo-preservation programs for maintenance of pre-embryos in excess of those transferred were recommended. With programs of this nature in place, the necessity of selective reduction would be reduced considerably since cryopreservation would also enable the transfer of a limited number of pre-embryos.

The American Fertility Society's Ethics Committee came out strongly against the use of a surrogate gestational mother for nonmedical reasons (e.g., the genetic mother's convenience). Even though it recognized the inherent controversy involved in the use of surrogation, the committee nonetheless concluded there is a definite role for surrogate gestation in reproductive medicine. Finding that the frequency of use for surrogation is low, and that the morality of the process is less an issue than the possible exploitation of the surrogates, it was urged that surrogate gestational motherhood programs should nonetheless have their protocol approved by a properly constituted ethics committee or institution review board. Furthermore, a full and voluntary informed consent must be obtained from the surrogate as well as the participating couple and those participating professionals should not receive any type of finder's fee for participating in the program; instead, they should only receive whatever customary fees allowed. It is preferable that surrogates, in turn, make no payment beyond compensation for their expenses and inconveniences with only rare cases being allowed for compensation beyond this standard.

Complex and unresolved ethical, social and psychological issues prevented the committee from endorsing fully the use of this new reproductive technology. Although finding its use appropriate where it offers the only *medical* solution to infertility for a couple of whom the woman has no uterus, is incapable of producing eggs, or is unwilling to pass on a genetic defect that she carries, it nevertheless cautioned against the potentially negative effects of the procedure on not only the surrogate gestational mother and the couple but the resulting child as well, the possibility of *in utero* bonding between the surrogate and the fetus, the need for thorough screening of the surrogate and the degree of appropriate care which must be exercised by her during the period of her pregnancy.

Summary

In exploring the noncoital reproductive sciences, a balance should be struck between the unfettered use of science for individual satisfaction and the promotion and maintenance of the social good. Thus, embryo research and experimentation which contributes to the goal of minimizing human suffering and maximizing the social good deriving therefrom must be pursued in a reasonable manner. As long as the central driving force in marital relationships continues to be procreation and the family unit remains at the core of a progressive society, efforts will be pursued which seek to expand the period of fecundity, combat infertility and ensure that inherited genetic deficiencies are not passed on to future generations. Genetic experimentation and planning, in conjunction with eugenic programming are more rational and humane than alternatives to population regulation through death, famine, and war or an abdication of genetic autonomy to the countervailing doctrines of gene sovereignty and biological determinism.

Socially responsible scientific inquiry should be restrained only when the scientist "is clearly able to foresee that the particular line of work is leading to a kind and scale of dangers" that would constitute a "limitation" or, in other words, presents "dangers of cataclysmic physical or psychological proportions for mankind as a whole".

While some would view research and experimentation in human embryology and reproductive biology as promoting a genetic disaster or cataclysm, the better view is that such work advances the goal of minimizing human suffering and maximizing the quality of purposeful and meaningful existence free of inherited genetic disabilities. Certain aspects of the new human reproductive biology (e.g., cloning) might well require greater degrees of reasonable self-restraint. By and large, however, the nature and degree to which restraint is mandated must be determined by the individual scientist.

Preemption of scientific work in human reproductive biology by the state is shortsighted and repressive of the principle of free scientific inquiry. Instead of developing a scientific regulatory scheme relying on legislative prohibition, rulemaking committees within the pertinent medical and scientific profession should be established to monitor and control scientific inquiry. Perhaps the best model would be a simple organization approached easily on a consultative and advisory basis and designed to assist biologists, scientists and medical researchers in making their own decisions.

Included in the Health Research Extension Act of 1985 were provisions to create a Biomedical Ethics Board and a Biomedical Ethics Advisory Committee to report on human genetic engineering and on the federal rules on human fetal research. If totally funded, the Committee would have also studied the ethical, social and legal implications of human genome mapping, genetic testing, eugenics and gene therapy. These bodies would have perhaps provided some continuity with the now defunct President's Commission for the Study of Ethical Problems in Medicine and Biomedical and Behavioral Research by advancing efforts to study, evaluate and organize responses to the new reproductive biology.

President Clinton renewed hope in the scientific community during the summer of 1996 by issuing an executive order creating a new National Bioethics Advisory Committee charged with studying ethical issues arising from experiments on human biology and behavior. More specifically, the commission will consider how best to use and manage genetic information derived from the Human Genome Project as well as explore the scientific, legal and ethical implications of patenting human genes. Whether the Commission's work will meet with greater success than its most recent precedessor depends in large part on the degree to which politics can be disengaged from the ultimate recommendations it will make.

It remains for lawyers to become more aware and indeed, educated to the challenges and complexities of these new scientific and technological advances in reproductive biology. If they fail to achieve this level of awareness and education, "they will increasingly lack understanding of the questions to be asked, let alone answers to be given." And, one such open-ended question remains: To what extent, if at all, is there a fundamental constitutional or international human right for procreative liberty, health assistance in biological reproduction, and the point in the biological developmental chart that mandates the state to extend its protection to "life"?

9

Malaria, Medicine and Meals

Introduction

The study of indigenous medicines commands a prominent position in medical anthropological study that seeks to comprehend, from multicultural and crosscultural perspectives, how people manage health and illness. Intellectually, such inquiry is most meaningfully cast in the theoretical idioms of a human ecology that explores not only the cultural and social construction of therapeutics but also the physiologic outcomes of health-seeking behaviors. Since the publication of pioneering research that revealed the extent to which the category "medicine" overlaps that of "food", studies of indigenous medicine increasingly include dietary and other contexts of plant use in order to assess the extent to which people are exposed to pharmacologically active plant constituents. Such investigations embody the biobehavioral perspective of medical anthropological inquiry.

Working in more narrow intellectual frameworks, phytochemists and pharmacologists are optimistic that the study of indigenous medicines will expand the biomedical pharmacopoeia, at the same time ironically that biological and cultural diversity are conserved. For their part, ministries of health in developing nations have formalized policies that champion indigenous medicine, both to accommodate the limited availability of biomedical resources and to serve political ends through the reaffirmation of traditional institutions. Compelled by a more applied agenda, international agencies such as the World Health Organization (WHO) have made explicit recommendations to study indigenous medicines. At present, more than 20 centers around the globe collaborate in the WHO Traditional Medicine Program, the primary objective of which is to conduct systematic investigations of efficacy and risk and to integrate local medicine into the provision of state health care.

All of those concerns are resonated in this chapter through a revised version of our contributions to earlier editions of this volume. We present data on Hausa medicine and diet, which are then interpreted through a unique model of disease adaptation. For the present version, we review findings from our research on plants used in both diet and medicine: the findings of two principal field sessions, 1975-1976 and 1987-1988, are compared and amplified by the results of continuing data analysis, including the laboratory investigation of plants used in the prevention and treatment of malaria. Additional observations/data that inform these analyses are regularly conveyed to us by the Nigerian member of our research team, Ibrahim Muazzamu of the Department of Medicinal Plants, National Institute for Pharmaceutical Research and Development, Abuja, Nigeria.

Comparing results of the two field studies suggests the temporal applicability of our model of disease adaptation: the seasonal fluctuation in consumption of certain plant foods/medicines that we invoked to explain low rates of malaria infection during the 1975-1976 period was no longer apparent during 1987-1988. This shifting perspective underscores the dynamic nature of the interrelationships among medicines, foods and illness, emphasizing that knowledge and understanding are emergent, that in science the "facts" and their configurations constantly undergo change. Longitudinal research such as described here offers the opportunity to retest and refine explanatory models to accommodate changing conditions as the physical and cultural landscapes are transformed over time.

Study Site and Data Collection

Our research was conducted among an agricultural Hausa-Fulani community located 50 kilometers southeast of the urban center

Kano, in northern Nigeria. The village core of Hurumi (a pseudonym) is a nucleated settlement of 400 residents, with dispersed compounds in the outlying hamlets raising the population total to approximately 4,000. The size of compounds in this rural settlement ranges from 2 to close to 40 occupants. These living units customarily include a compound head, his wife (or wives), his sons and their wives, and children. Not atypically, compounds are constituted by more than one "household" people who "eat from the same pot". This creates the potential for intracompound variability in access to resources, including, in the present context, knowledge of plants and composition of diet.

Hurumi's economy centers on intensive agriculture supplemented by the raising of livestock (primarily sheep, goat and fowl, with some cattle) and trade in locally produced and imported commodities. Although clearly less remote today than during our initial investigation, the village still is not served by paved roads and has neither electricity nor piped water. The greater part of subsistence labor from planting through harvest, supplemented by gathering in the "wild" is neither mechanized nor assisted by draft animals.

Hausa Medicine

Data on Hausa medicine, diet and health were first collected in the course of a 22-month investigation during 1975 and 1976, a time when Hurumi residents relied almost exclusively on an extensive botanical pharmacopoeia for all therapeutic and preventive measures. Information was collected regarding Hausa understandings of disease etiology and nosology in order to describe the most commonly perceived symptoms and their appropriate treatments. Extensive interviews were conducted with individuals who were identified by others and who perceived themselves, as most conversant in matters related to health. Five women and nine men constituted a core of principal respondents and included among them a woman whose knowledge of plant medicines, especially for spirit-caused illness, earned her districtwide recognition and clientele. Other respondents represented more narrow foci of medically related knowledge: a barber-surgeon, three midwives and authorities in such specific areas as venereal diseases, jaundice, weaning medicines, witchcraft and sorcery (predominantly ascribed to malfeasance among co-wives and jealousy). Other interviews and observations throughout the village revealed that most adults are familiar with at least several medicines for a variety of common disorders, including gastrointestinal complaints, fevers, children's illnesses and skin conditions.

Open-ended interviews were organized around the following: a catalogue of 637 plants, for which individuals described the physical attributes, availability and medicinal and other uses of each; and an inventory of 808 diseases, symptoms and related terms for which respondents described commonly used medicines, including source, preparation, additional constituents, approximate dose and schedule of administration, therapeutic objectives and alternatives for circumstances in which that medicine is not available or does not produce the expected results. Our data are more or less consonant with observations in other parts of Hausaland; differences are of a magnitude one would expect given temporal and ecologic variability and compounded by the varying methodologies (especially ethnographic depth) of other reporters for example, Adam et al. (1972), Busson et al. (1965), Dalziel (1937), Darrah (1980), Oliver (1986), Prietze (1913-1914), Stock (1980) and Wall (1988).

For the year-long follow-up study (1987-1988), we employed a more rigorous methodology in order to extend the depth of our inquiry, to understand better the antecedents and sequelae of plant use by Hausa and to collect additional antimalarial plants for further laboratory investigation. Plants still were the predominant medicines for prevention and therapy—this despite the dramatic incursion of biomedicine over the last decade and the marked increase in availability and widespread use of pharmaceuticals. Using the same plant and disease/symptom inventories, extensive interviews combined with observations of therapeutic and preventive events elicited the details of plant selection, preparation, application, and desired outcome. Two nonspecialists a man and a woman participated in the study as principal respondents; villagewide consensus identified them as most generally conversant regarding therapeutic and preventive objectives and plant identification. A representative, villagewide interview schedule (including 50 respondents) supplemented practitioner- and specialist-focused studies to provide a broader (exoteric rather than esoteric) base for compiling the knowledge that more accurately represents preventive and therapeutic modalities that affect the majority of villagers on a day-to-day basis. These data were supplemented by field and market surveys to assess plant availability, cost and so forth. The medical investigation was amplified by a monthly village health survey that recorded all disease episodes for all households. In addition, we conducted a two-month investigation at the recently opened biomedical facility located eight kilometers from Hurumi. Patients and staff participated in entry and exit interviews that explored, among other factors, reasons for clinic attendance and prior treatments, patient-physician encounters and "compliance" with prescriptive and other instruction topics that have potential influence on the continued viability and form of "local medicines".

During 1987 and 1988, villagewide interviews yielded nearly 5,000 medicinal preparations. Excluding replications, the number of remedies is 3,165. (A distinct remedy is defined by a unique combination of constituents, or each time that combination is used for another illness category.) Of those medicines, 89 percent (2,801) include a total of 374 plants. Three hundred forty-five of all plants are used for diseases that we have termed "overtly physiologic" (in application and in therapeutic objectives). These are illnesses whose etiology Hausa attribute to naturalistic phenomena such as dirt or disharmony along such axes as drywet, cold-hot, sweet-salty, bitter-sweet and permutations thereof and whose prevention and treatment include dislodgement or externalization of disease substance, palliation of pain or discomfort and, finally, symptom resolution.

Heeding the very inclusive Hausa definition of medicine magani, literally, anything that improves or repairs something necessitates attention also to plants used in the management of disorders attributed to human malfeasance or the intervention of extrahuman agency. Two hundred sixty-six of all plants are used for the mediation of sorcery, spirits and witches; this is accomplished largely through preventive measures but can be treated after the fact as well. To the extent that these intercessions include ingestion, topical application, fumigation, inhalation and other close contact with plant constituents, these contexts of use also have physiologic implications. We do not propose that the management of spirits, witches and sorcery entails a unique constellation of plants, for it does not. We draw attention to the issue here precisely because most researchers have not concerned themselves with plant applications whose rationale and objectives fall outside the context of disorders of naturalistic origin. Further, Hausa exposure to constituents of these plants increases dramatically because they actively engage these imperceptible threats to well-being on at least a daily basis and not just when the fact of illness is established.

Table 9.1. Most Common Categories for Hausa Medicinal Preparations

Hausa Nosology	General Analogue	A medicinal preparations
ISKAM	Spirit caused illness	104
SAMMU	Sorcery	103
CIWON CIKI	General GI disorders	94
CIWON CIKIN KABA	Acute GI disorders	90
SHAWARA	Hepatitis, malaria	72
KYANDA	Measles	70
MAYE	Witch caused illness	66
ZAZZABI	Febrile disorders	64
DANSHI	Pediatric malaria	59
MAYANKWANIYA	"Wasting" anemias	59

Hausa Diet

A dietary survey of eight households was conducted to understand the sources, distribution and preparation of foods and to document consumption. This was implemented for 24-hour periods, randomly selected twice per week per household, for 48 consecutive weeks to coincide with the end of one harvest and the beginning of the next, these being the most meaningful delineators of the annual agricultural cycle. Precise weight measures of unprocessed foods were augmented with extensive interviews and observations. The participating households contained a mean of 46 residents and were selected as a reasonable cross section of the larger hamlet, representing the relatively narrow range of economic, social and demographic variability in Hurumi.

For each of the three daily meals, all foods were weighed prior to cooking and other preparation. For all food preparers in the study, independent and repeated assessments of all food types and preparations included weight and volume measures for all ingredients, tabulated sequentially through all stages of preparation to final cooked (or otherwise modified) consumable form.

Table 9.2. Plant Medicines

	"Semi-Wild" Plants		**All Plants**	
Intended Use:	**n plants**	**n remedies**	**n plants**	**n remedies**
Physiologic	254	1854	345	2275
Other	215	452	266	526
TOTALS	272[a]	2306	374[a]	2801[b]

[a] Totals are less than the sums due to multiple plant uses.

[b] Excluded are five remedies that specify plant location or situation rather than a particular genus or species.

This permitted extrapolation from the unprocessed weight measures for each household to quantified approximations of nutrient values (for calories, protein, etc.) based on published food composition values. All foods, including snacks, consumed by adults and obtained from extrahousehold sources such as vendor, market, or gift were recorded in the same way, assessing step-by-step preparation and using collateral data such as cost per unit of prepared food, fluctuating market prices, and so on. Thus, the full food consumption cycle is accounted for, including seasonal variation, deviations related to illness or idiosyncratic disposition, celebratory meals ("feasting") and fasting (during Ramadan).

The dietary survey conducted during our follow-up study helped us to further understand the multicontextual use of plants. Building on the earlier investigation, the more recent survey replicated the methodology outlined above: the same eight households (54 residents) were monitored for a full 48-week harvest-to-harvest cycle. The range of items contributing to diet had expanded over the 12-year period as a result of increased interregional and international communication and trade. In both medicine and diet, more subtle changes were suggested by shifting environmental circumstances that affected the availability of medicinal and food plants. The changes in Hausa diet are discussed in greater detail elsewhere. We review only the yearly fluctuations in relative quantities of different food types, particularly with reference to grain-based foods (porridges and gruels, the mainstay of morning and evening meals) and foods that include "vegetables" (leafy and other herbaceous plants).

Selection of Plants for Study

Conventionally, investigations of indigenous medicines evaluate therapeutic efficacy on the basis of treatment for simple, discrete symptoms. Antimicrobial activity has been tested in plants used in the treatment of wounds, tooth and gum disease, dermatoses and gastrointestinal disorders. Antipyresis and analgesia are targets for medicines used in the treatment of fevers. Effects on platelet and phagocyte function and systemic arterial pressure generate most interest for plants used in the treatment of cardiovascular disorders. Studies of fertility-regulating plants deal principally with estrogen-modulating actions but also with effects on male fertility and abortifacient actions.

By contrast, our model for the empirical evaluation of plant medicines directs attention to the potential efficacy of therapies used in the treatment of disorders characterized by interrelated and superficially indiscernible symptom complexes. As we have discussed elsewhere, investigation of indigenous treatments of symptom-complex disorders such as malaria is particularly important in view of the associated high morbidity and mortality, and because it is in the prevention and treatment of those complex diseases that one confronts the most tension between biomedical and indigenous explanatory models.

Pharmacologic investigations of indigenous antimalarials tend to consider only those plants described specifically for the treatment of the malaria symptom complex in its entirety, a biomedical construct that not all medical paradigms recognize. Studies of antimalarials of which we are aware do not acknowledge the potential lack of concordance between biomedical and other nosologies and, so, do not include plants used only for one or some of the symptoms or for emically nonmedical purposes such as food, hygiene and cosmetics. (We do not count here wholesale screening of plants and compounds for antimalarial activity, since those studies tend to be informed by the paradigms of botany and phytochemistry and have virtually no bearing on ethnomedicine).

The plants that we selected for laboratory investigation following the 1975-1976 research are among the more common Hausa medicines used in the treatment of one or more components of what biomedicine understands to be the malaria symptom complex. These include the intermittent fevers that are the signature of malaria infection as well as more equivocal markers such as anemia, hemoglobinuria, spleno/hepatomegaly and jaundice. In this way, our analysis incorporates medicines used to treat the full range of symptoms, singly or in some combination.

Laboratory and Pharmacologic Studies of Hausa Plants

Rationale: Our first laboratory investigations drew conceptually on indirect measures of efficacy in malaria therapy, specifically perturbations of red blood cell oxidation-reduction (redox) equilibrium. That approach was an important departure from conventional pharmacologic studies of antimalarial activity, which until that time had been primarily constituent analyses probing for quininelike alkaloids or for compounds that approximate the structure and presumably the activity, of known synthetic antimalarials.

The significance of redox fluctuations in the course of malaria infection has been amply demonstrated over the last two decades. Recently other researchers also include redox phenomena in their investigations of antimalarial plants.The most salient point for the present discussion is that increased oxidation compromises host red cell integrity and interferes with *Plasmodium* metabolism to the extent that parasite maturation is impaired, resulting in the interruption of what would ordinarily be the regular, serial infection of new blood cells.

Red blood cell integrity is dependent upon suppression of chemical equilibrium with molecular oxygen. That equilibrium is offset in normal cells by redox reactions that are part of or integrally linked to the pentose phosphate shunt (PPS). This secondary pathway for glucose catabolism uses glucose to produce carbon dioxide (CO_2) and NADPH, a source of reducing (antioxidant) capacity and potential energy. This can link at three points with the primary, Embden-Meyerhof pathway, which metabolizes glucose to lactate and produces potential energy (ATP). Whereas ordinarily about 11 percent of red cell glucose passes through the PPS, that amount increases

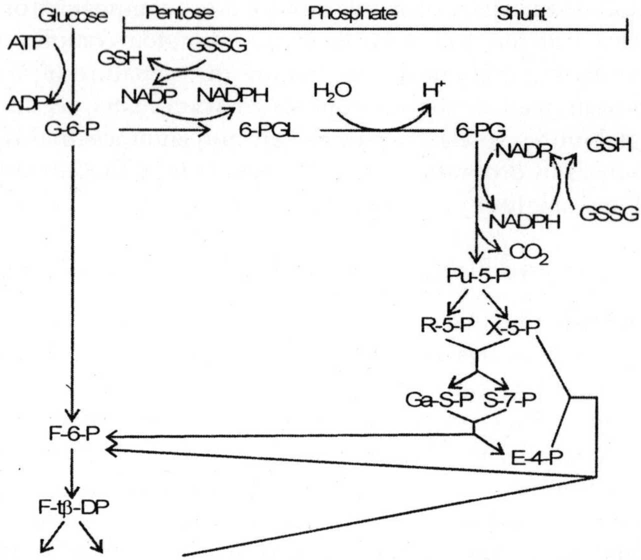

Figure 9.1. Glucose Catabolism through the Pentose Phosphate Shunt

Abbreviations relevant to the text discussion: NADP/NADPH and NAD/NADH = oxidized/ reduced forms of the enzyme cofactors nicotinamide adenine dinucleotide phosphate and nicotinamide adenine dinucleotide. GSSG/GSH = oxidized/ reduced forms of glutathione. Circled numbers correspond to enzymes. For the present discussion, note that 1 = glucose6-phosphate dehydrogenase.

When levels of intracellular oxidation are elevated. Such elevations occur in the course of normal metabolic fluctuations, in certain genetic anomalies, in the presence of infectious and other pathologies and as a reaction to some foods, drugs and other xenobiotics. The most salient point for the present discussion is that increased oxidation compromises the integrity of host red cells. This interrupts plasmodial development and leaves immature parasite forms that cannot transfer the infection to new red cells.

Evidence of oxidation during plasmodial infection includes elevated methemoglobin (metHb), coenzymes NAD and NADP and glutathione (GSSG) relative to their reduced counterparts (hemoglobin, NADH and NADPH, GSH); inhibition of catalase by aminotriazole (which requires the presence of the oxidant hydrogen peroxide, H_2O_2); lipid peroxidation; spontaneous generation of radical oxygen species; and parasite incorporation of host superoxide dismutase. These observations are understood to reflect both intraerythrocytic oxidation (of plasmodial origin and red cell response) and activation of leukocyte defense, including the release of reactive oxygen species among the immunomodulators.

The summary point is that *elevated intracellular oxidation, some of plasmodial origin, selectively renders infected cells more susceptible to hemolysis* through peroxidation of membrane lipids and decomposition of sulfhydryl-containing enzymes, hemoglobin and other key cellular constituents. Red cell destruction interrupts maturation of the plasmodium, which cannot survive extracellularly as an immature blood form. A range of circumstances that protect humans against fulminant malaria infection are thus explained: oxidant sensitivity in G6PD deficiencies (including "favism," a severe hemolytic reaction to the ingestion of the fava bean), some hemoglobinopathies (áand-ß-thalassemias, hemoglobins S and E), vitamin E deficiency, free-radical intermediates in the metabolism of certain pharmaceuticals and naturally occurring endoperoxides.

In view of that evidence, we investigated the oxidizing potential of Hausa plant medicines used to treat one or more symptoms of malaria. We hypothesized that the combined effects of plant and parasite-generated intraerythrocytic oxidation would overwhelm host cell oxidant defenses, resulting in lysis of infected red cells and release of immature parasites.

Conversion of Hemoglobin to Methemoglobin: Methemoglobin generation is a sensitive indicator of erythrocyte oxidant damage and is determined through standardized assays. Extracts were prepared from macerated plant materials in solutions of isotonic saline and neutralized to physiologic pH. Normal red call hemolysates in dilute hemoglobin suspensions were incubated at 37°Cin equivolume ratios with plant extracts, and metHb levels were determined after two hours' incubation. Control samples were identically prepared, sans plant extract. Data are summarized in Table 9.3, with two-hour metlib concentrations expressed as percentages of original Hb that was converted to the oxidized metlib.

In this study, *Guiera senegalensis* leaves appear to be the most potent oxidant generators, with 100 percent conversion of Hb ? metHb.

Glutathione Oxidation: Our second measure of oxidizing potential evaluated plant extracts for the ability to convert reduced glutathione (GSH) to its oxidized counterpart (GSSG). Extracts, hemolysates and controls were prepared as for the metHb studies, with starting GSH concentrations at 2.0 millimoles (mM). Samples were incubated for two hours at 37°C and residual GSH measured at 30-minute intervals (methods as reported in Etkin and Eaton).

Table 9.3. Methemoglobin Generation by Plant Extracts

Genus and Species	Hausa Name	Plant Part	%Hb ? MetHb
Acacia nilotica Del.	Gabaruwa	Root	56%
Fabaceae			
Azadirachta indica A. Juss.	Darbejiya	Leaf	42%
Meliaceae			
		Bark	9%
		Root	7%
Cassia occidentalis	Majamfari	Root	78%
Fabaceae			
		Leaf	68%
Cassia tora L.	Tafasa	Leaf	35%
Fabaceae			
		Root	29%
Cochlospermum tinctorium	Rawaya	Root	51%
Rich., Cochlospermaceae			
Guiera senegalensis JF	Sabara	Root	47%
Gmel., Combretaceae			
		Leaf	100%
Securidaca longipedunculata	Sanya	Root	29%
Fres., Polygalaceae			
Controls			0.5%

Results are summarized in Table 9.4, in which both relative rates of GSH depletion and glutathione residua for all samples are displayed. Highest oxidant activity is indicated for leaf extracts of *Guiera senegalensis, Azadirachta indica and Cassia tora,* which had the lowest final GSH concentrations.

The results of these preliminary investigations of methemoglobin generation and GSH depletion suggest that some Hausa plant medicines have oxidizing activity, indirectly recommending their efficacy in the therapy of malaria infection. On this basis we selected the best candidates for inclusion in direct in vivo tests of efficacy against an analogue of human malaria, murine *Plasmodium berghei,* studies of which represent most of the basic experimental work in human malaria therapy.

Table 9.4. Gluthatione Oxidation by Plant Extracts

Genus and Species	Hausa Name	Plant Part	0 min	30 min	60 min	120 min
Acacia nilotica Del.	Gabaruwa	Root	2.0mM	1.3mM	0.9mM	0.2mM
Fabaceae						
Azadirachta indica A. Juss.	Darbejiya	Leaf	2.0	1.2	0.7	0.1
Meliaceae						
		Bark	2.0	1.7	1.6	1.4
		Root	2.0	1.8	1.8	1.7
Cassia occidentalis	Majamfari	Root	2.0	1.9	1.7	1.5
Fabaceae						
		Leaf	2.0	1.9	1.6	1.0
Cassia tora L.	Tafasa	Leaf	2.0	0.4	0.4	0.1
Fabaceae						
		Root	2.0	1.5	1.3	0.9
Cochlospermum tinctorium	Rawaya	Root	2.0	1.8	1.7	1.2
Rich., Cochlospermaceae						
Guiera senegalensis JF	Sabara	Root	2.0	1.8	1.5	1.5
Gmel., Combretaceae						
		Leaf	2.0	0.5	0.1	0.1
Securidaca longipedunculata	Sanya	Root	2.0	1.8	1.7	1.5
Fres., Polygalaceae						
Controls			2.0	1.9	1.9	1.9

In vivo Studies: Malaria infection is maintained in laboratory animals by intraperitoneal (IP) injection of healthy subjects with plasmodium-infected red blood cells drawn from heavily parasitized animals. We interrupted this process with an incubation phase in order to expose parasites to extracts of the medicinals *Acacia nilotica* root, and leaves of *Azadirachta indica, Cassia tora* and *Guiera senegalensis.* After two hours' incubation, infected blood was injected into healthy subjects. We monitored time elapsed before the infection reached patency and the duration of infection prior to death, two standard evaluations used in the testing of antimalarial drugs. The toxicity of plant extracts was ruled out by a parallel series of investigations in which neutralized extracts were injected IP over a course of seven days. Results are summarized in Table 9.5. Exposure to extracts of *Acacia nilotica, Azadirachta indica and Guiera senegalensis* clearly suppressed infection, while *Cassia tora* extended survival only insignificantly.

Table 9.5. Effects of Plant Extracts on Plasmodial Infection

Genus and Species	Hausa Name	Plant Part	Parasitemia Day 7
Acacia nilotica Del.	Gabaruwa	Root	0%
Fabaceae			
Azadirachta indica A. Juss.	Darbejiya	Leaf	0%
Meliaceae			
Cassia tora L.	Tafasa	Leaf	83%
Fabaceae			
Guiera senegalensis JF	Sabara	Leaf	1%
Gmel., Combretaceae			
Controls			87%

The findings of these preliminary investigations of Hausa antimalarial plants could be clarified by more rigorous laboratory protocols to fractionate the specific constituents responsible for in vitro oxidant activity, establish whether ingestion of these oxidizing plants raises intraerythrocytic oxidation to levels that disrupt malaria parasite development and determine whether the apparent in vivo effects against Plasmodium berghei can be attributed to those other constituents. Our preliminary findings were sufficiently promising as a prototype study to sustain our investigatory energy. We reported those results in the first edition of this volume principally to highlight a unique methodology for the evaluation of antimalarial plants.

Investigations of Antimalarial Activity: Series 2

Rationale: In view of the growing body of literature confirming the role that oxidant sensitivity plays in protection against malaria (discussed above), the argument is still compelling that this feature should be explored in the continuing search for new antimalarial drugs. Other methodological advances need to be embraced as well, including two important advances that were developed since the late 1970s, when we began our antimalarial studies. Refinement of a continuous culture technique for Plasmodium falciparum has made possible the propagation and ever more intricate manipulation of human malaria parasites and long-term maintenance of cell cultures provides a system for the direct and quantifiable measurement of in vitro antimalarial activity.

We took advantage of this elaborated protocol to further assess the antimalarial potential of Hausa plants. Having expanded our original data base through the extensive follow-up study in 1987-1988, we tested 309 specimens representing 134 species for activity against P. *falciparum* cell cultures. This time, we further specified the sample by invoking the criterion of multicontextual use and selected from among 126 Hausa antipyretics 82 plants that are used in diet as well, thereby increasing people's exposure to any pharmacologic (and other) action. Primary aqueous/ ethanol extractions (I) of 23 specimens (22 species, 27%) demonstrated in vitro activity against P. *falciparum*. Differential extraction with saline (II NaCI) and chloroform (II Chlor), and finally extraction of the remaining insoluble residue with ethanol (III) revealed antimalarial activity in additional fractions. It is important to distinguish between this direct test for antiplasmodial action and the earlier, indirect assessment that probed for oxidant action. The two series of laboratory investigations employed different methodologies, but results are not mutually exclusive: failure to demonstrate oxidizing potential in some plants does not confirm lack of antiplasmodial action they may be effective through another mechanism of action; and efficacy demonstrated by plants in the later series may or may not be linked to their ability to increase intracellular oxidation. The methodological advances of the later series no doubt account in some measure for the disparity between the lists of "positives" that distilled from the two series of investigations; further testing will reconcile these differences.

Table 9.6. Activity of Plant Extracts against Plasmodium falciparum Cell Cultures

Genus and Species	Hausa Name	Plant Part	I	II	III	IV
				NaCl Chlor		
Acacia nilotica Del.	Gabaruwa	root	+	+	-	+
Fabaceae						
Agelanthus dodoneifolius P & W	Kauci	whole	+	-	-	+
Loranthaceae						
Artemisia maciverae Hutch.&Dalz.	Tazargade	whole	+	-	+	-
Asteraceae						
Cassia occidentalis L.	Majamfai	root	+	-	+	+
Fabaceae						
		leaves	+	+	-	+
Centaurea perrottetii DC.	Dayi	whole	+	-	+	-
Asteraceae						
Chrozophora senegalensis A. Juss.	Damagi	whole	+	+	-	+
Euphorbiaceae						
Cyperus articulatus L.	Kajiji	root	+	-	+	+
Cyperaceae						
Diospyros mespiliformis Hochst.	Kanya	leaves	+	-	-	+
Ebenaceae						
Erythrina senegalensis DC.	Minjirya	root	+	-	+	-
Fabaceae						
Feretia apodanthera Del.	Kurukuru	leaves	+	-	-	+
Rubiaceae						
Ficus ingens Miq.	Kawari	bark	+	-	-	-
Moraceae						
F. polita Vahl.	Durumi	leaves	+	+	-	+
Moraceae						
F. ovata Vahl.	Cediya	bark	+	-	+	+
Moraceae						
Momordica blasamina L	Garahunu	whole	+	-	-	-
Cucurbitaceae						

Genus and Species	Hausa Name	Plant Part	I	II	III	IV
Piper guineense Schum. & Thonn.	Masoro	fruit	+	+	-	-
Piperaceae						
Psidium guajava L.	Gwaiba	leaves	+	+	-	+
Myrtaceae						
Securinega virosa Baill.	Tsa	leaves	+	+	-	+
Euphorbiaceae						
Sorghum spp.	Dawa	root	+	-	-	-
Poaceae						
Syzium aromaticum Merr.&Perry	Kanumfari	clove	+	+	+	+
Myrtaceae						
Thonningea sanguinea Vahl.	Kulla	root	+	+	+	+
Balanophoraceae						
Xylopia aethiopica A. Rich.	Kimba	fruit	+	-	+	-
Annonaceae						
Zingiber officinale Rosc.	Cittar Aho	rhizome	+	-	+	+
Zingiberaceae						

A second strategic advance for research on antimalarial plants is access to NAPRALERT (NAtural PRoducts ALERT), a unique natural products relational database that distills the world literature on the chemical constituents, activity and pharmacology of plant parts and extracts. Its capabilities are vast and replace the type of literature search one used to do "by hand" or with weaker computer instruments. Ready access to those data greatly extends knowledge of the specific plants on which our studies center, helps us to understand more fully the physiologic outcomes of plant use and suggests direction for refining laboratory investigations.

Interrelations among Indigenous Medicines, Diet and Disease

In addition to pharmacologic assessment of these plants through laboratory study and literature review, it is important to consider the varied contexts in which they are used. Review of data collected during the first field study made us aware of the overlapping contexts in which individual plants are used. We and others have remarked that very little is known about the pharmacology of food plants and have argued that, given the blurred boundaries between medicines and foods, investigation of the pharmacologic qualities of medicines is not complete without attention to all contexts of exposure to those plants.

Diet is important additionally because plants consumed as food tend to be ingested regularly and in relatively large volume compared, for example, to use of those same plants as cosmetics or in occasional rituals. Further, we have argued elsewhere that Hausa knowledge of some plants as medicines has helped to identify those plants for inclusion in diet.

Nutrition and Disease

The bulk of clinical, epidemiological and biochemical evidence regarding interactions between nutrition and disease point to synergism between malnutrition and infection. This is recorded as increased susceptibility to infection secondary to diminished immune function; compromised skin integrity and reduced gastric acidity; exaggerated symptomatology; depression of nutrient intake due to anorexia; precipitation of frank nutrient deficits with increasing parasitemia; increased metabolic requirements (cellular hypermetabolism); fever-related pathologic changes leading to nutrient excretion via urine; and reactions linked to the mobilization of proinflammatory cytokines. These physiologic parameters are overlaid by such cultural variables as conscious underfeeding of ill children and therapeutically inspired food proscriptions.

Less is known of the antagonistic relationships between nutrition and infection, although a number of special cases have been described. Diets consisting almost entirely of milk suppress a variety of infections: rheumatic heart disease of streptococcal origin, likely attributed to the antimicrobial actions of oleic acid; malaria, due to low levels of PABA, riboflavin and vitamin E; *Giardia lamblia,* due to a human-specific lipase; and malaria, tuberculosis, *Entamoeba histolytica,* and others due to the presence in milk of partially saturated lactoferrin and transferrin in sufficiently high concentrations to compete with parasites for iron. In plants, naturally occurring chelators such as tannins, phytates, citric acid and other constituents of humic acid may sequester sufficiently large pools of serum iron to suppress some infectious agents, an effect that might be offset in the case of malaria by the antioxidant actions of phytate, or enhanced by simultaneous consumption of vitamin C. Similarly, low levels of iron and other nutrients have been implicated in suppression of those same infections among people experiencing temporary and long-term food shortages.

But what can one say of the pharmacologic effects of routine diets on the occurrence or expression of infection? There exists an atheoretical and disaggregated literature on "food pharmacology" that records physiologic activities for specific foods and projects that information onto populations whose epiderniologic circumstances may not be known but who consume those plants as food and/or medicine. For example, extracts of garlic *(Allium safiva L.)* and onion *(A. cepa L.)* are anthelminthic; West African black pepper (*Piper guineense* Schum. & Thonn.) has antiviral activity; ginger (*Zingiber officinale* Rosc.), cinnamon (*Cinnamomum verum* J. Presl), and turmeric (*Curcuma longa* L.) are antimicrobial. The difficulty lies in tying these observations to real populations with known disease history and rigorously testing such hypotheses. The edited volumes Plants in Indigenous Medicine and Diet and Eating on the Wild Side are organized explicitly around this goal and the studies reported therein provide direction for this type of inquiry. We use that same framework for reporting results of our investigations of Hausa plant medicines and foods.

Malaria in Northern Nigeria

Malaria is endemic throughout northern Nigeria and in Hurumi the risk of infection is greatest during August to October, a pattern typical of much of the sub-Saharan savanna, which is dominated by a unimodal pattern of rainfall. In this region the annual cycle includes 3 to 4 months of rains and an 8-9-month dry season. In most years the onset of rains in June is followed by the progressive development of microenvironments that support mosquito breeding, so that by August mosquitoes abound in numbers sufficient for the sustained growth of malaria parasites and their continued transmission to susceptible human hosts. Nonetheless, the reported incidence of fulminant and debilitating plasmodial infection is relatively low for this region. This apparent suppression of malaria infection may be ascribed to a number of factors, one of which the efficacy of indigenous antimalarials was discussed. The potential contribution of diet to malaria suppression is discussed below.

Malaria Epidemiology and Dietary Patterns: 1975-1976

Reflecting the dependence on local subsistence through the 1970s, dietary patterns in Hurumi were distinguished by marked seasonal fluctuations in the availability of foodstuffs. For example the principal staples, millet *(Pennisetum* spp.) and guineacorn (*Sorghum* spp.), were sown in early June, harvested from mid-September through November, and subsequently stored in granaries. The chief legumes cultivated are groundnut (*Arachis hypogaea* L.) and cowpea (*Vigna unguiculata* Walpers), generally sown in late June to early July and harvested the same time as the later-maturing sorghums. Maximum availability and lowest market costs for all of these products coincided with their harvest and their supplies gradually diminished through the end of the dry season and beginning of the rainy months, with market prices for their replacement increasing commensurately. The exception to this pattern of fluctuating availability for the primary foodstuffs was cassava (*Manihot esculenta* Crantz), which was available year-round (protected from livestock, it can endure as a transannual, providing edible rootstock for as long as three years).

The patterning of types and quantities of foods consumed in Hurumi corresponded closely to fluctuations in availability and costs. Variability was greatly diminished immediately following the harvest, when grains were readily available for consumption in the form of thick porridges favored by Hausa as the appropriately energy-dense base around which the primary (evening) and some other meals are contrived. Dietary elaboration was increasingly pronounced through the progression of the dry season and commencement of rains. This took the form of an increased variety of foods eaten and of their sources and preparation styles. Figure 9.2 depicts the frequency with which nongrain foods contributed to total caloric intake and illustrates increasing dietary reliance on nongrain foods as the next harvest approached.

This dietary elaboration is explained by both ecological and cultural features; its implications are multiple. The depletion of staples stored from the previous harvest contributed to greater reliance on market purchases of raw grains and on foods purchased from extrahousehold sources, typically market vendors and village women who sell prepared main dishes and snacks. These sources amplified the range of variability in the household's diet beyond what would otherwise have been only those products reaped during the previous harvest. Moreover, the frequency and duration of market attendance increased during the dry season. The population was thus exposed to a greater array of foods from other areas and increased purchases beyond necessities for household meals. Another factor that encouraged dietary variability toward the end of the dry season is a larger number of ceremonies that, in the public celebration of life-cycle events, involve intra and inter-village food exchanges and redistributions. Although grains predominated in the diet throughout the year, the steady increase in market costs which reached a maximum during the latter part of the rainy season dissuaded many people from replacing their diminished grain stores. Instead, they relied on other, less-preferred but readily obtained foods.

Table 9.8. Food Uses of Local Semi-Wild Medicinal Plants

FOOD TYPE		Plants (n=61)	% age
MEALS	soups	20	32.8
	gruels	7	11.5
	misc. midday secondary	12	19.7
	misc. midday primary	10	16.4
SNACKS	prepared mixture	12	19.7
	raw	5	8.2
	sweet beverages	2	3.3
	milk	4	6.6
EMERGENCY		7	11.5

Another feature of dietary elaboration that characterized the rainy season is the increased availability of "semi-wild" plants. We refer to these as "vegetables" to underscore their role in Hausa diet, for which they are marked primarily by their foliage (although young stems, calyces, buds, fruits and flowers are indicated in some cases). These are to a large extent "free goods", since those growing on public grazing land, paths and other nonprivate property can be collected without permission or obligation. Tables 9.2 and 9.8

document the significance of semiwild plants for Hausa medicine and diet. These plants were most prominent in diet during the last two months of the rainy season (only some are dried for consumption throughout the year). That timing can be explained by three interrelated factors. First, these plants were more readily available then; compared with grains, they matured and were available for collection or market purchase earlier and were less expensive. Second, these vegetables, added to cereal-based mixtures, helped to extend remaining grain stores during the period of shortest supply. Third, they provided a welcome substitute for cassava, which was itself a substitute for the declining grains and had become, by Hausa standards, tedious. Cereal-based dishes were augmented by the addition of vegetables and by the substitution of cassava for at least one meal, usually at midday, in order to reserve grains for the most important, evening meal. The aggregate effect of these seasonal changes was increased consumption of vegetables through the progression of the rainy season.

The leaves of some species were especially favored as centerpiece for several popular dishes, including, from Table 9.7, *Amaranthus hybridus, Cadaba farinosa, Cassia tora, Hibiscus sabdariffa, Momoradica balsamina, M. Charantia,* and *Moringa oleifiera.* Other leaves that figure more prominently for soups and as seasonings include, from Table 9.7 *Adansonia digitata, Atremisia maciverae, Corchorus ttidens, Celosia trigyna, C. isetrii, Ficus ovata, F. polita, Guiera senegalensis, Parkia filicoidea, Sesamum radiatum* and *Tamarindus indica.* Figure 9.3 demonstrates this increased use of vegetable foods in household diet as the annual cycle approaches the next harvest.

Further, most of the plants listed in Table 9.7 are also used medicinally, other than for malaria. Notable in this regard is Guiera senegalensis, one of whose Hausa names, "mother of medicines" (uwar magunguna), reflects its use as both principal and vehicle in various medicinal preparations. The likelihood that the use of several of these plants would influence malaria infection is heightened by their indication for the prevention and treatment of other rainy season diseases such as sanyi and raba, complex symptom clusters whose etiology is ascribed to dampness and the chill of wet clothing and house floors.

As noted earlier, during 1975 and 1976, the period of highest malaria risk coincided with the end of the rainy season, when increases in vegetable consumption and decreases in grain utilization were most marked. We suggest that these interrelated aspects of dietary patterning may have antagonistic effects on malaria infection, thereby helping to explain why, despite the high risk, plasmodial infections that occurred tended to be relatively moderate.

Malaria, Medicine and Meals

From a pharmacologic perspective, dietary and other uses of antimalarial plants should be interpreted as additional exposure to constituents of potential therapeutic efficacy. That is, the consumption of oxidizing and otherwise antiplasmodial plants in both medicinal and dietary contexts during a time when risk of malaria infection was highest may have had a compound effect in limiting this infection.

Additionally, the reduction in grain consumption that coincided with increased use of vegetables may curtail parasitemia. We draw here on the observations of Murray, who noted recrudescence of plasmodial infections among populations in famine-relief programs. It is possible that the apparent protection against malaria occurred because of deficits in vitamin E (an antioxidant), and that this balance was overturned on supplying those populations with vitamin E-rich grains. Or iron may be the critical nutrient. In any case, the observation holds that the circumstances of grain deprivation coincide with suppressed malaria infection.

We proposed that what appeared to be paradoxically low levels of fulminant malaria in Hurumi could be attributed at least in part to the combined effects of decreased consumption of grains rich in vitamin E and iron and increased consumption of vegetables and medicines that generate oxidants and/or otherwise impede plasmodial development.

Dietary Update, 1987-1988

During our follow-up study in Hurumi we noted marked diminution in the seasonal constraints on resources that had characterized dietary patterns 12 years earlier. This is due in part to increased availability of a range of foodstuffs through expanded regional markets, attendant upon the growth of transportation networks and other infrastructural developments. There was substantial evidence of increasing participation of Hurumi residents in the larger economy more took part in short-term migration to urban areas, bringing back to Hurumi cash and new food preferences; a greater number were selling and buying foodstuffs, both more often and more regularly throughout the year. Further, cassava cultivation and consumption declined dramatically for the most recent period; whereas cassava provided as much as 14 percent of all calories consumed during its peak consumption period in 1975-1976, it represented no more than 2 percent of all calories consumed during the 1987-1988 period (the respective weekly means being 6.1% and 1.6%). This reflects changes in food preference as well as such environmental variables as unfavorable growing conditions and plant diseases. The full impact of these dietary shifts is beyond the scope of this chapter, but we do need to underscore two aspects that are relevant to our earlier model of a seasonally changing diet and its potential impact on malaria.

The first aspect of changing diet pertains to grain consumption. Although there were no marked cyclical reductions for the 1987-1988 research period, the overall yearly consumption of grain was relatively low, in fact comparable to the diminished rates of grain consumption that characterized the 1975-1976 high-malaria-risk season. (The 48-week mean was 450 grams per capita for 1987-1988.) The lower consumption of grain was accounted for in part by the year-round substitution of legume-based midday meals and the more frequent inclusion of imported and costly, polished rice.

The second aspect of dietary change is of greater concern for the continued relevance of our model. Here, we note for 1987-1988 a marked reduction in the quantity of semi-wild vegetables consumed. This decrease, particularly during the period of malaria risk, can be partly attributed to replacement of cassava-based dishes with more favored legume and grain-based dishes and a concomitant reduction in vegetable-based dishes. It is interesting that while the quantity of vegetables in the diet diminished, the incidence of population exposure to at least some of these products was comparable for the two research periods, illustrating the continued importance of vegetables as dietary supplements. Whether this dietary change that attends economic and infrastructural changes portends a trend that may affect malaria expression is at this stage only conjecture. Indeed, most recent reports from our Nigerian colleague suggest an ever more complex environment characterized both by the wax and wane of regional markets, creating conditions in which people actually rely more on foods from local sources and the expansion of antimalarial programs that include the widespread but sporadic use of biomedical prophylaxis. While the exploration of this dynamic awaits further fieldwork, the dietary and medicinal pharmacologic model suggested by our earlier work continued to inform our investigations through the most recent field research and helps to shape future inquiry as well.

Conclusion

A model that integrates features of disease ecology and plant pharmacology was applied to investigate how certain foods and medicines might interact with malaria infection. Elsewhere, we used this framework to investigate how foods and medicines might influence gastrointestinal disorders, as well as to expand the number of overlapping contexts beyond the two considered here (including also plants used as cosmetics and for personal hygiene). Collectively these studies illustrate how the pharmacologic potential of botanicals is extended through their use in various contexts. By focusing on these plants for investigations of biocultural adaptations to disease, we conceptualize them broadly as ingestible plants rather than exclusively as "medicines", "foods", or something else.

This chapter evaluates the continued utility of our model for dietary shifts as adaptations to both the fluctuating availability of plants and the seasonal occurrence of malaria infection. In sum, we note that a number of Hausa medicinal plants used to treat malaria infection are also important dietary constituents. Laboratory investigations of Hausa antimalarials suggest their efficacy. Moreover, the plasmodiostatic activity demonstrated for some of these plants might be amplified by a diminished consumption of grains. An examination of local diets during 1975 and 1976 revealed that both increased use of medicinal plants as food and diminished consumption of grains coincided with the period of greatest risk of malaria infection. From our more recent study, we document changes in the local diet most significant, a decrease in the quantities consumed of plants that provided the focus of our earlier investigations. These observations, cast in a broad ecological framework, provide a basis from which we can explore the potential implications of other dimensions of change.

10

Medical Care and Diagnosis

Introduction

A complete medical history and an adequate physical examination are vital to the diagnosis and effective management of your or your child's asthma. To get a proper basis for treatment and possibly to find out what is causing your asthma your doctor should do three main things: take a careful history, conduct a thorough physical examination and order some laboratory tests, including an X ray.

Frances, 67, suddenly develops a persistent cough, pains in the right side of her chest and a wheeze. Because of the wheezing she is convinced she has asthma. She goes to the drugstore and buys Primatene Mist. After using it for 10 days with no success she decides to see a doctor. By that time Frances is very short of breath. Her doctor listens to her chest and, because he does not hear air movement, orders an X ray. The X ray shows a collapse of part of her right lung. A bronchoscopy is done. During the procedure the doctor extricates a cherry pit that was apparently taken into the lung some time before. Frances does not recollect the event. "I hardly ever eat cherries", she says. "I don't even *like* them".

Medical History

The medical history is the most important element in the process of finding out whether or not you have asthma and if you do, what causes it. A good, thorough, well-taken history can and often does establish the validity of the diagnosis of asthma and its causes. You should be prepared to answer the doctor's questions accurately, fully and honestly. (This is also a good way to check on how thorough and careful the doctor is in trying to help you. Where important areas are neglected if your family background goes unchecked, for instance, or if you are not asked about changes in your environment that occurred about the time of your first attack you should take note). The doctor will be especially interested in the nature of the onset of your asthma. Was it sudden and unexpected or slow, gradual and progressive? Was it associated with a fever or infection? Did it show up when you moved or changed your environment at work, home, or school? Do you have any pets? Any new pets? Does your asthma get worse at particular times of the year? Do you smoke? Do some foods seem to trigger your asthma or make it worse? What are they?

Physical Examination

Your physician should give you a *complete* physical examination. You can get some idea of the caliber of your doctor by taking note of how careful and thorough the physical is. A good doctor (or staff) will carry out the routine steps, such as recording weight, height, pulse and blood pressure. If you are over 40 the doctor should do a rectal examination; women should have their breasts examined.

Then come the steps that tie in more closely to asthma, beginning with carefully listening to your chest with a stethoscope. (Many physicians believe that, for asthmatics, the stethoscope and what lies between its ear pieces is the most powerful diagnostic tool!) If the doctor doesn't listen to your lungs at all or does it in a perfunctory way, you've been short-changed. The lungs are vital to maintaining all systems in your body and asthma starves the lungs by cutting off the air flow. Thus, asthma can affect the heart, the kidneys and the skin. Your physician, by combining direct inspection and laboratory testing of these organs and sites, can determine if they have been affected by chronic lack of oxygen, for example.

Next, an X ray should be taken. This will reveal what your lungs look like and will show up any damage or the presence of other conditions emphysema, for example which may be mistaken for asthma. Unfortunately, there are many people who dread and balk at the idea of having a chest X ray, fearing the possibility of cancer. It is true that exposure to a radioactive source can be dangerous and harmful. However, the amount of exposure nowadays is much smaller than it was even a few years ago when the equipment was less sensitive and efficient. The small risk that radiation carries has to be weighed against the real dangers that respiratory problems carry. Tragic errors have occurred because of refusals to have a needed X ray.

Anthony had had asthma all his life and was used to wheezing, which he controlled adequately by taking over-the-counter medications. His doctor frequently advised him that there were much better drugs available, but Anthony paid no attention. He did not like the thought of taking prescription drugs, believing that the over-the-counter remedies were less harmful to him a surprisingly common error. Even so, at age 40 he was able to live fairly comfortably with his complaint. Then, one afternoon at work, he began to experience aches and chills. He went home, thinking he had the flu. His wife took his temperature, which registered 101.5°. He also noticed that his wheezing was getting worse. That didn't surprise him because it almost always got worse when he had a virus. Next morning his temperature was 102°.

Anthony went to his doctor, who listened to his chest and concluded that Anthony might have pneumonia. He told Anthony he ought to have an X ray and be placed on antibiotics. Anthony refused. The doctor tried to insist and became angry when Anthony refused to comply. Anthony, too, lost his temper and stormed out. That night his fever suddenly shot up to 104° and he became confused and disoriented. His wife called an ambulance and Anthony was taken to the emergency room where an X ray was finally taken. The picture showed severe diffuse bacterial pneumonia. Anthony was admitted to the hospital and started on antibiotics, but not soon enough. He died two days later.

The doctor, by losing his temper and not insisting more determinedly, was just as foolish as Anthony was in his stubborn refusal. A calm and reasoned approach entails weighing the implications of both actions. You have to decide open-mindedly if the risk of an X ray outweighs that of developing an undiagnosed and possibly treatable disease. Doctors now are much better informed and careful about ordering X rays than they were 20 years ago. If you're nervous about the X ray, speak up and listen carefully to your doctor's reply. If you're pregnant, or think you might be, tell the doctor *and* the X-ray technician. They will shield your pelvis during the process.

Laboratory Tests

The doctor may order some laboratory work. In addition to a urinalysis, which can point to any one of a large number of conditions, you may have blood samples drawn. Many individuals find this experience upsetting and painful, but it is useful in detecting anemia or infections. It can also establish the presence of immunoglobulin E (IgE), a strong indicator of an allergic base for your asthma. A tuberculin skin test, to determine if you have been exposed to tuberculosis, may be administered because this disease, once a rarity, is making a determined comeback. Finally, the doctor will consider and discuss with you the possibility and advisability of having allergy skin tests. Skin tests and other tests for allergies and their place in diagnosing asthma are discussed.

Choosing a Physician

There are a number of things to look for in a physician and they apply regardless of the source of your medical care independent, private physicians or a large health maintenance organization. Most important, you should feel comfortable with your physician and have solid reason to believe that he or she is well trained and competent. When you first call for an appointment, inquire where the doctor received his or her training. You may find the following guidelines useful:

1. Is the doctor a graduate of an American medical school?

Levels of training and standards of performance demanded in medical education vary greatly around the world. U.S. schools enforce fairly consistent standards and their graduates perform better in medical qualifying examinations.

2. What is the doctor's specialty and does he or she have board certification to back it up?

Upon graduating from medical school, the brand new doctor who has merely completed his medical school courses is awarded a license to practice "medicine and surgery". This occurs before undergoing any intensive clinical experience (internship) or specialized training (residency) and does not really signify that its holder is competent to practice. Having an M.D. degree alone does not qualify its holder to go out and practice allergy or any other specialty.

There are a number of medical groups that have acquired the special training and background that qualify them to treat asthma. These are pediatricians, internists, chest or pulmonary physicians and allergists. Depending on your age, your first asthma visit should probably be to a pediatrician (for children or youth) or an internist (for adolescents and older). Most patients with asthma are adequately treated by pediatricians and internists. Make sure, however, that your prospective physician is board certified in pediatrics or internal medicine. If the receptionist or office nurse does not know about certification, the doctor is probably not certified. Insist until you get a definite yes or no answer to the question of board certification.

You can also start with a family practitioner (not the same as the old time general practitioner), who has had special training in family medicine. Family practitioners can manage most routine medical problems efficiently and competently, but for serious asthmatic symptoms you should be referred to an internist, a pediatrician or either a chest physician or an allergist for consultation.

3. Choose a doctor when you are healthy.

Too often, people moving to a new town put off finding someone to take care of them. Then, when they get sick, they no longer have the freedom or time to choose carefully. For them it's the emergency room and pot luck. It is also hard on a new doctor to examine you during a crisis, having to make decisions without knowing you, your history, or your physical exam results.

If you are new in town and have no idea where to go, call the county medical society or the nearest medical school. Ask what internists or family practitioners are located near your work or home. Then, check on board certification and training, as discussed earlier. Shop around. Ask the receptionist for names of neighbors who are patients of that doctor and solicit their opinions about the quality and cost of the care they receive. Visit the doctor's office and arrange to have your medical records transferred. If you are not satisfied with the doctor's attitude or work schedule, then it's time to go shopping again.

4. Having a family practitioner, an internist or a pediatrician in addition to any specialists you require.

Just because you have asthma does not mean that you should only see an allergist or a chest physician. Have someone available who cares about your whole body, someone you can consult about your headache or your infected toe, someone who can answer questions about how good a job your allergist may be doing.

5. Choose a doctor who asks about the "healthy things" you are doing, who cares about prevention, not just doctoring you when you are sick.

A healthy life-style depends on prevention. Your doctor should want to see you periodically, even if only once every year or two, for a physical examination. Select someone who inquires about your diet and your use of vitamins, who cares about your weight and your smoking and drinking habits. These questions point to a doctor who cares about maintaining your good health, not just treating your disease.

6. Do you feel comfortable with your doctor?

This is by far the most important feature. Doctors are people too. They get sick and have to see doctors themselves. They can be hurried, harried, and sometimes unsure of themselves. A good bedside manner in the old days was largely a matter of knowing you as a person. It meant being willing to stop, listen and respond honestly and fully to your questions. This openness should exist between you and your physician. When it is absent you should try to establish it. Physicians sometimes do not question or probe; if they are brusque and devote less time to the human side of illness the confusion, the fear, the misunderstanding, the pain then they are not providing the best possible medical care.

Consult a Chest Physician or Allergist

Both chest physicians and allergists are thoroughly trained and experienced in the care of patients with asthma. Yet, surprisingly, the chest physician will often express negative opinions about the allergist, while the allergist may declare that the chest physician has it all wrong. The animosity between these two groups of physicians has much to do with their different opinions about the value of skin tests and allergy shots. Most chest physicians believe that asthma is best managed by medications and that allergy shots have little if any valid role in treatment. Allergists, on the other hand, think that skin tests and allergy shots may be extremely important and helpful in caring for asthma.

If you have extrinsic asthma, you should certainly consult an allergist at some point in your care. On the other hand, if your asthma is intrinsic, with no seasonal aggravation and no obvious pollen or environmental triggering factors, a workup by an allergist is unnecessary. Good allergists recognize this and following history, physical exam and perhaps skin tests will return the non-extrinsic asthmatics to the care of their original internist or pediatrician or perhaps refer them directly to a chest physician.

The matter of referral brings up another important point. Choose a physician who will not hesitate to seek a second opinion or to obtain special consultative help for you. It is your life and your health. If your physician has the kind of ego that makes it hard to seek help and guidance from other physicians, then you should get somebody else.

Other Factors to Consider Coverage

When you seek out a physician, find out if round-the-clock coverage is provided. If your doctor relies on the Emergency Room and the doctor on call there for backup, then find someone else. Good physicians offer full coverage for their patients. While it is impossible for physicians to be on call 24 hours a day for all of their patients, they can work out sharing arrangements with similar groups of specialty physicians. Thus a group of internists may share "on call" with one another; so may a group of allergists. This assures that their patients will be adequately covered in an emergency. It also means that the physician on call has access to your medical records and knows where to reach your physician, should that be necessary.

Fees and Hours

A physician needs to earn a living like any other individual, but money should not be his or her sole reason for treating you. We are weary and a bit distrustful of physicians who require cash payments up front before treatment. Money is important to patients too, and you should not be afraid to ask the doctor what the charges are and what mode of billing and payment applies. If the doctor gets touchy about money and treats you like a second-class citizen because you are concerned about money, then you are seeing the wrong person. If the doctor refuses to accept you as a patient because your resources are inadequate or your insurance coverage is unacceptable, ask to be recommended to someone else. Good physicians accept responsibility for finding alternative care for people they are themselves unwilling to treat especially when the reasons are purely economic ones.

Don't choose a doctor with 10 patients in the office, all of them with one o'clock appointments. Such a practitioner will probably be too harried, rushing from one patient to another, to give you the time and personal attention you need and deserve.

What about a Second Opinion?

Second opinions are a way of life in medicine. If you want a second opinion, ask your doctor to recommend someone. Sometimes you may be referred to an associate in the same office; often you may be sent to a medical school or a large clinic. However, do it openly and seek your own doctor's cooperation. Don't go around "doctor shopping". looking for good news. It helps the second doctor if you bring all your records after all, you paid for them and can legitimately insist they be provided. Without them, it's like starting to run the race all over again from the beginning. Time and money are wasted.

Dr. Francis has been Pam's physician for more than 20 years. In fact, he delivered her. Pam has been seeing him for asthma for nearly 10 years. She is concerned that the treatment he recommends for her asthma may not be the most current or the best. Generally, she feels well, but on occasion she has bouts of wheezing which are not as readily controlled as she would like. She wants to ask Dr. Francis to recommend someone for a second opinion but is afraid of offending him. Instead, she goes across town and sees a specialist, Dr. Gray. She does not plan to give the specialist Dr. Francis's name, but somehow it slips into the conversation. The specialist reviews the medication she is on and makes some minor changes and suggestions. About six weeks later Pam sees Dr. Francis for her regular checkup. She is surprised when he says he is glad that Pam saw Dr. Gray. He explains that the specialist had been courteous enough to give him a phone call and had sent a letter describing what his results and recommendations were.

Dr. Oliver is an outstanding chest physician, one with enough board certificates and diplomas to fill an entire wall. He also has an ego to match. At a medical conference, a colleague, Dr. Madison, told Dr. Oliver that he had seen Lou R., one of his patients. In fact, Lou had called and made an appointment without a referral. Lou also requested that Dr. Madison not inform Dr. Oliver. Dr. Madison thought Lou was being too concerned about Dr. Oliver's feelings and said that he would mention it the next time they happened to meet. Dr. Oliver's reaction to the disclosure astounded Dr. Madison. Dr. Oliver went into a rage. He said that he did not want his patient seen by other doctors unless he approved it. Then, to make matters worse, he was extremely rude to Lou on his next visit. Unfortunately, Lou, like many others, considers doctors to be above reproach and continues to see him.

Being a Good Patient

We emphasize how you must take charge of your asthma and be ultimately responsible for yourself and your disease. To do this you obviously need information, understanding and the willingness to look, listen and make decisions, some of them risky. A very important part of being able to take charge of your asthma is being a responsible patient. Be prepared to describe everything to your doctor as carefully and in as much detail as you possibly can. When you consult your doctor, write down what bothers you before you get there. Be specific. Often the doctor may start out the conversation by asking you how everyone is at home and how you are enjoying the weather. The doctor is doing this to relax you, not invite you to chat. This may divert attention from your problem and get in the way of talking about what is troubling you, which should be the focus of your visit.There are a number of specific questions that you should be prepared to ask and to note the answers. For asthmatics, they might include the following:

1. What are the types of drugs being prescribed?

2. What are the harmful side effects or risks of these drugs?
3. How soon should the drugs work?
4. How long should I take the drugs?
5. Should I call the doctor if the treatment does not help? How soon?
6. When should I see the doctor again?
7. Is a second opinion appropriate in my case? Will the doctor recommend someone?

Establishing an honest, open relationship with your (or your child's) doctor makes coping with the illness considerably easier. It will help you both to weather the crises and enjoy the periods of remission.

11

Asthma: Precautions and Treatment

Introduction

Asthma may turn up at any age, although it is likely to occur for the first time before the age of five. In childhood it is three times more common and more severe in males, but after puberty the incidence in the sexes is about even. It is more often found in urban, industrialized settings, in colder climates and among the urban disadvantaged, especially blacks.

Asthma may take many forms, from mild and short-lived exercise induced wheezing to severe, life-threatening attacks that require emergency hospital treatment. There are few if any ailments that have terrified sick persons and their families more and more often, than asthma.

Asthma is among the most common of diseases and accounts for more absences from work and school than any other chronic illness. It is a leading cause of visits to the doctor's office. It is a serious disease the death rate during hospitalization attributed to asthma is under 1 percent in children but rises to 2–4 percent in adults; from 1980 to 1987 the asthma death rate increased by 31 percent.

Individual members of every culture in the world have asthma; there are no areas that are asthma-free. Yet there are striking differences in its incidence and severity among different populations. Presumably these differences are genetic. Asthma is extremely uncommon among West Africans and American Indians. In other parts of the world Trinidad Island, for instance 20 to 30 percent of the population has asthma.

Asthma is most common in childhood. Although the predominant feature that determines its presence is inheritance, environment is important. Atopic (allergy-prone) individuals are more likely to be worse if they live on farms with farm animals and crops nearby than if they live in the city. Similarly, there are certain ethnic groups who seem particularly vulnerable. There is an especially high prevalence of severe asthma among African-Americans; black Americans have a much higher rate of hospitalization than white Americans. Asthma is a serious condition, not to be dismissed as a minor psychological disorder, but it has at least two redeeming features. First, its symptoms are quite likely to become less severe or to vanish altogether as the sufferers grow older. Second, there is a great deal that can be done for asthmatics or that they can do for themselves to control, lessen the frequency of and minimize the severity of their attacks. Furthermore, asthmatics do not, as many authorities mistakenly and carelessly believe, just wheeze or pant their way into old age.

Symptoms of Asthma

Asthma (a medical term which originally meant "shortness of breath") is a collection of respiratory symptoms. The most important ones are :

- Shortness of breath
- Wheezing
- Coughing
- Increased production of mucus

Shortness of Breath

Shortness of breath (which can develop with amazing rapidity) and wheezing are produced by "twitchy" or spastic, airways.

Everybody who suffers with asthma has twitchy air passages. The twitchiness affects the layer of muscle that sheathes the air tubes. In asthmatics this muscle layer is oversensitive; when affected, it contracts, causing the air tubes to constrict. Breathing air, like delivering water through pipes, is more efficiently done through larger tubes.

As air is inhaled it flows through a series of airways. These airways hollow tubes, really begin in the throat and descend all the way down to the base of the lungs, branching and proliferating as they go. At the level of the throat and upper chest they are fairly large. The uppermost and largest is called the trachea. About a third of the way down into the chest it branches into two somewhat smaller airways known as main stem bronchi. Each of these main stem bronchi supplies air to one of the lungs.

As the bronchi extend deeper and deeper into the chest, the air tubes divide and proliferate so that they become smaller and smaller. The result is a complex maze of small tubes airways which resemble the root structure of a tree.

The surrounding layer of smooth muscle maintains the size and shape of the airways. When the smooth muscle sheath goes into spasm it chokes or constricts the airways, thus making less room for the air to move in and out of the lung. It is this restriction of air flow that produces the high pitched wheezing and the struggle to breathe that characterize asthma.

This tendency to twitchiness is usually inherited. In some it is apparent from the moment a child takes its first breath; in others it shows itself on only a handful of occasions during an entire lifetime. It now seems clear that airway inflammation is the key factor in hyper- responsiveness. However, the tendency for spasm can be made worse by a number of factors. A majority of cigarette smokers, even those unaware of problems with their lungs, have this increased twitchiness of their airways. The twitchiness caused by smoking is in addition to the other lung damage that tobacco wreaks. The most important substances or conditions that aggravate twitchiness are :

- Allergies (to foods, pollens, animal dander, etc.)
- Upper respiratory infections of all kinds including ordinary colds
- Cigarette smoking

- Tobacco smoke in a room (secondhand smoke)
- Dust
- A heavy concentration of particles in the air (wood-burning stoves or fireplaces often trigger asthma)
- Exercise or hyperventilation
- Cold air
- Air containing sulfur dioxide, ozone or smog
- Ingestion of aspirin and the many drugs used to treat arthritis
- Certain food dyes
- Foods containing metabisulfite
- Intense emotion, including laughing and crying
- Household or occupational chemicals, vapors, fumes or dusts
- Nighttime

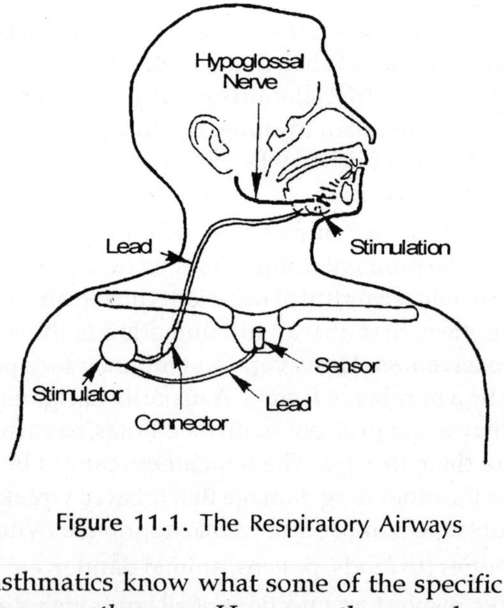

Figure 11.1. The Respiratory Airways

Most asthmatics know what some of the specific factors that trigger their own asthma are. However, they may be aware of only the major or obvious causes and do not notice minor or incidental contributors. In most people there are several such triggers.

Kevin has had asthma since early childhood. Although he had a rough time when he was younger, the symptoms gradually eased. He still had occasional episodes but could manage them comfortably by avoiding cigarette smoke, dust, and other airborne triggers and by using an Alupent inhaler when he would start to wheeze. He didn't worry much about being asthmatic, though, because he felt he had things under control.

But Kevin was in for a rude awakening. One night he was partying with a few friends and suddenly began to experience serious trouble breathing. He used his Alupent inhaler, but it didn't help; in fact, despite the medication his breathing worsened. Soon he was literally struggling for breath. A friend drove him to the emergency room and there he was given epinephrine and antihistamines. These kicked in quickly and brought relief.

Kevin went to his physician to report the incident and to try to establish its cause. He had not had any symptoms that day and, apart from the partying, had done nothing unusual. No one at the party was a smoker. The doctor asked Kevin if he had eaten anything out of the ordinary that evening. "I had a few glasses of wine and some snacks", Kevin answered.

"What were the snacks?" the doctor asked.

"The usual. Peanuts. Crackers. Cheese. Chips. Salsa."

"Probably something you ate," the doctor said. "Ever have any trouble with any of those things before?"

"Never."

Even though Kevin said he had had no problems with the foods he'd eaten, the doctor instructed him to be careful when he ate those foods in the future. Kevin had a second, milder attack a few weeks after the first one. The circumstances were much the same except that he had eaten only tortilla chips with salsa. Playing a hunch, the doctor asked Kevin to identify the foods' brand names. She then checked the lists of ingredients on the packages. There were no common allergens listed; still, she asked an old friend and colleague at the local medical school to run a series of tests for possible triggers. She found that the salsa, though labeled as fresh, contained an enormous dose of the preservative metabisulfite. The doctor gave Kevin a challenge test with the salsa and he reacted positively to it.

She and Kevin concluded that the sulfite-laced salsa combined with sulfite-laden wine had produced his symptoms.

Kevin's case is typical of individuals suddenly affected by a previously innocuous agent. Although he had eaten foods containing metabisulfite in the past, he had not experienced the massive dose he got from the heavily treated salsa plus the wine.

Wheezing

Most people know what wheezing is, even when they hear it for the first time. It sounds like a breathy whistle or the noise made by an accordion. To test for wheezing, breathe in and out as deeply as you can to clear your throat. Then take a deep breath by inhaling as quickly as you can for as long as you can. Then exhale as fast as you can for as long as you can. While you do this, listen very carefully to the sound you are making. If you do not have asthma all you should hear is the movement of air in and out of your mouth. No sound or noise occurs below the level of the throat, long as you can. Then exhale as fast as you can for as long as you can. While you do this, listen very carefully to the sound you are making. If you do not have asthma all you should hear is the movement of air in and out of your mouth. No sound or noise occurs below the level of the throat. Have someone with asthma do the same maneuver. You will hear a high pitched, reedy sound if you put your ear against the back of their chest. Sometimes, when people with asthma feel relatively good, you can hear this wheezing only during expiration (breathing out) and only when they exhale quickly and deeply.

It is important to distinguish wheezing from the ordinary sounds associated with breathing. Children with asthma often develop significant swelling and inflammation of their adenoids as well as congestion of nasal passages. These children may seem to snore when they sleep, or their nose may sound squeaky. It is usually easy to distinguish between the noise produced by their nasal obstructions and chest wheezing. Putting your ear to their chest will permit you to make the distinction easily.

Mucus

In addition to the spastic muscle tissue surrounding the airways, mucus producing cells called *goblet cells* are important contributors to asthma symptoms, particularly the persistent, deep cough. Everybody, asthmatic or not, has these mucus-producing cells.

Mucus is important because it transports the enzymes and chemicals that help the lungs fight infection. Asthmatics have many more of these mucus-producing cells than nonasthmatics, and those with severe asthma have the most goblet cells of all. These cells produce an excess of mucus which clogs airways and obstructs the flow of air, especially in the small airways at the bottom of the lungs.

Mucus is the major lurking problem in asthma. Chronic asthmatics build up large amounts of mucus in their airways. If it is not cleared, it can cause severe breathing difficulties and even death.

Different Types of Asthma

The symptoms of asthma do not vary no matter what is producing them, only their severity. Asthma has so many different causes that it is difficult to catalogue them neatly. One old-fashioned but still useful way to do this is to think of asthma as having three types of causes extrinsic, intrinsic, and mixed. Your doctor may use one of these words to describe your asthma.

1. *Extrinsic* ("from without") asthma refers to attacks that follow exposure to substances in the environment — dusts, pollens and the like. It is usually associated with high levels of IgE (immunoglobulin E) and represents a true allergic reaction. Extrinsic asthma, which generally can be reliably diagnosed by skin tests or provoked by challenge tests, ordinarily shows up in childhood, often associated with eczema and hay fever. Curiously, people with extrinsic asthma are also likely to wheeze following exertion or exercise.

Mary's asthma began at about age 8 and lasted until she reached 13. It always showed up in the springtime and was invariably worse on windy days. She began listening to the weather report and soon realized that her symptoms were worse when the pollen count was high. Although Mary's asthma proved difficult to manage during the pollen season, she was symptom-free the rest of the year.

2. *Intrinsic* ("inherent") asthma, found in both children and adults, follows or can be made worse by infection, psychological or emotional stress and changes in environment or climate. Skin tests are not as useful here, but the typically close correspondence between wheezing and other activities or events makes it easy to spot the

cause.

Arthur's asthma began suddenly, eight years ago, when he was 18. It hasn't let up since. He has to take a lot of drugs to remain comfortable and must see his physician several times a year. Although many factors make Arthur's asthma worse, the one thing that always triggers it and makes him extremely sick is viral infection. Arthur was once admitted to the hospital for asthma following a bout of sinusitis and any common cold will send him to the emergency room. Unfortunately, he now has asthma 12 months a year. He went through an extensive battery of allergy skin tests and they were all negative.

3. *Mixed* asthma may have both extrinsic and intrinsic elements.

Jim had eczema in infancy but it went away around age 4. However, at age 6 he began to show signs of hay fever and at age 7 signs of asthma. His asthma, like his hay fever, always came on during the spring and fall. His mother learned to keep the windows closed and kept him indoors on windy days. Jim also wheezed whenever he exercised. As Jim grew older his seasonal symptoms gradually abated. Although they did not vanish, the wheezing was never as bad as it had been when he was in elementary school. However, when he was in his early 20s he began to wheeze when exposed to cigarette smoke and on occasion, during a cold. Thus, his asthma, which was seasonal in childhood, now occurs year-round and has other factors besides pollen associated with it.

This is the most common question asthma sufferers ask. The answer is related to certain genetically determined characteristics that may include a predisposition to develop allergies and to have twitchy airways. You can have allergies without asthma, or asthma without allergies. However, the two often go together.

Although more than two-thirds of asthmatics can point to a close family member who has or has had asthma, the complaint is complex and not completely understood. Some individuals from families riddled with asthma never show the disease; others from seemingly clear backgrounds inexplicably turn up with it.

Arthur, the intrinsic asthmatic we discussed earlier, has absolutely no family history of asthma. He is one of seven brothers and three sisters; none of them nor either parent is asthmatic. We do not know why Arthur developed asthma; in Arthur's case the hereditary basis seems not to be a factor.

Jim, who has mixed asthma, is an altogether different story. Jim has two brothers and one sister. One brother and one sister have asthma, which started at almost the same age as Jim's. In addition, the asthmatic sister has had severe eczema all her life. Jim's mother has asthma but his father had no allergies whatsoever. Jim's asthma is clearly familial.

In addition to the genes that make you more likely to develop allergies, there may be other genes that determine how severe these allergies may be. However, it is clear that anyone who is *atopic* genetically disposed to manufacture large amounts of immunoglobulin E (IgE) is likely to develop allergies to many things. Being atopic is a complex hereditary condition and allergies and asthma are closely tied to it.

Panic Can Make Asthma Worse

Panic may intensify the spasms of the airway muscles, which worsens the condition and may impel family members to suggest or supply remedies that only compound the difficulty. Counseling the asthmatic to "breathe deeply and slowly" is a mistake. It causes the asthmatic to hyperventilate, further constricting the airways and worsening the wheezing and shortness of breath. Encouraging coughing does the same thing. It also forces mucus into the airways, blocking them even more. *The acute shortness of breath that defines asthma attacks usually appears to be much more dangerous than it actually is.* If you or someone in your family has asthma, it helps to remember this.

Having asthmatics take tranquilizers (a common and *extremely* dangerous treatment, growing out of the mistaken belief that asthma is due to excitement or emotional upset) only makes things worse. Moreover, severe asthmatics have to keep awake just to breathe harder and more often in order to get the air they need. Sedation taking tranquilizers can bring on a sleep that may end in suffocation and death.

Asthma Look-alikes

There are a number of complaints whose symptoms closely resemble those of asthma. These look-alike complaints are not treated the same way as asthma; to mistake them for asthma can be extremely dangerous. That is why a physician's careful differential diagnosis of wheezing and shortness of breath is absolutely essential.

Emphysema is a loss in elasticity of the lung tissue brought on, most often, by cigarette smoking or long-time exposure to polluted air. Its external symptoms are shortness of breath, which gets progressively worse, accompanied by a persistent, dry cough. Emphysema hardly ever affects children and is most commonly seen in middle-aged smokers.

John began to smoke at age 16 and soon developed a pack-a-day habit. At about age 45 he noticed that whenever he got a cold it settled in his chest and seemed to last longer. Still he continued to smoke. At age 50 during what started out as an ordinary cold he became acutely short of breath, turned blue, and collapsed. His wife called the rescue squad, who brought him to the emergency room. John was breathing very rapidly and, while listening to his chest, the emergency room doctor heard some wheezing. John was admitted to the hospital and a chest X ray was done. It revealed a tremendous amount of swelling of the air sacs in his lung. Further studies disclosed that his air tubes were damaged and large air-filled cysts had formed in his lung.

Treatment for emphysema entails respiratory therapy, which may include regular inhalation of oxygen. It is a severely disabling disease and is reaching near-epidemic proportions. Although people with emphysema may wheeze, and although their wheezing is treated much like asthma, the similarity between the two diseases ends there. *Unlike emphysema, asthma is reversible.* Between bouts of symptoms, pulmonary function and airways virtually always return to normal. Moreover, unless there is some infection present, the lung stays intact and even in the most severe cases, the lung tissue remains normal. Such is not the case in emphysema, where there is actual destruction of the lung itself.

Chronic bronchitis also mimics asthma. Like emphysema, it is frequently found in people who smoke. Workers in certain industries or residents in areas with heavy air pollution often develop bronchitis. For this reason it is more common in large, pollution-plagued cities like Los Angeles.

Carl has bronchitis. He smoked heavily for about 20 years. He also worked off and on in the coal mines of Pennsylvania. Because of an injury he gave up the mines and moved to be with his daughter in Los Angeles. There he noted that his chronic cough always got worse when he drove on the freeways. When the doctor listened to Carl's chest he sometimes heard wheezing. Unlike people with asthma, though, Carl's bronchitis and cough was always evident. He was never symptom-free. All he can hope for is that his condition will not deteriorate further and that, after flare-ups, he will always return to his borderline status.

Gastroesophageal reflux (GER) is a disease much more common in children than adults. This reflux of the stomach's contents into the esophagus leads to stimulation of the nerves in the esophagus; presumably the nerves precipitate the wheezing. Most patients have symptoms of burping, belching and heartburn.

Jimmy, age 3, wakes up every night with wheezing. His mother has frequently complained that he belches a lot. Jimmy's pediatrician recognized that he might have GER and suggested raising the head of his bed 6 to 8 inches. He also told the mother to avoid feeding Jimmy between dinner and bedtime. Jimmy's reflux got much better and his wheezing stopped.

Surgery for GER is possible but is not recommended unless the condition is very severe.

Cystic fibrosis, a tragic disease affecting children, is sometimes mistaken for asthma. Cystic fibrosis runs in families and occurs in both boys and girls. We do not know what produces cystic fibrosis, but we do know that it is characterized by a tremendous increase in the quantity and the thickness of mucus in the airways as well as by an increase in mucus in all body secretions. Even the sweat of cystic fibrosis victims is thicker than that of other people, and sometimes little crystals of salt can be seen to form on their skin. Children with cystic fibrosis experience severe, recurrent bacterial infections which gradually destroy the lung; survival beyond age 20, even with aggressive medical care, is uncommon. These children also often have asthma so often in fact that, when asthma starts in early childhood, physicians consider the possibility of cystic fibrosis and may order a sweat chloride test to rule out that diagnosis.

Penny had her first bout of pneumonia when she was only five months old. She was hospitalized, given antibiotics and recovered without incident. When she was one she was admitted again for pneumonia and recovered. At age 18 months she developed a cold which was accompanied by severe wheezing. That put her in the hospital again. At this point the doctor grew suspicious because Penny had had several episodes of serious respiratory disease in less than two years. He ordered a sweat chloride test and it came back positive. Penny had cystic fibrosis. Even though she had a difficult future, it was extremely important for the doctor to confirm this diagnosis early in her life. It meant that she could have earlier and more aggressive treatment for infections when they occurred.

Foreign objects in the lung can produce asthmalike symptoms. Usually victims of this kind of accident suck in small objects, especially bits of candy or peanuts. However, the variety of foreign bodies doctors pull out of lungs is astonishing peanuts, M&M's, nails, hair balls, paper clips, seeds, cigarette butts. Even when an object is not picked up by X ray, the affected lung will show inflammation. Or the doctor's exam will disclose that the wheezing is confined to only one lung. Foreign-body wheezes in only one lung are not due to asthma.

Six-year-old Robin ate too many peanuts. She felt fine, but after three or four days her mother (who did not know about the peanuts) noted that she was coughing and her skin seemed a little blue. She also had a wheeze. Robin was taken to her doctor, who listened to her chest and thought she could have asthma. Still, it didn't sound quite right. To be on the safe side he ordered an X ray. The X ray showed that the lung had collapsed in one of the lobes on her left side. This suggested an obstruction in the airways. He hospitalized Robin and had a pediatric chest specialist examine her. The chest specialist did a bronchoscopy (inserted a long, flexible tube into her mouth and down her windpipe) and in the process saw and was able to retrieve the peanut without an operation.

12

Allergies, Asthma and Its Precautions

Introduction

The word *allergy* conjures up a host of meanings. To those of us who suffer from them, allergies can be anything from a minor nuisance to a frightening, ever-present threat to life. The causes are not as well understood as those of most other medical conditions and so treatment sometimes appears to be little more than educated guesswork.

To many, the word *allergy* seems strange and exotic, which may help to explain its careless and widespread application. It has even taken on nonmedical connotations: "Maybe I'm allergic to my desk", states Peppermint Patty, the cartoon strip character, to explain her poor grades.

Those fortunate enough to be free of allergies are inclined to regard an allergic person as a mystery, a crank, a hypochondriac, a malingerer or a pitiable weakling. They have little understanding of the misery wrought by allergies and cannot sympathize with the millions who suffer from a staggering variety of allergic complaints. They cannot fully comprehend the anxiety and dread of a mother who does not know the cause of her child's allergy or even if allergy is involved; the acute discomfort and self-consciousness of an adult who endures hives and chronic itching; the agony of a teenager trying to live through the maddening discomfort and disfigurement of persistent eczema; the sense of failure experienced by a student with severe hay fever whose grades suffer because of the sedation produced by antihistamines.

Even people who treat allergies have wide-ranging views of what an allergy is. To the more medically conservative practitioner it is a specific set of conditions verified by rigorous laboratory tests. To others it is any of a broad and ill-defined series of reactions that almost everyone has at one time or another.

Medical authorities generally use the word *allergy* to refer to the hypersensitivity of the body to a specific substance, usually termed an *allergen* or *antigen*, that results in any of a wide variety of reactions. Some allergic reactions are eczema, hives, hay fever, vascular problems and, most important to us here, the wheezing, shortness of breath, and mucus production that attend asthmatic attacks.

Your asthma is more than likely to be the result of, or at least made worse by allergies. Out of a population of roughly 250 million in the United States, an estimated 37 million (15 percent) have some sort of allergic disease; about 10 million (4 percent of the total population and over 25 percent of all allergy sufferers) have asthma.

Allergy: Definition and Meaning

Many authorities believe allergies originated millennia ago with the human body's evolution of mechanisms to rid itself of invading worms and parasites. The body fights these invaders by producing a special antibody called immunoglobulin E — IgE, for short. This antibody, a chemical released into the blood, helps the body attack and destroy foreign materials, especially those in the gut or lung.

Most parasites enter and live either in the lung or in the intestines of the host. Lining the interior surface of the lung and the intestine are special groups of lymph nodes. These lymphoid tissues harbor the cells that have the machinery to make IgE. The production of IgE was once perhaps essential to man's attempt to survive the threat of parasites. However, as civilization (and hygiene) advanced, the prevalence of human parasites declined and the need to fight worms with IgE became less important. For most of us in the Western world, these special IgE-producing cells are no longer needed.

Nonetheless, these redundant cells continue to exist and although they are not ordinarily called on to fight parasites, they continue to react to the presence of other foreign substances in the body. And, because they are found in the lung and the gut, they are among the first tissues to encounter those things that enter the body from the outside world; they monitor everything inhaled and eaten. Some people have a predisposition, probably inherited, to manufacture large quantities of IgE. This higher level of IgE does no apparent good; worse, it is associated with most forms of allergic disease. Individuals with this genetic tendency are often called *atopic*, a word that connotes people with allergies.

Allergy, then, is nothing more than a reflection of the individual's production of this special antibody known as IgE. Those who make lots of it generally have allergies; everyone else has levels that are either irrelevant or too low to provoke an allergic reaction. Accurate diagnosis and efficient management of allergic symptoms rest on the detection and measurement of IgE.

Body to Trigger an Allergic Reaction

Most of the air we breathe and the food we swallow contain pollens and chemicals considered foreign by the body. Our bodies process these foreign materials in one of two ways either by routinely processing and degrading the allergen or antigen and excreting it or by degrading the antigen but also producing IgE to react against it. Production of IgE appears to be an attempt to accelerate the elimination of the allergen. Unfortunately, the process of manufacturing this antibody also activates an entire new battery of body immune machinery.

The process is easy to understand. The IgE antibody that is produced binds onto certain white blood cells in the body. These white cells are known as mast cells and basophils. The IgE antibodies are constantly on guard, like a sentry, looking out for foreign bodies or chemicals (allergens) while attached to these white cells. If the allergen enters the body, as when a grass pollen is inhaled or a particular food eaten, it is quickly detected by these sentry IgE antibodies. The sentries, as soon as the allergen touches them, shoot holes in the white cells. The white cells, because they now have holes in their walls, release stored chemicals, the most important of which is histamine. It is the release of this histamine and the other stored chemicals that causes allergic symptoms such as flushing, wheezing and hives. Unhappily, the white cells are not content to stop at that point. Once the sentry has made the holes, the white cells begin to synthesize a whole new group of chemicals in the body. Some of these chemicals include substances known as prostaglandins and leukotrienes. These materials may require from several hours to as long as several days to be produced by the white cells. However, once they are manufactured and released, they may cause persistent, severe and stubborn allergic symptoms. Thus, the elements that combine to produce allergic symptoms include the presence of the allergen (a substance you are allergic to), the IgE antibodies, and the white cells.

Danger of Allergies

Sometimes it is impossible to predict the severity of an allergic reaction. For example, two young men, each 18 years of age, may see the same doctor for a strep throat. Each has received penicillin many times before. Both are given the same prescription for penicillin. One takes the penicillin for 10 days, clears the strep infection and goes his merry way. The other takes the penicillin and, within a few minutes of swallowing the first pill, breaks out in hives, begins to wheeze, has acute shortness of breath and experiences a serious drop in blood pressure. Without immediate emergency treatment this man could die.

Fortunately, of the millions of Americans who suffer from allergies, most experience only minor inconveniences. They are troubled by hay fever during the pollen season, or they may have an occasional bout of hives or eczema as a child. For most of these individuals antihistamines purchased over-the-counter, coupled with an occasional visit to a physician, enable them to manage their symptoms comfortably.

Exposure makes Allergies Worse

It is common practice in childhood to immunize against diphtheria, whooping cough, tetanus, polio, and measles. These vaccinations are extremely effective.

The process of immunization usually involves a series of injections, or shots. Pediatricians know that there are certain ages and intervals between shots that make immunization most effective. For example, a child may require several doses of a polio virus before developing adequate immunity. With each dose of the vaccine the body makes a better and better antibody response. This process is known as sensitization; and when the child is adequately sensitized, sufficient antibodies are on hand to fight off the disease.

This same process of sensitization is also required for the appearance of IgE antibodies. The body must encounter allergens over a long enough period of time before they set off an adequate IgE response. Many people have to be exposed to an allergen scores of times before even small amounts of IgE are seen. To people who are known as atopic, IgE antibodies may show up after brief or casual exposure.

Jack, a 43-year-old carpenter, had lived in New York City all of his life and had hardly ever ventured out into the country. Jack had been essentially healthy and had never suffered from any allergies. For business reasons he moved to Sacramento, California, sometimes called the Queen City of Allergies.

The first year he resided in Sacramento Jack's health remained good. The second year he began to experience some springtime hay fever. The third year, however, Jack developed severe hay fever, chronic sneezing, and itchy red eyes in springtime. For the next several years spring meant suffering for Jack. He finally made the allergy connection one May when he left the Sacramento area to visit his family in New York. Within a few days of arriving in New York his symptoms abated. Jack's business was doing well in Sacramento so he returned there, although he now requires the care of an allergist to hold his symptoms to manageable levels.

Jack had the predisposition to develop allergies all along but needed two years of exposure to the pollens in Sacramento for his symptoms to appear. He did not have hay fever in New York because New York is not as rich an agricultural area as is Sacramento and has fewer and different pollens.

Dr. Pierce is an oral surgeon. He is an active jogger who stays in good shape. He neither smokes nor drinks. During childhood he suffered from scarlet fever and was given an injection of penicillin. The scarlet fever improved, but he remembers that for several weeks after the injection he had hives. It has been more than 20 years since the scarlet fever and Dr. Pierce has not had to take penicillin since. One morning he wakes up with a severe sore throat. His doctor diagnoses a strep infection. Accordingly he gives Dr. Pierce a prescription for penicillin. Dr. Pierce reminds the family physician of the hives he suffered from as a child. The physician is rightly concerned that Dr. Pierce might be allergic to penicillin and prescribes an antibiotic known as Keflex. Dr. Pierce takes the Keflex and within minutes collapses in his study wheezing and desperately short of breath – an anaphylactic shock reaction. He is rushed to the emergency room and immediately given an injection of Adrenalin and recovers without incident. Dr. Pierce is in fact allergic to penicillin; his family doctor forgot that a small percentage of patients who are allergic to penicillin also have a cross-reactivity to other antibiotics, among them Keflex.

It is important to know not only what you are allergic to but whether there are other substances that share enough characteristics with the offender to produce a cross-reaction. Peaches, for example, are in the same food family as almonds. If you are allergic to peaches you are also likely to be allergic to almonds.

If a person lives in the same area for a long time, the sensitization process occurs with every season. And, as the seasons roll around, the amount of IgE produced by the atopic person may go up and up. In fact, if you measure the quantity of IgE in the blood of a hay fever sufferer regularly over a period of 12 months, you will find that the level rises with the onset of the pollen season and is often at its lowest before the beginning of the next season.

One common treatment for allergies perhaps the most popular medically administered one is to deliver injections that introduce the offending antigen into the body in a series of gradually increasing dosages. This procedure, if appropriate for your condition and if it works, often succeeds in desensitizing you to the offending substance. In effect, it modifies the process by which your allergy established itself in the first place.

13

Chemical and Occupational Asthma

Introduction

It has been known for more than 250 years that asthma may be caused by materials other than pollens, animal danders and house dust. In 1713 an Italian physician named Ramazzini described asthmalike symptoms occurring in men who worked in flour mills. Ramazzini believed the coughing and wheezing these men suffered was due to a reaction between the grain and their lungs. Since then, chemicals have literally saturated the workplace, the home and the environment. Chemicals not only are more sophisticated but also have multiplied ten thousand-fold in the last century. It is impossible to avoid exposure to chemicals: our clothes, our food, the air we breathe are all contaminated with them. We do not imply that exposure to chemicals always makes asthmatics worse; however, many chemicals can produce allergic and asthmatic reactions and thousands of others can cause nonallergic sensitivity reactions.There are three ways chemical sensitivity can make asthma worse:

1. Exposure to some chemicals, like toluene, stimulates the production of IgE, which can cause asthma.
2. Other chemicals, like IVP (the dye used to take kidney X rays), can cause body mast cells or white cells to degranulate

and release histamine directly, even without IgE. Chemicals and drugs having this tendency include codeine and polymyxin.

3. Some chemicals are such harsh irritants that they can make your bronchial muscles go into spasm. Prominent among these irritants are plastics, gasoline fumes and some glues.

Reactions to Chemicals

A true allergy, as we have noted, is a reaction mediated by the antibody immunoglobulin E. There are other types of reactions occurring in many people that some physicians interpret as allergic, when in fact they represent sensitivity. The difference between allergy and sensitivity is an important one.

Peter and Sam have been partners in a house painting business for nearly 15 years. Peter has always maintained that he likes the smell of fresh paint, even though he knows that the fumes and the paint itself contain chemicals. Sam, on the other hand, has always hated the smell of paint. Almost from the very beginning he developed nausea and headaches whenever exposed to paint. He continued to work as a painter despite these complaints. Recently, his headaches and nausea have gotten worse and he has also developed dizzy spells. Medical tests showed that Sam does not have a true allergy to paint; yet it is quite clear that his symptoms are real and that he is very sensitive to its fumes. His doctor advised him to give up house painting and find other work. Sam believed that the only way he could give up painting was to have his condition diagnosed as an allergy, thus qualifying him for disability.

There are many other materials with strong odors that make people develop nausea, giddiness or headaches. Most of these materials will not produce asthma, but certain ones, if they show up in the air you breathe, do have the potential to trigger asthma or to make it worse without any allergic (IgE) involvement.

Particulate matter and smog provoke chemical sensitivities and along with sulfur dioxide and ozone in the air, aggravate asthmatic symptoms by increasing the twitchiness of airways. Strong odors can also make asthma get worse in this same way. The table lists odor-producing substances or materials that can have this effect.

Table 3.1. Sources of Asthma-Provoking Odors or Fumes

aerosols	formaldehyde (formalin)
alcohol (rubbing)	incense
ammonia	ink
bubble bath or oils	insect repellents
camphor	moth balls
candles	paints
castor beans (flour or oil)	perfumes
cleaning fluid	phenol
coal, gasoline, kerosene, oil	polyurethane
cosmetics	smoke
creosote	soaps
deodorants	tobacco
detergents	toluene
floor wax	turpentine

Occupational Asthma

There are a myriad of materials found in the workplace that have the potential to make asthma and allergies worse. The symptoms may include everything from hay fever with sneezing, nasal congestion, runny nose, watery eyes and hives to asthma. The given table lists industries that use these materials.

The histories of individuals having occupational asthma are often very similar to Joe's:

> *Joe shows up for work Monday morning at 8:00 feeling great. He gets off work about 5:00 and stops off at a local bar for a beer on his way home. At 8:00 P.M., so punctually that Joe can set his watch by it, he begins to cough and wheeze. He coughs and wheezes throughout the evening and almost into the night, relieved only by medication. By morning he is fine and goes back to work.*

At first Joe's doctor thought that Joe might be allergic to beer or something at home. Despite numerous tests they could not find the probable cause. Moreover, Joe pointed out that nothing ailed him at home on weekends. His doctor then concluded that something on the job was bothering Joe. Joe worked in a processing plant that converted whole to powdered milk. Joe explained that he loathes milk and he doesn't even eat ice cream because it gives him diarrhea.

The doctor, intrigued, had Joe avoid all milk products for a few days and then drink a glass of milk. Nothing happened. The doctor concluded Joe was not allergic to milk, but asked Joe whether there are fumes or odors of powdered milk at work. "Everywhere", Joe replied.

Joe was referred to an allergist who found Joe had high levels of antibody directed at milk proteins. He also had Joe inhale a very small quantity of powdered milk. Four hours after the inhalation challenge test, Joe began to wheeze.

This delayed daily reaction, with asthma developing several hours after work, is typical of what occurs in many individuals who have occupational asthma. Other patterns include progressive deterioration during the week, with the worker rebounding over the weekend or sometimes a gradual decline week by week, in pulmonary function.

Table 3.2. Industries Linked to Chemically Induced Asthma

• Communications and electronics
• Detergent manufacturing or distribution
• Dyeing and photocopying
• Food production, processing, and packaging
• Lacquer and rubber manufacturing
• Metal refining and plating
• Oil production, refining, or distribution
• Paint, plastics, and coatings, especially ones using polyurethane
• Pharmaceuticals and drugs
• Printing
• Textile weaving or finishing (natural or synthetic fabrics)

Specific Causes of Occupational Asthma

People who are sensitive (or allergic) to wheat, rye, or other flours suffer from what has long been called "baker's asthma". Dust from coffee or castor beans can also be a problem, even affecting people who live near plants that disperse these materials into the air. Asthma has been noted frequently in occupations that entail exposure to trimellitic anhydride (used in making plastics, epoxy resins and paints) or isocyanide (involved in producing polyurethane insulation, paint and adhesives). Formaldehyde, which can appear in plywood, insulation, wallpaper, carpeting, furniture and other products associated with the building industry, is a major trigger of asthma. The symptoms it provokes are acute, a direct and immediate response to the insult offered by the chemical itself, and they should disappear after one leaves the contaminated environment. In addition, asthma has turned up in individuals who work in "tight" office buildings.

Do You Have Occupational Asthma?

The procedures to follow in determining if you have occupational asthma are essentially the same as those used in nailing down other causes for the appearance of the disease. First, maintain a careful record or history of the onset of the attacks and their relationship to other activities in your life. Then if you suspect occupational asthma consult a physician, either your own doctor or, if it has one, the company's. The doctor should help you determine if your asthma results directly from exposure to substances you encounter at work or is due to other reasons. In the case of hard-to-diagnose symptoms, you may be in for a long series of tests, which would include a good physical examination and skin testing, particularly effective in spotting asthma caused by trimellitic anhydride, coffee beans and enzymes or detergents. Pulmonary function tests in the workplace before and after exposure to potentially triggering substances may be conducted and a laboratory-based series of inhalation challenge tests may also be carried out. This last should be done only if the suspected agent can be accurately measured and administered in dosages below the acute irritant level and if there are no contraindications like heart disease. If carried out, a physician should be present because, as with all respiratory challenges, there is an element of serious risk. Such tests require a preliminary period of preparation, and the actual tests may extend over a period of up to six days.

Hypersensitivity Pneumonitis and Occupational Asthma

If something on your job provokes persistent, recurring asthma, even mild, you have only one recourse avoid the insult and immediately remove yourself from that workplace. Continued exposure can make the asthma much worse and may lead to the development of a serious syndrome called hypersensitivity pneumonitis.

This condition, most often resulting from exposure to agents encountered at work, is a distant cousin of asthma. People with it virtually always display sensitivity or allergy to chemicals or airborne allergens generally found in specific occupations. They may include farmers allergic to moldy hay, office workers sensitive to mold growing in office air conditioners, or lumber mill workers sensitive to redwood or maple dust. In addition to wheezing, these people develop an inflammation in the lung itself, which, if unchecked, leads to severe lung damage. If you suspect that something in your work environment is impairing your health, we strongly urge you to seek medical attention and to avoid further exposure on the job until the issue is resolved.

Treatment of Occupational Asthma

Occupational asthma is treated much like any other asthma. It commonly results from substances entering the respiratory system. If exposure is absolutely unvoidable, reduce the risk with a special face mask, even though it is cumbersome and uncomfortable. Workers who handle chemicals to which they are sensitive often find special hoods helpful.

Table 3.3. Causes and Conditions Associated with Hypersensitivity Pneumonitis

Cause	Conditions
Bacteria (actinomyces) resulting from fermentation of organic matter	Farmer's lung, mushroom worker's lung, fog fever
Molds or fungi	Cheese-maker's lung, humidifier lung, sauna-taker's disease
Dusts or other airborne allergens or contaminants	Bird fancier's lung, wood dust disease, coffee worker's lung, ventilation system pneumonitis
The list of conditions is illustrative only and not intended to be complete or definitive.	

Drug therapy for occupational asthma is the same as that for ordinary asthma. However, medications do carry side effects, which may render the work environment more hazardous; this risk should be kept in mind.

Allergy shots are hardly ever used in individuals with occupational asthma because the allergen or antigen may be unknown, the appropriate dosages (concentrations) have not been worked out, or because they are potentially dangerous. The only exceptions are veterinarians with extreme sensitivity to animal danders.

In some instances the prognosis for occupational asthma may be very poor. A good deal depends on the length and severity of your exposure. Remember Sam, the house painter we discussed earlier? Sam's symptoms, although not due to IgE and non-diagnosable by conventional tests, are nonetheless real. Sam's body is extremely sensitive to and irritated by chemicals or paint fumes. He cannot totally avoid these chemicals, which are contained in paint as well as floor polishes, the ink in some newspapers, mimeograph machines and so on. Despite the obviousness of his distress and the clear cause of it, Sam has a hard time convincing anyone that his problem has physical rather than emotional roots. This is often the plight of individuals with occupational asthma and one that needs understanding and clarification.

Environmental Safeguards

The growing prevalence of chemicals in the environment and their ability to provoke asthmatic symptoms have led some physicians and hospitals to devise heroic procedures for providing facilities or environments that are chemically free. These tactics are sometimes recommended for individuals either for whom treatment has proved ineffective or whose reactions are so severe that they cannot live a normal life. The more extreme cases are called "universal reactors" and their condition is sometimes referred to as "twentieth-century disease".

This development in treatment procedures, an outgrowth of the widespread concern with ecological issues, has been enthusiastically adopted by a group of practitioners who refer to themselves as clinical ecologists. Recent observations of this drastic treatment found that most of the individuals studied, who manifested diffuse reactions to toxic chemicals, actually suffered from psychosomatic ailments and that the stringent environmental measures taken to remedy their complaints were ineffectual in almost all cases.

We have no doubt that there are those whose symptoms do ease when they are freed of chemical influences, but there are others whose symptoms would have cleared regardless of steps taken. The complex and virtually unknown relationship between allergic (and asthmatic) complaints and the emotional status of the individual certainly needs further study. Your doctor should be expected to listen carefully to your complaint, be it allergy or sensitivity and to pull out all the stops in doing what is best for you.

14

Diabetes: Definition and Meaning

Introduction

Diabetes is a permanent change in your internal chemistry, which results in your blood containing too much glucose. The cause is a deficiency of the hormone 'insulin'.

> *"I just started feeling lousy, losing weight, always thirsty it seemed like I could never get enough to drink. And there I was diabetic! I thought my life was ruined. And then I said: 'No, dammit, this is the way I am now and I'd better learn to live with it, 'cos all of those feelings, the anger, the frustration aren't going to take it away.'"*
>
> *"One of the most difficult things I found that I had to come to terms with when you are newly diagnosed is that diabetes is for life".*

Diabetes is one of the oldest known human diseases. Its full name, 'diabetes mellitus', comes from the Greek words for 'siphon' and 'sugar' and describes the most obvious symptom of uncontrolled diabetes: the passing of large amounts of urine, which is sweet because it contains sugar. A proper understanding of the condition has only developed over the last hundred years or so. In 1921, two Canadian scientists, Frederick Banting and Charles Best, discovered that a mysterious substance was produced in small groups of cells, known as the *islets of Langerhans* within the pancreas. They named this substance 'insulin' (after the Latin name for 'islet' which is *insula*), and it was probably the most important discovery in the history of diabetes. When insulin became available as a treatment for diabetes after 1922, it was seen as a medical miracle, transforming the lives of many young people who would otherwise have died after a painful 'wasting' illness.

The cause of diabetes is a deficiency of the hormone 'insulin'. A hormone is a chemical messenger that is made in one part of the body (in this case the pancreas; see Figure 14.1) and has an effect on more distant parts when it is released into the bloodstream. In type 1 diabetes there may be complete failure of insulin production. In type 2 diabetes, however, there is usually a combination of a partial failure of insulin production and a reduced body response to the hormone. This is known as *insulin resistance.* This chapter will discuss what diabetes is and what goes wrong with normal blood sugar regulation, the different types of diabetes, what causes it, what the main symptoms are, who gets it and how it is diagnosed.

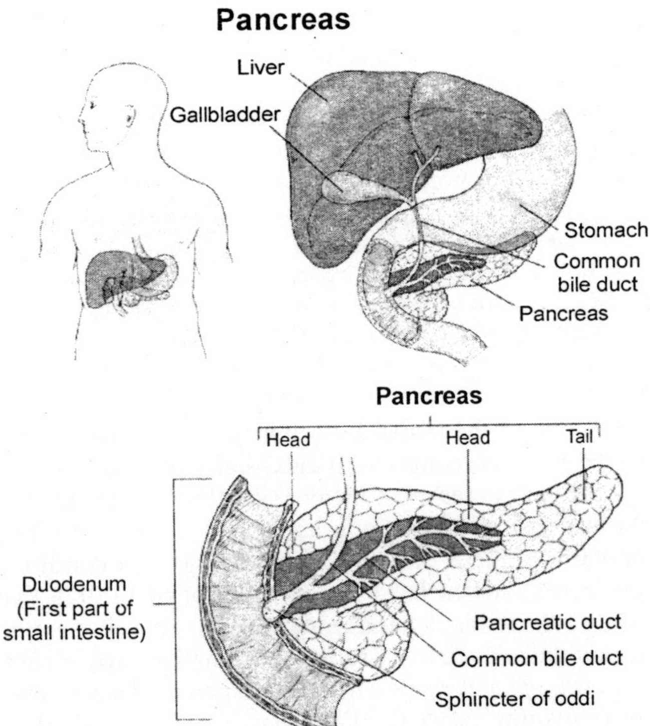

Figure 14.1

The glucose in your blood comes from the digestion of food and the chemical changes made to it by the liver. Some glucose is stored and some is used for energy.

Insulin has a unique shape that plugs into special sockets or receptors on the surface of cells throughout the body, and by plugging into these receptors, insulin not only makes cells extract glucose from the blood but also prevents them from breaking down proteins and fat. It is the only hormone that can reduce blood glucose and it does this in several ways:

- By increasing the amount stored in the liver in the form of glycogen.
- By preventing the liver from releasing too much glucose.
- By encouraging cells elsewhere in the body to take up glucose.

Other mechanisms in the body work in conjunction with insulin to help to maintain the correct level of blood glucose. However, insulin is the only means available to the body of actually lowering blood glucose levels, and when the insulin supply fails, the whole system goes out of balance. After a meal, there is no brake on the glucose absorbed from what you have eaten, so the level of sugar in your blood continues to rise. When the concentration rises above a certain level, the glucose starts to spill out of the bloodstream into the urine. Infections such as cystitis and thrush can develop more easily when the urine is sweet as the germs responsible can grow more rapidly.

Another consequence of rising blood glucose is a tendency to pass more urine. This is because the extra glucose in the blood is filtered out by the kidneys, which try to dispose of it by excreting more salt and water. This excess urine production is known as *polyuria* and is often the earliest sign of diabetes. If nothing is done to halt this process, the person will quickly become dehydrated and thirsty. As previously mentioned, as well as regulating blood glucose, insulin acts to prevent weight loss and helps to build up body tissue so a person whose supply has failed or is not working properly will inevitably lose some weight.

Symptoms

The severity of the symptoms and the rate at which they develop may differ, depending on the type of diabetes.

Type 1 (IDDM: Insulin-dependent diabetes mellitus)

This type starts most commonly in younger people who have to have regular injections of insulin to remain well. As the person is not producing any insulin, the symptoms can come on very rapidly as blood glucose control is lost. Insulin has a very important role in maintaining stability in the body by preventing breakdown of proteins (found in muscle) and fats. When insulin fails, the by-products of the breakdown of fat and muscle build up in the blood and lead to the production of substances called *ketones.* If nothing is done to stop this, the level will rise until eventually it causes the person to go into what's known as a *ketoacidotic coma.* This is much less common these days as diabetes is usually diagnosed long before coma develops. However, when it occurs patients need urgent hospital treatment with insulin and fluids into a vein. This is not the same thing as a coma induced by low blood sugar (or hypoglycaemia).

Type 2 (NIDDM: Non-insulin-dependent diabetes mellitus)

Type 2 diabetes, also sometimes known as age-related or maturity onset diabetes, is more common in middle or later life and can be controlled by tablets or just by dietary modification. As the supply of insulin is reduced or is not quite as effective as normal, the blood glucose level rises more slowly. There is less protein and fat breakdown so ketones are produced in much smaller quantities and the risk of a ketoacidotic coma is low.

Who gets it?

Around 2 per cent of people in this country have diabetes, although as many as half of them may not realise it. The vast majority have type 2 diabetes, which affects more men than women. As the age of the population as a whole is rising, type 2 diabetes is likely to become even more common during the coming years. Among schoolchildren, about 2 in 1000 have diabetes. The prevalence of diabetes is much greater in ethnic minorities, so that, for example, more than 16 per cent of Asians in the UK may be affected.

Causes of Diabetes

There are several known reasons why insulin secretion may be reduced and any individual might be affected by one or more of them. There are many other explanations that people believe, but they are not based upon scientific evidence.

Genetic Factors

Researchers studying identical twins and the family trees of patients with diabetes have found that heredity is an important factor in both kinds of diabetes. With type 1 diabetes, there is about a 50 per cent chance of the second twin developing the condition if the first one has it and a 5 per cent chance of the child of an affected parent doing so. With type 2 diabetes, it is virtually certain that if one of a pair of identical twins develops the condition, the other will also do so.

It is difficult to predict precisely who will inherit the condition. A small number of families have a much stronger tendency to develop diabetes and scientists have identified several genes that seem to be involved. In these circumstances, it may be possible to test family members and determine their risk of developing the condition. For the most part, however, it is difficult to identify the genes involved and this makes it different from some other conditions such as cystic fibrosis, where a single gene is operating. So even if a close member of your family has diabetes, there is no certainty that other members of the family will develop it, or if you have it, it does not follow that your children will develop it. Some people who inherit a tendency to diabetes never actually contract the condition, so there are obviously other factors at work.

Infection

It has been known for some time that the onset of type 1 diabetes in children and young people is more likely to occur at certain times of the year when lots of coughs and colds are circulating. Some viruses, such as mumps and Coxsackie, are known to have the potential to damage the pancreas, bringing on diabetes. As far as individual patients are concerned, however, it is very rare that doctors can link the onset of their diabetes with a specific bout of infection. A possible explanation for this is that the infection may have begun a process that only comes to light many years later.

Environmental Factors

People who develop type 2 diabetes are often overweight and eat an unbalanced diet. It is interesting to note that people who move from a country with a low risk of diabetes to one where there is a higher risk have the same chance of developing the condition as the locals in their new country. Dramatic changes in lifestyle can also make it more likely that a person will succumb to diabetes.

A good example of this is shown by the Pacific Islanders of Nauru who became very wealthy when phosphates were discovered on their island. As a consequence, their diets changed dramatically, they put on a lot of weight and became much more prone to developing diabetes.

All this points to important connections between diet, environment and diabetes. However, there is no precise link between developing diabetes and the individual consumption of sugar and sweets.

Secondary Diabetes

There are a small number of people who develop diabetes as a result of other diseases of the pancreas. For example, pancreatitis (or inflammation of the pancreas) can bring on the condition by destroying large parts of the gland. Some people suffering from hormonal diseases, such as Cushing's syndrome (the body makes too much steroid hormone) or acromegaly (the body makes too much growth hormone), may also have diabetes as a side-effect of their main illness. It can also be a result of damage to the pancreas caused by chronic over-indulgence in alcohol.

Stress

Although many people relate the onset of their diabetes to a stressful event such as an accident or other illness, it is difficult to prove a direct link between stress and diabetes. The explanation may lie in the fact that people see their doctors because of some stressful event and their diabetes is diagnosed opportunistically at the same time.

How is diabetes diagnosed?

"It really scared me. My uncle had diabetes and he died when he was 40..."

"Finding out I had diabetes was a complete shock. There were times in the beginning when I panicked and thought I would never be able to cope..."

Diabetes may or may not be accompanied by obvious symptoms. In some cases, a number of symptoms become apparent very rapidly and are impossible to ignore.

Measurement of Blood Glucose Levels

The amount of sugar concentrated in the blood is measured in units called milligrams of glucose per 100 millilitres of blood. The normal 'fasting' level of sugar in the blood usually before breakfast or after another length of time when no calories are taken in by eating ranges from 60 to 115 mg/dl in a person who does not have diabetes. After eating, the concentration of blood sugar increases, although it usually does not rise above 180 mg/dl in a healthy person. Over a period of 2 to 4 hours, blood sugar returns to the body's normal baseline. There is no such thing as a constant blood sugar level; it is normal for the concentration of glucose in the blood to vary. However, the variations that occur in people without diabetes are not as marked as the variations in people with diabetes.

What blood tests are used to diagnose diabetes?

Diagnostic tests are used to confirm a diagnosis of diabetes if there are symptoms or other indicators of the disease. For diagnostic tests, the doctor draws one or more samples of blood and sends them to a laboratory for analysis. Diagnostic tests vary according to cost, accuracy, and ease of administration.There are a number of different types of blood tests that can be used to diagnose diabetes.

- The *fasting plasma glucose test*— (FPG) —is given after the patient has fasted for at least 8 hours, usually overnight. 'Fasting' means not taking in any foods or drinks that contain calories. A blood sample is taken in a laboratory or in the doctor's office to measure blood glucose levels.
- The *random plasma glucose test*—for which the patient does not have to fast—measures blood glucose levels at any given time. This is the simplest test for diabetes because it can be administered whether or not the person has had anything to eat or drink.
- The *oral glucose tolerance test* (OGTT)—which requires fasting and is administered after the patient has ingested a special glucose-containing solution—measures blood glucose levels

five times over a period of 3 hours. First, an initial blood sugar is drawn to measure fasting plasma glucose levels and the person being tested is then given 75 grams of glucose (or 100 grams for pregnant women) in a sweet-tasting solution. Blood sugar levels are measured at 30 minutes and at 1, 2 and 3 hours after the solution is given. In a person who does not have diabetes, blood sugar levels rise after drinking the glucose solution but quickly fall back to normal as insulin enables body cells to absorb glucose from the bloodstream. In a person with diabetes, on the other hand, glucose levels rise higher than normal and take a much longer time to decrease.

- In addition, the *glucose challenge test* is used to determine if a woman has diabetes in pregnancy (known as 'gestational diabetes'). It is given between the twenty-fourth and twenty-eighth weeks of pregnancy. The woman being tested is given a glucose solution to drink, and her blood glucose level is measured 1 hour later. An OGTT is usually required to make a definite diagnosis.

Conclusion

- Diabetes develops when an individual cannot make enough insulin or the insulin that he or she does make is either insufficient or is ineffective at controlling blood glucose levels.
- Insulin is a hormone (chemical messenger) that is critical for maintaining a healthy life.
- Symptoms of diabetes are weight loss, passing large amounts of urine, thirst and feeling run down.
- There are several causes including genetic predisposition, infections, environmental factors and stress, and any or all of these may be important in each individual case.
- Around 2 per cent of people in this country have diabetes, the vast majority of whom have type 2 diabetes.
- The prevalence of diabetes is much higher in people of Asian or
- African-Caribbean origin.
- The only certain way to determine if a person has diabetes is to have his or her blood sugar levels measured by a doctor.

15

Labeling Theory and Biological Psychiatry

Introduction

A vast number of studies of functional mental disorder, there is as yet no substantial, verified body of knowledge in this area, comparable, say, to medical knowledge of infectious diseases. At this writing, there is no rigorous and explicit knowledge of the cause, cure, or even a coherent classification of the symptoms of functional mental disorders (such as schizophrenia, depression, or anxiety disorders). Clinical knowledge in psychiatry and the other mental health therapies is large and impressive, but so far has not been formulated in a way that would be subject to verification by scientific methods.

During these five decades, most research on mental illness has sought to establish three main contentions:

Etiology (causation)	1.	The causes of mental illness are mainly biological.
Classification	2.	Types of mental illness can be coherently classified (DMS-IV).
Treatment	3.	Mental illness can be treated effectively and safely with psychoactive drugs.

My argument about these claims will be based on a highly selective review of the relevant literature. My emphasis, for the most part, is on those studies that raise questions about the validity of the biopsychiatric approach. My review is probably as unrealistically negative as the biopsychiatric literature is unrealistically positive.

Many people have the impression that all three of the biopsychiatric goals have been reached. Articles by journalists usually assume as much. Indeed, most of the articles published in psychiatric journals at least imply that these three goals are already established or that they will be established shortly. They are taken for granted. Certainly in psychiatric practice it is now a truism that most cases of mental illness should be treated with psychoactive drugs. Indeed, many psychiatrists argue that it is unethical not to. Their effectiveness and safety is assumed not only by the majority of psychiatrists, but also by health maintenance organizations, which in insuring medical care, have come to have an enormous say in the practice of psychiatry. Needless to say, advertising by drug companies continuously brings these alleged truths before the public.

But these assumptions still have not been proven. The true picture is much more complex. In a recent editorial in the *American Journal of Psychiatry*, a biological psychiatrist complained about the three goals. He argues that the system of classification developed in psychiatry (DMS-IV) does not actually fit many patients, and that it has only succeeded in distracting attention from the patient as a whole. His main objection, however, is that the syndromes outlined in DMS-IV are free-standing descriptions of symptoms. Unlike diagnoses of diseases in the rest of medicine, psychiatric diagnoses still have no proven link to causes and cures. As Tucker says, making a point about both classification and causation: "All of this apparent precision [in DMS-IV] overlooks the fact that as yet, we have no identified etiological [causal] agents for psychiatric disorders". This particular sentence exactly explodes the biopsychiatric bubble.

This article is especially noteworthy because it appears in the flagship journal of the American Psychiatric Association, the main psychiatric association in the United States, the home country of biological psychiatry. The most widely read of all psychiatric journals, until 1998 it relentlessly promoted the threefold objectives of biological psychiatry. This direction now seems to have slightly shifted, however, suggesting that the dominance of biological psychiatry may be coming to an end.

A second article challenging the position of biological psychiatry was published in the same journal soon after the Tucker article, reviewing studies that support interpersonal causation in the origins and outcome of mental illness. Lewis proposes ten central premises of the interpersonal school of psychiatry, and reviews studies that show the effectiveness of secure adult relationships in undoing the adult consequences of destructive childhood experiences, and the role of well-functioning marriages in decreasing depression. The appearance of the editorial and the special article in the AJP that challenge fundamental tenets of biological psychiatry may signal the beginning of the end of its dominance.

Even during the years of biological dominance, there has been a steady stream of studies that raise crucial questions about each of the three major strands. The status of claims of biological causation and systematic classification have always been ambiguous. Obviously there have been significant advances in knowledge about the interaction of biological and nonbiological factors in mental illness. A representative study of rates of occurrence of schizophrenia in Finnish twins can serve as an example. Tienari and Wynne found that the rate of schizophrenia in the "adopted-out" twin born to a schizophrenic mother was manyfold greater than in the population at large, suggesting a genetic factor. But on the other hand, even though the rates were high, still most of the adopted twins with a schizophrenic mother were not diagnosed as schizophrenic, suggesting a nongenetic origin.

To confirm a genetic cause, even for only one part of those diagnosed as schizophrenic, the deficit gene would have to be isolated. Although studies of DNA report promising areas of exploration, this step has yet to occur. Like the claim earlier in the century that psychoanalysis was on the threshold of a breakthrough, the claim of genetic causation seems premature.

The classifications of psychiatric disorders that have been organized into the succeeding DSM versions appear to be little more than attempts to confirm current psychiatric practices, rather than empirical studies. Empirical studies usually show broad discrepancies between diagnostic categories and patient symptoms. An example is the study of symptom clusters by Strauss, a widely respected research psychiatrist. He compared the actual cluster of symptoms that each of 217 first-admission patients displayed with the diagnostic syndromes. He concluded that the clusters of "the vast majority [of the patients] fall between syndromes". That is to say, the symptoms of the large majority of actual patients do not cohere the way the DSM organizes them, suggesting that, in this fundamental respect, the problems that psychiatrists treat do not seem to fit into the medical model of disease.

Researchers from social work have published two books suggesting that the DSM classifications are determined much more by the politics of psychiatry than by evidence. In the first book they show that evidence that would confirm the DSM classifications is vanishingly small.

The strongest strand of the biological revolution in psychiatry has always been treatment with psychoactive drugs. In the early years of their use, these drugs were seen as ways of controlling and dispelling the symptoms of mental illness, if not as absolute cures. Especially when compared to psychological and social measures, drugs were seen as being cheap, quick, safe and effective. There is still no question about how quick, cheap, and easy to administer the drugs are. But in the last twenty years evidence that contradicts the effectiveness and safety of psychoactive drugs has been becoming available. There are also indications that these drugs may be administered to manage or control certain categories of patients, rather than to help them.

Effectiveness of Psychoactive Drugs

There are a vast number of systematic studies that seem at first glance to testify to the effectiveness of psychoactive drugs. These are almost all what is called randomized clinical trials (RCTs), carried out using the standard design for scientific experiments. A group of patients with similar diagnoses are divided randomly into two subgroups. One subgroup, the treatment group, receives the drug, the other, the control group, gets an inert substance disguised as a medication, a "placebo". The design requires that the administration of the substances be "blind", that is, neither the patients nor the doctors know which are the drugs and which placebos. If the subgroups are set up at random, and if the participants are "blind", then any change in the treatment group larger than the control group can be confidently ascribed to the effects of the drug.

The usually positive results of these studies are thought to demonstrate two points: (1) that psychoactive drugs are more effective than the placebos used in the control groups, and (2) that their effectiveness is due to the correction of biological deficits in the patients. However it is important to note that even if these results are accepted at face value, the average difference in effect between the drug and the placebo group in the typical study is not large and is often short-lived, as shown in studies over time. Typically, in repeat studies done from four to eight months after the initial one, the average advantage of the treatment group over the control group has decreased or even disappeared. Since we are dealing with averages among many patients, this is not to say that there aren't strong positive and negative, and even no effects on individual patients. To summarize: even accepting the validity of the RCTs, most psychoactive drugs are only slightly and briefly more effective than placebos. The decreasing effectiveness over time is suggestive of a placebo effect.

In recent years many studies have challenged the standard interpretation of the RCT studies, that psychoactive drugs, in themselves, are more effective than inert substances and that their effectiveness is due to the correction of biological deficiencies. It now appears that most RCTs are not truly blind, because most of the participants can make accurate guesses as to whether the patient is receiving a psychoactive drug. Shapiro and Shapiro reviewed 27 studies that asked doctors, patients and "raters" (outside observers) to guess who was receiving the drug.

On average, 93% of the doctors, 73% of the patients and 67% of the raters could accurately guess the active agent. Doctors, patients and raters can use physical effects, taste, color, texture, and dissolvability to guess. Especially for the patient, the physical effects on the body often reveal the active drugs, since many of them are powerful stimulants, sedatives or emotion blockers. The drug companies who conduct most of the RCTs seldom try to make a close match between the drug and the placebo, because they think it is not sufficiently important to warrant investing in the complex task of precise matching. In a scholarly review of this issue, Healy is also critical of the use of RCTs in evaluating the effects of antidepressants.

In my opinion, even a careful attempt at precise matching would face an insoluble dilemma. If the placebo were precisely enough matched to the medication, then its own effects on the patient would make the results of the experiment ambiguous. I think that experimental designs that necessitate blind administration of medicine and placebo are inappropriate for human beings. Case studies are more appropriate. Although they also involve reliability problems, they are nearer to the surface. The RCTs hide validity and reliability problems behind the mask of hard science. For a proposal to apply the case study method to the problem of evaluating drug effects, see Jacobs and Cohen.

If the great majority of the participants are not truly blind, then the validity of the entire method of research is thrown into question. The purpose of the RCT design is to rule out all explanations other than the biological effect on the patient. If most of the patients and doctors in the studies know which medications are active, the possibility arises that some or even most of the effects are psychological and/or social.

Placebo Reactions

This possibility is known as "the placebo effect". It has been documented that all substances prescribed by a physician, even if they are inert, can have powerful effects on the patient. The processes that give rise to this effect are not well understood. It is believed, however, that the social psychology of hope, both in the doctor and in the patient, plays an important role.

Even in physical illness, the loss of hope can lead to deterioration of health independently of the disease process. For example, one study of 2,400 middle-aged men found that hopelessness was the best predictor of death from heart disease and cancer. Six years after the initial interview, the 11% of the men with the highest level of hopelessness had died at three times the rate of the men who were hopeful. Hopelessness was the best predictor of death or illness even in those men who had no prior history of heart disease or cancer.

In mental illness, the effect of hope is probably still greater. Anything that can increase the patient's hopefulness can be potent medicine. In understanding the effects of psychoactive drugs on doctors and patients, it is important to remember that before "the tranquilizer revolution", many psychiatrists believed that there was nothing they could do to help their patients, especially their psychotic patients. Perhaps the chief effect of these drugs, particularly the anti-psychotic ones, has been on the psychiatrists, restoring their confidence in their own competence, and therefore their hope for the patients. The doctor's hope, quickly sensed by their patients, could increase the patient's own hope and improve the relationship between doctor and patient, and therefore the whole social psychology of treatment of mental illness.

Of course many, many patients are themselves convinced that they have been helped by psychoactive drugs; they feel that the drugs they were given were instrumental in controlling their psychosis, depression, or anxiety. What is the harm to them if the help they got, in most cases, was entirely due to the placebo effect? This issue brings up the question of side effects of psychoactive drugs.

Safety of Psychoactive Drugs

It has been known for many years that some of the widely used anti-psychotic drugs (neuroleptics), such as Thorazine, cause neurological damage, even in small doses, if they are administered regularly. It is possible that all psychoactive drugs, including the mildest tranquilizers, have potent side effects. The side effects, unlike drug effectiveness, have not received enough direct research attention. Since the actions of most psychoactive drugs are complex and not understood, patients receiving them are being experimented on.

There are now many studies that demonstrate adverse effects of psychoactive drugs in a sizable minority of patients. Tardive dyskinesia is caused by Thorazine and other similar neuroleptics. If administered for as little as three months, even in low dosages, these medications will sooner or later cause severe neurological damage, tardive dyskinesia. In this syndrome, the patient loses control over his body, leading to involuntary spasms and tics that impair motor functions. Surprisingly, although this side effect is widely known, and many new neuroleptics have been introduced that are supposed to be less likely to cause it, Thorazine and the other offending drugs are still used widely.

Antidepressants have also been shown to have adverse side effects. One study showed that these drugs led to profound apathy and indifference in 11% of the patients who receive the drugs. A second study reported that 20% of 207 consecutive admissions to a psychiatric hospital had psychoses caused by withdrawal from antidepressants. Surely in physical medicine any treatment that had such severe and frequent side effects would be peremptorily suspended from use. It is no longer clear that the benefits of psychoactive drugs outweigh the costs, even though a majority of psychiatrists, and all drug companies and HMOs, have persuaded themselves that this is the case.

In my own observations of persons who take psychoactive drugs, the reactions have been variable. In mental hospitals, by the middle of the eighties, virtually all of the patients were being given psychoactive drugs. Most of the patients were receiving at least two different drugs, some as many as five. Most of the patients I interviewed complained about adverse effects, hinting that they discarded the drugs. Some showed me how they were able to evade the drugs even if they were given them by nurses, by "mouthing" the drugs so that they could later dispose of them.

Some of my outpatient subjects were ambivalent about their drugs. Two of them had a quite similar reaction to lithium carbonate, a mineral still widely used to control mood swings in bipolar (manic-depressive) illness. Both reported that the mineral brought considerable relief from their mood swings, but also interfered with their mental and creative capacities. Both elected to discontinue.

On the other hand, a few of the hospital patients and a majority of the people I knew as outpatients, told me that they were undoubtedly helped by their drugs, often spectacularly. In questioning them closely about drug effects, I usually found that these subjects were convinced to the point that they were impatient with my detailed questions. Some reminded me of persons who had had a religious conversion. They sang the praises of their drugs, and were not cooperative in responding to questions.

The psychiatrist Aaron Lazare found that many patients in the outpatient clinic he directed requested tranquilizers, even in cases when the psychiatrist thought other treatments were indicated. In response, Lazare developed a protocol he called "the negotiated approach to outpatient treatment", and trained his staff to use it.

First the psychiatrist elicits a request from the patient, with a choice of 14 categories: advice, confession, succorance, ventilation and so on. If the patient requested drugs, the psychiatrists were taught to give the patients brief demonstrations of alternative treatments, such as psychotherapy. Using this method, Lazare's clinic managed to reduce the number of patients on drugs to a level far lower than the average.

There is one further problem connected with the biological approach: the way it is used with vulnerable populations. It seems likely that it is frequently being used to control or manage children, confined aged persons and women, rather than to help them. It is clear that the drug Ritalin is being used widely to control children whom teachers find difficult to manage. Even a physician who prescribes their use admits that they are vastly overused. Although not condemning the cautious use of Ritalin, Diller, like Breggin, DeGrandpre and Walker, proposes that there is an epidemic of indiscriminate use for problems that are social or psychological rather than biological.

There is also scattered evidence that psychoactive drugs are administered indiscriminately to a majority of the elderly who are confined in convalescent and board and care homes: "Neuroleptic medications are used in 39% to 51% of elderly institutionalized patients". These figures refer only to anti-psychotic drugs. If antidepressants and other tranquilizers were included, the figures would be much higher. It may be that psychoactive drugs are being used as chemical straitjackets for a large majority of the confined elderly.

A sizable number of books and articles have protested the way in which psychiatric diagnosis and treatment systematically discriminates against women. It would appear that what would likely be called symptoms of mental illness if they occur in women are apt to be ignored when they occur in men. Since the vast majority of psychiatrists, until quite recently, have been men, feminist commentators argue that male psychiatrists have usually discriminated against women in their diagnoses and treatment. They also argue that the DSM classification series has discriminated against women. For example, sexual behavior that would probably be ignored in men has been classed as psychopathy or hypersexuality in women:

> *The concern over female autonomy that was implicit in the category of hypersexuality helps explain why psychiatrists considered failure to engage in heterosexual courtship whether simple lack of interest or overtly lesbian behavior just as psychopathic as a woman's too vigorous exercise of her seductive powers.*

Although Lunbeck's comment concerns diagnostic practices earlier in this century at the Boston Psychopathic Hospital, evidence provided by Brown, Lerman and Tavris suggest that it is still relevant to current practices.

Challenging the Rule of Biopsychiatry

Biopsychiatry so dominates the whole field of mental illness that it is difficult to view the field from a different perspective. It is not easy to locate descriptions of practice that do not assume the three central principles of classification, causation, and treatment described above. To give an alternative view, I call upon a report by a psychiatrist who substituted for a vacationing regular at a managed care mental health clinic. This psychiatrist has asked that he not be identified for fear of retaliation:

The clinic was privately run, but it had the state contract to provide the local community mental health. I chose not to speak openly about my views, but to lay low and keep quiet. I did manage to lower the dose or discontinue the medications on most of the patients I saw. I was also able to get the court-ordered treatment rescinded on one patient, so all in all I was able to do some good.

Here's what I learned: The whole mental health system seems to be relying almost exclusively on medications. If a patient requests medications, he is given it freely. If he requests any kind of counseling or therapy, he has to present his request before a review panel that will in most cases deny the request. When a patient was not doing well, everyone looked to me immediately to "adjust his medications". If the patient was already adequately medicated, then the assumption was that the patient must not be "compliant". No one ever seemed to consider the possibility that the medicines may not work, even if taken. Nearly every patient I saw was on multiple medications.

The majority of patients on Lithium and Depakote were not being adequately monitored with the required blood tests (I diagnosed 4 cases of lithiuminduced renal impairment that should have been detected long before). Tardive Dyskinesia was very prevalent but frequently undiagnosed or misdiagnosed. Even in diagnosed TD, the offending agent was not discontinued, except in a few cases. Most patients had no idea what medicines they were taking or why. They take the medicine because everyone wants them to, or in some cases because their continued SSI, housing, and other benefits depended on it. The whole system is infantilizing. Those people who take well to being infantilized, thrived in it (i.e., they became fully infantile). Those who didn't were considered difficult.

I was hailed by the clinic staff and by many patients as a good psychiatrist, mostly because I was the first psychiatrist they had seen who bothered to talk with patients about their real problems. Apparently all other psychiatrists focus exclusively on medications and "symptoms". The progress note and psych eval forms they gave me to complete were fill-in-the-blank checklists that were exclusively symptom-oriented. If I wanted to note any sort of psychosocial issue (like the patient going through a divorce, etc.). I had to write it in the margin! I thought that pretty much said it all. I did a lot of scribbling in the margins in hopes that maybe someone would read it and be inspired to think of the person as a person, and not just as a set of symptoms.

Although this particular observation, based only on one clinic, may not be universally relevant, it is alarming enough to warrant at least some skepticism about biopsychiatry. It could well be the promised breakthrough or it could also be a mere house of cards. It is too early to tell.

Given the lack of substantial knowledge of drug actions and effects, an attitude of patient study and observation would seem to be fitting for biopsychiatry at this time. All too often, however, mere hype is hidden by terminology. One example is the naming of the antidepressant drugs called SSRIs (systemic seratonin re-uptake inhibitors), like Prozac, Zoloft and other similar drugs. A more modest procedure for naming would be to use the chemical class these drugs belong to, because the name SSRI prejudges the issue. Although there is substantial evidence that the amount of seratonin (a neurotransmitter) available to the brain is increased by these drugs, it is also known that they have many other complex effects, none of which are understood. It is conceivable that the positive drug effects are not due to seratonin or at least not solely, but to one or more of the other effects.

Given the overall picture of the lack of proof of genetic causation, the chaos of diagnosis, the small average efficacy and dangerous side effects of psychoactive drugs and their abuse in vulnerable populations, why hasn't the biological approach been overthrown? The economics of drug use supplies part of the answer. It has been extremely profitable for drug companies to exaggerate the efficacy of psychoactive drugs, and to play down their brief effectiveness and destructive side effects. It has also been profitable to the HMOs and to many of the psychiatrists who administer them.

The main alternative to drugs is psychotherapy, which is lengthy and extremely costly in comparison, and whose outcome is uncertain. HMOs much prefer paying $50 to $100 a month for medications than the at least $500 a month that four sessions of psychotherapy would cost. Similarly, the psychiatrist who dispenses drugs can schedule four patients an hour, rather than taking a whole hour for each psychotherapy patient. Being a psychotherapist rather than a pill prescriber also takes more skill, considerably more patience and exerts more emotional wear and tear on the therapist. Identifying the emotional and relational tangles in a patient's life is not an easy task, requiring experience, patience, and self-confidence. Finally, psychoactive drugs give psychiatrists a competitive edge over other professionals who treat mental disorder, since only psychiatrists can prescribe them.

But independently of these incentives, there is also a powerful demand for drugs from patients and from their families. Drug treatment upholds the social and emotional status quo; individual and group psychotherapy can threaten it. Psychiatric approaches to the causes and treatment of mental disorder that focus on biology have been embraced wholeheartedly by the families of mental patients who support the National Alliance for the Mentally Ill (NAMI). To them, biopsychiatry seems to dismiss the possibility of familial causes and changes in the family system that might, be required by social and psychological approaches. These families have bitterly rejected the idea that family relationships may be a cause of their relatives' mental disorder. Biological psychiatry, as they interpret it, seems to relieve them of dealing with shame and guilt, and indeed from any concern with their own behavior, emotions and relationships. It leaves their family systems, no matter how slightly or extremely dysfunctional, inviolate.

Emotional/Relational World

The emotional/relational aspects of Western civilization are usually hidden from view. Western societies are highly oriented toward individualism and individual achievement (rather than toward groups and toward tradition, as in Asian and other traditional societies). Perhaps the clearest exposition of this doctrine was voiced by the American philosopher Emerson, in his philosophy of self-reliance. In one of his many paeans to the individual, he said: "When my genius calls, I have no father or mother, no brothers or sisters". This idea is exactly opposite to the ruling idea in traditional societies, that *nothing* comes before family, clan or nation.

Unwittingly, Emerson's idea has become one of the main driving forces in Western societies. It prepares children for individual careers, enabling them to be social and geographically mobile so that they can avail themselves of opportunities for achievement, no matter at what personal and interpersonal cost. It has been one of the main forces leading to the suppression of emotions and the ignoring of personal relationships. One's feelings and the quality of one's personal relationships do not show up on résumés; they are dispensable. The relational world and its accompanying emotions have become virtually invisible in the Western middle-class world.

A classic example of the role of emotional/relational tangles in generating psychiatric symptoms was provided by a psychiatrist/sociologist team in their study of patients in a mental hospital. Using case histories of symptom flare-ups, they demonstrated that each and every one was due to events in the patients' social environment. The feature common to all of their cases, they found, was covert disagreement among the staff about the patient. To unearth the actual cause of the flare-up took, in each case, patient and sometimes lengthy investigations. Even then, in the pretranquilizer era, there was considerable pressure to attribute the flare-up to the patient's illness, and to treat it with medication. The identification and correction of emotional/relational tangles is not a simple task, especially since it sometimes results in collisions with the egos of the participants and with the emotional/relational status quo in the organization or family.

Another example of social/emotional causation of symptom flare-up can be found in Retzinger microanalysis of a psychiatric examination of a woman who had been previously diagnosed as schizophrenic. Taken from a widely used textbook on the initial psychiatric examination, the flare-up of the patient's delusions is usually interpreted as an unpredictable outcome of the patient's illness. But Retzinger's close examination of the transcript tells a different story. She shows that the psychiatrist's (Fritz Redlich) manner initially was so warm and sympathetic that the patient responded to him in a patently sane and human way. The turning point comes when she notices that he has been glancing at the clock. Apparently threatened by being caught out by a supposedly insane patient, or perhaps worried about who is in control, Redlich's manner abruptly shifts. Without warning, he changes from a friend to a relentless diagnostician. He repeatedly probes and leads, trying to unearth the delusions reported in her record, to the point that she relapses into a delusional state. Retzinger calls Redlich's maneuver "reverting to technique", a subtle labeling and rejecting of the patient as a person. In this instance, the psychiatrist unwittingly shamed the patient into a delusional state.

The labeling that goes on in "Rhoda's" family is also subtle. In the dialogue between her and her mother that Rhoda reports in the therapy session, the mother never says directly that Rhoda is mentally ill, but she repeatedly implies that Rhoda is not a responsible person. Rhoda must understand this implication, because her emotional reactions are intense each time it occurs. The transcript on which this chapter is based is taken from another well-known text, an early microanalysis of a therapy session.

Labov and Fanshel's reaction to their own analysis illustrates the elusiveness of the emotional/relational world in our civilization. At the end of the book, they note that if their analysis of the family dialogue reported by Rhoda is to be believed, then conflict is perpetual in that family: every line bristles with covert hostility, rejection, or withdrawal. But this idea troubles the authors, because it is also clear from the dialogue that Rhoda and her mother are both completely unaware of their emotional conflict; they recognize only physical violence (Rhoda is anorexic). Labov and Fanshel raise an astounding question: how could there be conflict if the participants are unaware of it? Opting to believe the participants rather than their own data, Labov and Fanshel disown their work, the emotional/relational world they themselves uncovered.

Biological approaches to mental illness support and help perpetuate the hiding of the emotional/relational world. This is a Durkheimian idea that I will discuss further later in this book. Preserving the inviolability, the sanctity of our avoidance of emotions and relationships can help explain the intensity of the societal reaction to mental illness. Biological psychiatry, in its crude popular form, is a collective representation that serves to maintain the emotional/relational scheme of things in our society.

Gove's Critique of the Labeling Theory of Mental Illness

In the seventies and early eighties, Walter Gove published several articles and two highly influential critiques of labeling theory. He proposed in these critiques that the evidence was so overwhelmingly negative that the theory should be abandoned. At least in mainstream studies in sociology and in related disciplines, his recommendation was nearly carried out. As a result of both the ascent of biological psychiatry and Gove's and other critiques, the great majority of researchers in social and medical science have virtually dismissed labeling theory as a fad of the sixties and seventies.

Since Gove's critique has been so influential, I will critique it in turn, in light of the evidence since the time that it was published. I cannot much criticize his review of the evidence at the time that he wrote. With some exceptions, the studies that sought to apply the theory found little or no support for it, just as he said. A clear and explicit general theory that is testable is a rarity in the social sciences. The survival of general theories like those of Marx and Freud are due, in least in part, to their vagueness. Quantitative researchers, whose forte is entirely given over to testing hypotheses, rather than generating them, fell upon labeling theory ravenously. They were encouraged also by the hubris of the original theorists, who overstated the importance of labeling.

By now, however, the situation has changed. In the last twenty years, a steady stream of studies has given a much more mixed picture. On the one hand, there are still plentiful studies that ignore labeling hypotheses, reject them on a conceptual basis, or, in some cases, once more find negative evidence. On the other hand, there are by this time a large number of studies that consistently report labeling effects. The best-organized series has been conducted by

Bruce Link and his colleagues. For the period 1980 to 1990, Link and Cullen report eight of Link and his colleagues' own published studies, as well as those of others; they all show labeling effects in mental illness. More recent studies continue in the same vein.

To be sure, the continuing evidence for the labeling theory of mental illness is still sparse and mixed: a mixture of positive and negative findings. However, we now know that the evidence relevant to biological psychiatry is also mixed. As already indicated, there are now many studies that at least raise questions about the validity of genetic causation, the effectiveness and safety of psychoactive drugs, and the reliability of diagnostic classifications. There are also reasons to doubt the validity of the many studies of effectiveness and safety of drugs that were produced or sponsored by drug companies.

Even acknowledging the initial spate of studies that failed to support the labeling theory of mental illness, Gove's recommendation that it be abandoned also arose out of the unfavorable comparison he made between labeling and psychiatric theory. Although his assessment of the evidence available at the time of his critique was mostly sound, his assessment of the validity of the psychiatric approach was not. He far overrated the coherence of diagnosis, the effectiveness and safety of drugs and indeed, the validity of the entire psychiatric approach. Given what we now know, Gove's view of psychiatry was naive. For this reason, it seems to me that the labeling theory of mental illness is still in the hunt. Of course, I am not suggesting that the other theories should be replaced by labeling theory, but only that mental illness and indeed all human behavior, is still pretty much a mystery; competition between viable theories is still needed.

Bibliography

Amos, A. (1996) 'Women and smoking: a global issue', *World Health StatisticsQuarterly* 49:127-33.

Annandale, E. (1998a) 'Health, illness and the politics of gender', in D. Field and S. Taylor (eds) *Perspectives in the Sociology of Health and Illness*, Oxford: Blackwell Scientific.

Bloor, M. and McIntosh, J. (1990) 'Surveillance and concealment', in S. Cunningham-Burley and N. McKeganey (eds) *Readings in Medical Sociology*, London: Routledge.

Bond, J. (1991) 'The politics of care-giving: the professionalization of informal care', paper presented at the British Sociological Association conference, Manchester.

Brykczynska, G. (1992) 'Caring: a dying art?', in M. Jolley and G. Brykczynska (eds) *Nursing Care: the Challenge to Change*, London: Edward Arnold.

Bukatman, S. (1993) 'Gibson's typewriter', in M. Derv (ed.) *Flame Wars: TheDiscourse of Cyberculture*, Durham, NC: Duke University Press.

Bunting, S. (1993) *Rosemarie Parse: Theory of Health as Human Becoming*, Newbury Park, CA: Sage.

Callari, A., Cullenberg, S. and Biewener, C. (1995) 'Marxism in the new world order', in A. Callari, S. Cullenberg and C. Biewener (eds) *Marxism in thePostmodern Age*, London: Guildford Press, 1-10.

Chollat-Tracquet, C. (1992) *Women and Tobacco*, Geneva: World Health Organization.

Cornell, D. (1991) *Beyond Accommodation*, New York: Routledge.

Crawford, R. (1984) 'A cultural account of "health": control, release, and the social body', in J. McKinlay (ed.) *Issues in the Political Economy of Health*, London: Tavistock Publications, 60-103.

Gardner, K. (1992) 'The historical conflict between caring and professionalisation: a dilemma for nursing', in D.A. Gaut (ed.) *The Presence of Caring*, New York: National League for Nursing Press.

Goldstein, J. (1984) 'Foucault among the sociologists', *History and Theory* 15: 170-92.

Graham, H. (1979) 'Prevention and health: every mother's business', in Harris, C. (ed.) *The Sociology of Family*, Keele: Keele University Press.

Gray, G. and Pratt, R. (eds) (1991) *Towards a Discipline of Nursing*, Melbourne: Churchill Livingstone.

Griffin, G., Hester, M, Rai, S., and Roseneil, S. (1994) 'Introduction. Stirring it: challenges for feminism', in G. Griffin, M. Hester, S. Rai and S. Roseneil (eds) *Stirring It: challenges for Feminism*, London: Taylor & Francis, 1-7.

Hatt, S. (1997) *Gender, Work and Labour Markets*, London: Macmillan.

Hennessy, R. (1993) *Materialist Feminism and the Politics of Discourse*, London: Routledge.

Holton, R. (1996) 'Has class analysis a future?', in D. Lee and B. Turner (eds) *Conflicts about Class*, London: Longman, 26-41.

Holton, R. and Turner, B. (1989) *Max Weber on Economy and Society*, London: Routledge.

Leonard, D. and Adkins, L. (1996) 'Reconstructing French feminism: commodification, materialism and sex', in D. Leonard and L. Adkins (eds) *Sex in Question:French Materialist Feminism*, London: Taylor & Francis, 1-23.

Levin, D.M. and Solomon, G.F. (1990) 'The discursive formation of the body in the history of medicine', *Journal of Medical Philosophy* 15:515-37.

Lowe, D. (1995) *The Body in Late Capitalist USA*, London: Duke University Press.

Lynaugh, J. and Fagin, C. (1988) 'Nursing comes of age', *Image* 20:184-90.

Lynch, K. (1989) 'Solidary labour: its nature and marginalisation', *SociologicalReview* 37:1-14.

Marshall, B. (1994) *Engendering Modernity*, Cambridge: Polity Press.

Marshall, M. (1991) 'The second fatal impact: cigarette smoking, chronic disease, and the epidemiological transition in Oceania', *Social Science and Medicine* 33:1,327-42.

Oakley, A. (1997) 'A brief history of gender', in A. Oakley and J. Mitchell (eds) *Who's Afraid of Feminism?*, London: Hamish Hamilton, 29-54.

Ortiz, G.M., Pierce, A.M., and Wilson, D.F. (1996) 'Palatal changes associated with reverse smoking in Filipino Women', *Oral Diseases* 2:232-7.

Pakulski, J. and Waters, M. (1996) *The Death of Class*, London: Sage.

Parse, R. (1987) *Nursing Science: Major Paradigms, Theories and Critiques*, Philadelphia: W.B. Saunders.

Parse, R., Coyne, A.B. and Smith, M.J. (1985) *Nursing Research: QualitativeMethods*, Bowie, Maryland: Brady.

Parsons, T. and Fox, R. (1952) 'Illness, therapy and the modern American family', *Journal of Social Issues* 8:31-44.

Piha, T., Besselink, E., and Lopez, A.D. (1993) 'Tobacco or health', *WorldHealth Statistical Quarterly* 46:188-94.

Plant, S. (1993) 'Nomads and revolutionaries', *Journal of the British Society forPhenomenology* 24:88-101.

Popay, J., Bartley, M. and Owen, C. (1993) 'Gender inequalities in health: socialposition, affective disorder and minor physical morbidity', *Social Science andMedicine* 36:21-32.

Saltonstall, R. (1993) 'Healthy Bodies, social bodies: men's and women's concepts and practices of health in everyday life', *Social Science and Medicine* 36:7-14.

Savage, M., Barlow, J., Dickens, P. and Fielding, T. (1992) *Property, Bureaucracyand Culture*, London: Routledge.

Shrock, R.A. (1982) 'Is health visiting a profession?', *Health Visitor* 55:104-6.

Sims, S.E.R. (1991) 'The nature and relevance of theory for practice', in G. Gray and R. Pratt (eds) *Towards a Discipline of Nursing*, Melbourne: Churchill Livingstone.

Stacey, M. (1988) *The Sociology of Health and Healing*, London: Unwin Hyman.

Thomas, J. and Dolan, B. (1993) 'The changing face of nursing 2000 and beyond' in B. Dolan (ed.) *Project 2000: Reflection and Celebration*, London: Scutari.

Tuckett, D., Boulton, M., Olson, C. and Williams, A. (1985) *Meetings betweenExperts*, London: Tavistock.

Twinn, S.F. (1991) 'Conflicting paradigms of health visiting: a continuing debate for professional practice', *Journal of Advanced Nursing* 16:966-73.

Zalewski, M. (1990) 'Logical contradictions in feminist health care: a rejoinder to Peggy Foster', *Journal of Social Policy* 19:235-44.

Index

C

D

E